Skin Microbiome Handbook

Scrivener Publishing
100 Cummings Center, Suite 541J
Beverly, MA 01915-6106

Publishers at Scrivener
Martin Scrivener (martin@scrivenerpublishing.com)
Phillip Carmical (pcarmical@scrivenerpublishing.com)

Skin Microbiome Handbook

From Basic Research to Product Development

Edited by

Nava Dayan

Dr. Nava Dayan L.L.C.

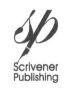

Scrivener
Publishing

WILEY

Wiley Global Headquarters
111 River Street, Hoboken, NJ 07030, USA

For details of our global editorial offices, customer services, and more information about Wiley products visit us at www.wiley.com.

Library of Congress Cataloging-in-Publication Data

ISBN 978-1-119-59223-5

Cover image: Pixabay.Com
Cover design by Russell Richardson

Set in size of 11pt and Minion Pro by Manila Typesetting Company, Makati, Philippines

10   9   8   7   6   5   4   3   2   1

*This book is dedicated to my one and only ever and forever,
my husband and partner, and to my two amazing children.
My husband was the one who seeded in me the idea to edit this book.
He and my children teach me, every day, the practice of unconditional love
and support and, as such, they are my mentors to connect to God.*

Contents

Part 4: Skin's Innate Immunity 217

Part 6: Regulatory and Legal Aspects for Skin Microbiome Related Products 303

Preface

I belong to those scientists who believe in the existence of God and as such I know we are here to connect to Him, love and cherish Him and His creation. Exploring nature through research is merely a way of understanding the Creator. While humans can invent extraordinary creations, these are only a revelation and exploration of His work. It also means that we are extremely limited. Humility is at the core of our work.

Our senses dictate to a great degree the reality we live in. Yet, as educated human beings in the scientific era, we acknowledge the fact that the existence of another entity or power in our life, even if not sensed or seen, can be real. The microbiome is a dimension of our reality that is alive and vibrant but cannot be seen by the naked eye. An entire microcosmic universe of activity affects every aspect of our being, from the planet to our bodies to our spirit and back. With the invention of high-resolution techniques, such as microscopy, we began to learn about these entities. With the immense advancement in genomic research, we are now making progress in exploring their nature and identity.

Our ability to sequence the genome in a faster and more economically savvy fashion has been greatly promoted by the human genome project, which gave rise to this new level of exploration of entities with genomic material that is different from humans, such as the microbiome. In the end, we are all connected.

Of more importance is the profound acknowledgment of the power and influence that the microbiome holds over our health and well-being. These microorganisms can make the difference between life and death, health and disease, depression and mania... The list goes on! This book is written at a time when the research is still shaping our knowledge, and as such, it can be perceived as a milestone at a stage where we know the basic nature of the players but are still at the edge of exploring the interplay in the scene. Bacteria, viruses and fungi communicate. They communicate with one another and they communicate with us at the cellular and sub-cellular levels when on us or inside us. This cross talk is what I believe the next era of research will focus on. In a sense, the identity of the communicator (bacteria or human cell) is mute when compared to what it conveys and why. In research we call it "functionality." Take for example a bacterium that contains genetic material of about 2500 protein encoding genes. In theory, it has the potential to generate 2500 proteins that will function as receptors, toxins, enzymes and other biomarkers. These can be recognized by human cells that will respond in accordance to the message carried with the biochemistry produced. The environment is the compass for the bacteria to act in one way or another. This is the epigenetics of the human body as an ecosystem that contains both human cells and microorganisms.

If there is an imminent safety threat, it will create a protection *weapon* in the form of toxins. If it is well nourished and safe, it may facilitate a beneficial immune response that will strengthen our bodies.

From a practical evolutionary point of view, the microbiome that resides in a healthy human body would have an agenda of survival and proliferation, and as such, would strive to protect the body and maintain its health so that symbiosis persists.

The idea of good and bad, protection and nourishment, health and disease, survival and death are all God's creation embedded in us at a molecular, cellular, and sub-cellular level. In a sense, every part of us, however big or small, is on a journey to explore the higher levels of conciseness. After a decade of studying the skin microbiome, I am convinced that we limit our understanding because we attribute to it aspects of human nature. Humans are the only entity in this world that have been created with an ego. As generations advance, the ego has now grown to monstrous dimensions. Bacteria, on the other hand, does not hold these same aspirations. Rather, it is busy with the very basics of survival. Adopting this understanding may allow us breakthrough revelations.

This book, similar to my other books, is a compilation of knowledge and experience of good colleagues. They are all experts in the field and I am extremely thankful for their hard work and dedication.

It covers various aspects in observational and interventional studies, health and disease conditions, testing techniques, human body response, as well as legal and regulatory outlooks.

I can only hope that you, the reader, will experience the same joy of learning as I did while editing this book.

Nava Dayan
June 2020

Part 1

HEALTHY SKIN MICROBIOME AND ORAL-SKIN INTERACTIONS

The Microbiome of Healthy Skin

Samantha Samaras[1]* and Michael Hoptroff[2]†

[1]Beauty & Personal Care Science and Technology, Unilever, United States
[2]Beauty & Personal Care Science and Technology, Unilever UK Limited, UK

Abstract

Over the last decade, radical advances in sequencing technologies have provided the tools with which to characterize microbial communities with unprecedented completeness and the consequent adoption of the term microbiome to describe the totality of microorganisms associated with a particular ecological niche. The application of these techniques has driven a renaissance in microbiology and nowhere is this truer than in our rapidly advancing understanding of the human-associated microbiome in all its complexity.

The work of the Human Microbiome Project and numerous other research groups has led to characterization of the skin microbiome in healthy and pathological skin, across body sites and populations. The emerging picture is one of a holistic association between skin and microbiome where healthy skin is the foundation of a balanced microbiome and where a balanced microbiome contributes to maintenance of healthy skin.

Keywords: Antimicrobial lipid, antimicrobial peptide, commensal microbe, microbiome, pathogen

1.1 Introduction

1.1.1 Retrospective

From the 1950s, pioneering microbiology studies began to reveal more about the composition of microbes on human skin. During this time much was

---

*Corresponding author: Samantha.Samaras@Unilever.com
†Corresponding author: Michael.Hoptroff@Unilever.com

Nava Dayan (ed.) Skin Microbiome Handbook: From Basic Research to Product Development, (3–32) © 2020 Scrivener Publishing LLC

learned regarding the identity of the dominant skin resident microorganisms under normal conditions and their association with disease. Typically, skin resident microorganisms are classified as those whose lifecycles are near permanently wedded to the skin (often referred to as skin resident or skin commensal microorganisms) and those which use the skin as a temporary conduit or transport mechanism by which to complete an aspect of their life cycle (the transient microbial population; for example, the role of hands as vectors for fecal or oral transmission of enteropathogenic *Escherichia coli*).

As the title of this chapter suggests, the focus will be on those resident or commensal microorganisms for which skin is their permanent home. These microorganisms derive their nutrients from skin, such as skin and sebaceous lipids or from other community members and the skin microenvironment determines local ecology and growth rate and limitation.

As will be discussed in more detail later, the ever-increasing accessibility of next generation sequencing techniques and their application to the field of microbiology continues to transform our understanding of the skin microbiome at a taxonomic and functional level. As this understanding grows, so does the need to embed those insights in an understanding of how local skin conditions (nutritional, microenvironmental, physical, chemical and immunological) impact the local microbial ecology, which may vary from the centimeter scale of occluded, non-occluded, sebaceous or non-sebaceous, hair or non-hairy body sites to the micron length scales of an individual hair follicle, eccrine gland or skin squame.

Pioneering work in the 1960s by Donald Pillsbury and Mary Marples laid essential groundwork for our understanding of how ecological constraints, such as the fundamental aridity of skin, affects what skin microorganisms. Later, work was done on the importance of skin lipids as nutrient sources and as natural antimicrobials [1–3]. This work helped to ground our understanding of how the normal processes of healthy skin modulates its microbiome by maintaining its local environment within narrow windows of pH, sebaceous activity, aridity, osmolarity and desquamation and how differences in these parameters help to explain the normally occurring differences in the microbiome between body sites [4–7].

That this is a two-way relationship, with microbes impacting skin condition and vice versa, was confirmed through seminal investigations by Roger Marples, Mary Stewart and others. These authors demonstrated how commensal skin microorganisms contribute to the normal functioning of healthy skin through the hydrolysis of sebaceous triglycerides into free fatty acids and glycerol, thereby contributing to the maintenance of normal skin acidity and hydration [8–13]. Such insights into the relationship between human lipids, their role as microbial nutrients and the impact on microbial localization to skin invaginations, such as hair follicles, were confirmed in light microscopy work by Montes [14]. More recently, the application of fluorescence *in-situ* hybridization (FISH) [15, 16] and cryosectioning scanning electron microscopy (SEM) techniques [17] have provided researchers with an unprecedented ability to visualize the spatial localization of microorganisms at the micron scale (Figure 1.1).

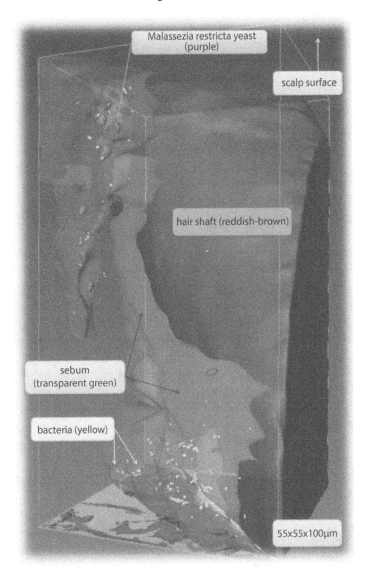

Figure 1.1 Use of an SEM image stack to visualise localisation of bacteria and yeast in a hair follicle. Reprinted with permission © Unilever.

However, despite the undoubted contribution of this work, it suffered from the limitations of laboratory culture techniques which restricted the organisms that could be detected and quantified to those that could be reproducibly cultured under laboratory conditions, and failed to capture the true diversity of the skin microbiome [18, 19].

1.1.2   Next Generation Sequencing

The advent of next generation sequencing techniques and advances in bioinformatics have transformed our understanding of the skin microbiome by tackling the reliance of the researcher on the agar plate as their sole tool in elucidating the composition of the skin's microbial ecosystem.

Consequently, rather than simply culturing and examining a few microbial species at a time, it is now possible to examine the entire skin microbiome in a single experiment and the advent of affordable, assessible sequencing has led to a rapid expansion in our understanding of the human skin microbiome [18, 20–23].

The NIH funded Human Microbiome Project (2007-2014) and subsequent Integrative Human Microbiome Project (2014-2016) collected keystone information on the taxonomic composition of the vaginal, oral, skin and gut microbiomes and subsequently, through the iHMP, insights on host-microbiome interactions [24–27].

Although the work of the HMP played an essential contribution to kick-starting large-scale cohort studies of the human microbiome, the job is far from done. Significant work is needed to expand the clinical space (the iHMP focused on preterm birth, inflammatory bowel disease and type 2 diabetes) and our understanding of the normal cross-sectional and longitudinal variance of the health-associated microbiome.

Whilst the HMP focused primarily on taxonomic characterization, it is likely that future investigations will focus more on functional characterization through the application of metagenomic and combined microbiome/metabolome analysis. This trend is already apparent in gut research where gut microbiome studies, such as MetaHIT in Europe, ElderMet in Ireland, the Canadian Microbiome Initiative and Japanese Human Metagenome consortia, all focused on elucidating function [28].

Application of such functional characterization techniques to the skin microbiome is already happening [29, 30] and their use in large-scale cohort studies focused on the skin microbiome and the derivation of this data into a holistic, ecological perspective on host/microbiome looks likely to represent the next new frontier for skin microbiome research [31].

1.2   The Skin Microbiome in Health

1.2.1   Composition

As an ecological substrate, human skin varies enormously across different locations over the body. Sebum-rich sites are found on the face, chest, back and groin. Hair density similarly varies with higher densities on the scalp, underarm and genital areas. Consequently, it should be no surprise that the composition of the human microbiome similarly varies and that body site, by virtue of these ecological differences, plays a key role. This gives rise to the notion that the skin microbiome may be more properly considered as a composite of the interrelated but distinct microbiomes of the scalp, leg, axilla, face, etc. [22, 23, 32, 33].

Comparing across certain body sites, we see that a niche of specific microbial ecology characteristics may be observed that is driven by the physiological conditions present at each site (Figure 1.2). The skin microbiome of all body sites is expected to contain representatives from the genera *Cutibacterium*, *Staphylococcus* and *Corynebacterium* and when mean relative abundances are summed together these three genera may typically comprise between 45 and 80% of the overall skin microbiome and thus

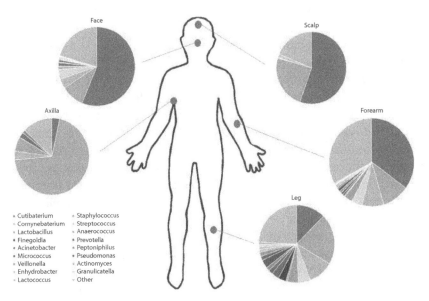

Figure 1.2 Genus level bacterial composition of different body sites as characterised by 16S rRNA gene sequencing (or metataxonomics).

may be considered as being good candidates for any consideration of what a "core" skin microbiome might look like.

However, even within these "big three" genera, important differences in microbiome profile between body sites are apparent. In the axilla moist, occluded sites staphylococci dominate, comprising over 70% of the microbiome in terms of mean relative abundance whilst lipophilic cutibacteria comprise less than 4% of the total bacterial microbiome.

In contrast, in sebaceous body sites the situation is, if not quite reversed, then certainly more favorable to cutibacteria. On both the face and scalp, cutibacteria are the dominant genera, comprising over 50% of the microbiome in terms of mean relative abundance and staphylococci less than 25%.

These changes serve to illustrate the importance of the local microenvironment, particularly the importance of skin sebaceous lipids, skin pH and occlusion/hydration in creating the conditions which define the "normal" or "steady state" microbiome balance which is characteristic of a particular cutaneous niche.

Such changes impact not only the balance of cutibacteria and staphylococci but also the overall diversity of these niche specific microbiomes with sebaceous and occluded sites being more likely to possess an individual genera comprising more than 50% of the microbiome in terms of relative abundance, whilst drier sites appear to be more refractive to any individual genera achieving dominance, which is likely to contribute to the greater microbial diversity observed in these sites.

A similar trend is apparent when the skin microbiome is examined at the species level with generally more species represented (principle genera being *Cutibacterium*, *Staphylococcus* and *Corynebacterium*) in the microbiome of body skin relative to sebaceous or occluded sites (Table 1.1A, B).

Examining the species composition in more detail, we also observe that just as *Cutibacterium*, *Staphylococcus* and *Corynebacterium* are compositionally dominant at the genus level that within these genera the microbiome profile is also skewed to one compositionally dominated by a relatively small number of species with *Cutibacterium acnes* the dominant cutibacteria, *Staphylococcus epidermidis* and *Staphylococcus hominis* the dominant staphylococci.

Although the majority of studies focus on the bacterial microbiome due to the relative maturity of methods, databases and bioinformatic analysis of bacterial 16S rRNA gene sequence data, the fungal microbiome (also referred to as the mycobiome) should also be considered [34].

In comparing the bacterial and fungal skin communities a striking observation is one of diversity. In the case of bacteria it is frequently observed that, for a given body site niche, that one, two or three genera are numerically

Table 1.1 Species level bacterial microbiome of healthy skin (A) Leg, (B), Axilla.

(A)

Cutibacterium		Staphylococcus		Corynebacterium	
Cutibacterium acnes	91%	*Staphylococcus hominis*	32%	*Corynebacterium striatum*	19%
Cutibacterium acidifaciens	5%	*Staphylococcus epidermidis*	28%	*Corynebacterium pseudogenitalium/ tuberculostearicum*	18%
Cutibacterium granulosum	2%	*Staphylococcus haemolyticus*	9%	*Corynebacterium kroppenstedtii*	8%
Cutibacterium propionicum	1%	*Staphylococcus capitis/caprae/ epidermidis*	8%	*Corynebacterium urealyticum*	6%
Cutibacterium avidum	1%	*Staphylococcus equorum*	6%	*Corynebacterium lipophiloflavum*	5%
Other Cutibacteria	1%	Other Staphylococci	17%	Other Corynebacteria	43%

(B)

Cutibacterium		Staphylococcus		Corynebacterium	
Cutibacterium acnes	68%	*Staphylococcus epidermidis*	78%	*Corynebacterium_sp*	100%
Cutibacterium acidifaciens	32%	*Staphylococcus hominis*	13%		
		Staphylococcus lugdunensis	4%		
		Staphylococcus haemolyticus	1%		
		Staphylococcus sp	3%		

dominant and that there is a "long tail" of genera that are less abundant but still frequently observed at greater than 1% when measured in terms of mean relative abundance. In contrast, the fungal skin mycobiome is, almost regardless of body site niche, overwhelmingly dominated by a single genus, *Malassezia*, a basidiomycete yeast. Whilst other fungi may be detected, including *Candida*, *Trichophyton*, *Rhodotorula* and *Epicoccum*, they are, in healthy skin, a very small part of the overall skin fungal mycobiome [35].

The most comprehensive study of the human skin mycobiome available at the time of writing, conducted by the U.S. National Institute of Health [36], suggests that nearly all cutaneous sites are overwhelmingly numerically dominated by *Malassezia* yeasts, with this species often accounting for more than 90% of the skin fungal mycobiome as measured by mean relative abundance [36], confirming the numeric dominance of *Malassezia* observed by earlier work conducted using qPCR [37]. Indeed, the only body sites where *Malassezia* was not overwhelmingly numerically dominant were the feet (planter heel, toenail and toe-web space), an exception that may be attributed to the dependency of nearly all species of *Malassezia* on an exogenous supply of metabolizable fatty acids [38].

The genus *Malassezia* currently comprises over 14 cultured species [39, 40], of which *Malassezia restricta*, *Malassezia globosa*, *Malassezia slooffiae* and *Malassezia sympodialis* are the predominant species found on human skin [36]. The ratios of these organisms can vary between body sites with *M. slooffiae* and *M. sympodialis* being more abundant on less sebaceous sites [36, 41], potentially due to their less stringent requirements for exogenous lipids [42]. In contrast, *M. restricta* and to a lesser extent *M. globosa* are specialists which thrive in body site niches, such as the scalp and face, rich in sebum and capable of supporting their lipophilic metabolism [40, 43, 44].

To date, the majority of microbiome research has focused on the bacterial community and to a lesser extent, the fungal community. Completing our understanding of microbiome composition is likely to require characterizations of the viral community or virome [45–47]), as well as that of higher organisms such as *Demodex folliculorum*. However, although the microbiome jigsaw is not complete without these elements, we should caution against the belief that without them we are unable to draw useful conclusions, as to do so would be an unnecessary impedance to scientific research.

1.2.2   Diversity

The diversity of any microbiome is typically measured through a combination of alpha diversity (diversity within communities) or beta diversity

(diversity between communities) metrics or by analysis of the number of observed operational taxonomic units (OTUs) [20], and the same measures can be readily applied to analysis of skin microbiome data.

Examinations of skin microbiome diversity in non-compromised skin indicate reproducible differences in microbiome diversity between body sites and also show how local changes in skin ecology, such as changes in oiliness, or barrier integrity can help to explain person to person differences in the same body site.

In their analyses of body site differences, Shibagaki *et al.* [48] demonstrated that the cheek, forehead and scalp typically display lower microbiome diversity than the forearm, and in our own analysis of body site differences (Figure 1.3) our team observed that, in healthy skin, the forearm and leg are typically more diverse than the forehead.

Such observations are consistent with the interpretation proposed in the previous section that sebaceous skin sites are, under normal conditions, less diverse habitats than non-sebaceous sites [49].

This analysis can be taken one step further through the work of Mukherjee *et al.* [50] by looking at diversity differences within an individual body site and comparing that data to person-to-person differences in skin oiliness.

In this study of 30 healthy female subjects, we see not only that a significant positive correlation is observed between *Cutibacterium* sp. and sebum

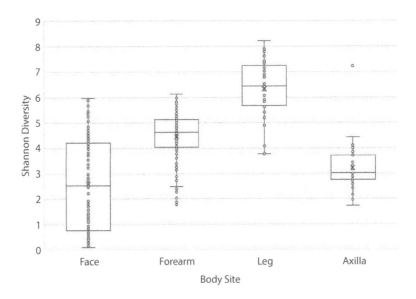

Figure 1.3 Body site differences in microbiome diversity.

levels (Sebumeter, Courage + Khazaka electronic GmbH), but also a step-wise reduction in microbiome diversity as facial sebum levels increase (Figure 1.4).

These insights taken together nicely show not only how the local micro-environmental conditions of different body-site niches act as key drivers in determining normal microbiome diversity but also cautions against the assumption that higher microbiome diversity is inherently "better" than lower microbiome diversity.

A more considered interpretation would be to base conclusions first on an assessment of the normal level of microbiome diversity associated with an individual body site niche under the healthy conditions of non-compromised skin, and then to determine if changes in the diversity of that microbiome, either an increase or decrease in diversity is associated with changes in the underlying skin condition. A deeper level of understanding may be to probe the functional behavior of the various species, meaning judging "health" and "disease" by biota functionality and ideally correlation to clinical manifestation and not by its identity, diversity or distribution.

When such analyses are undertaken, sensible conclusions can be drawn, be they the increase in body site specific microbiome diversity observed in aged skin [48], the conflicting data on changes in microbiome diversity in atopic skin which may either be unchanged [29] or reduced [51] or the lack of significant changes in diversity when comparing normal skin to mild dry skin [52].

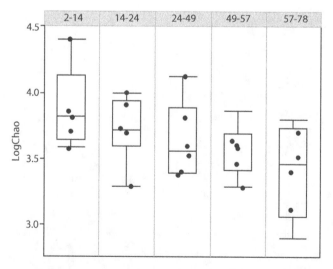

Figure 1.4 Increased skin sebum associates reduced microbiome diversity.

1.2.3   Uniqueness

The uniqueness of each person's individual microbiome is a frequently cited perspective in the scientific and popular press [53–56], and indeed this very uniqueness is being explored for practical application in personalized medicine and forensics [57–61].

However, whilst every person's microbiome may be unique they are not totally dissimilar from one another, indeed much of the core elements of the skin microbiome are common between individuals and populations and the very fact that one can conduct clinical investigations which can characterize the "average" microbiome of a population or which can compare the microbiomes of different body sites [32] supports the hypothesis that, although unique, the differences between the microbiomes of individuals are not so great nor so variable as to confound our attempts at clinical or epidemiological analysis.

Superficially, the notion that an individual's microbiome can simultaneously be unique and sufficiently similar to other people as to permit population-based analyses may appear to be a contradictory one; however, in reality these concepts are able to coexist quite happily.

Perhaps a useful analogy at this point is that of the fingerprint, wherein the unique pattern of whorls, ridges and valleys is, through complex analysis, quite capable of identifying one individual within a population of

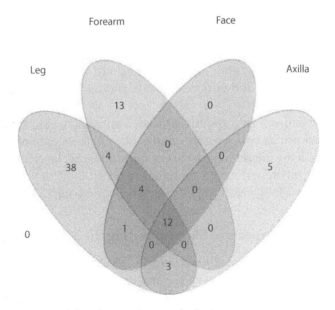

Figure 1.5 Unique and shared genera between body sites.

billions. However, despite their uniqueness in the fine details, fingerprints still remain sufficiently generic for a lay person without any specific training to identify a fingerprint as being "a fingerprint."

Similarly, in the fine details of the microbiome there are unique, abundant patterns spanning potentially many hundreds or thousands of individual genera or species capable of identifying individuals and potentially highlighting therapeutically important changes in microbiome composition or function. However, by stepping up a length scale one can observe the commonalities between individuals and body sites (Figure 1.5) which are characteristic of the healthy human population.

1.3 Healthy Skin is the Foundation of a Balanced Skin Microbiome

To the skin microbiome the skin is the primary source of nutrients, the primary determinant of microenvironmental conditions such as pH, water availability, temperature and osmolality, the key determinant of physical stability through desquamation and the major source of naturally derived antimicrobial peptides and lipids. Through these processes skin is the curator, shepherding microbiome development and maintaining normal processes of healthy skin development and is the foundation of a balanced skin microbiome.

The skin is composed of several layers, the living tissue of the dermis and epidermis and the outer facing layer of terminally differentiated desquamating keratinocytes called the stratum corneum. Inlaid into this landscape are the many thousands of specialized secretary integuments comprised of eccrine and apocrine glands and terminal and vellus hair follicles [62–64].

The architecture of skin and the associated microbiome are increasingly being viewed not as two separate entities but rather as part of a holistic whole wherein the microbiome forms an outward facing layer atop normal healthy skin, which performs a range of important biochemical and protective functions [65] which will be discussed in more detail later.

1.3.1 Physical Aspects of Skin Impacting the Microbiome

The terminally differentiated keratinocytes comprise the "bricks" of the brick and mortar construction of the stratum corneum, with the mortar comprised of lipids such as ceramides, fatty acids and cholesterol organized in lamellar structures [66, 67].

Although the primary role of the stratum corneum is to prevent water loss from the body and protect the skin by creating a physical barrier to water, the structure is also a key pillar in how healthy skin manages its microbiome, discouraging pathogens and maintaining the presence of commensal organisms [68].

As keratinocytes move outward they undergo a process of terminal differentiation, expressing specialized keratins such as K1 and K10, and late differentiation markers such as involucrin, loricrin and filaggrin, followed by the breakdown of intracellular organelles and conversion of filaggrin into a mixture of filaggrin-derived natural moisturizing factors (NMFs) [69]. Finally, in the last stages of keratinocyte differentiation a finely controlled balance of desquamatory proteases cleaves the protein "rivets" or corneodesmosomes linking stratum corneum cells (squames) together, leading to the controlled shedding of dead skin cells, matching the rate of new cell production and thereby maintaining a constant thickness of stratum corneum [70–72].

This fundamental process, which is so characteristic of normal skin, also has profound implications on the skin microenvironment and thus on the skin microbiome.

The process of desquamation, wherein one layer of skin cells are effectively shed each day means that any adhered microorganisms are similarly shed, creating a biological chemostat selecting for those specialized skin commensal organisms capable of both adhering to skin cells and reproducing at a sufficient rate to maintain a stable community [73]. This process may help to explain why persistent skin-associated biofilms are usually confined to invaginations such as hair follicles [15].

In addition to desquamation, as keratinocytes differentiate free water already localized to the cell interior becomes nearly completely bound by lipids and, importantly, by amino acids including the natural moisturizing factors (NMFs), creating a highly arid environment that is functionally devoid of free water [74].

The exceptionally low water availability of the skin surface combined with high concentrations of stratum corneum and eccrine amino acids (up to 0.3M) [75] combine to create an environment with high osmolarity [73], further increasing the risk of desiccation posed to any resident microorganism.

Potentially as a result of the low availability of free water on the surface of normal healthy skin changes in skin hydration can have a significant effect on the human microbiome [76]. Studies have also demonstrated that skin hydration, as measured by corneometer, impacted the proportions of cutibacteria and staphylococci on the face [50] and aerobic bacteria on hands [77].

Thus, maintaining the physical microenvironment of the stratum corneum of healthy skin creates powerful selective pressures which help to tailor the skin microbiome by permitting those organisms specialized to survive in such conditions the opportunity to flourish whilst discouraging non-commensal opportunists.

1.3.2   Biochemical and Defensive Aspects of Skin Impacting the Microbiome

1.3.2.1   The Acid Mantle

Healthy skin maintains a mildly acidic pH through a combination of releasing polycarboxylic acid from filaggrin, the liberation of free fatty acids endogenously from phospholipids and via hydrolysis of sebaceous triglycerides by the commensal microbiome and the release of lactic acid from eccrine glands, all of which contribute to the skin's ability to maintain a remarkably stable acidity [78, 79].

This acidic layer helps to discourage non-commensal species with commensals evolving numerous strategies to facilitate survival, including the use of arginine deiminase pathways to generate ammonia through the conversion of ornithine to arginine [80].

Typically, skin pH values range from 4.0 to 6.0, with normal healthy pH around 5.0. Microbes on the skin are dependent on the slightly acidic pH of the skin. For example, experimental studies show that the commensal *S. epidermidis* grows well under acidic conditions (low pH), but an increase in pH may lead to it being outcompeted by potentially pathogenic species such as *S. aureus* [81].

Changes in skin pH can also impact the balance between commensal species, as has been observed with skin staphylococci and corynebacteria with species of the latter genera being less tolerant of more acid skin pH and tending to be most abundant in body sites like the axilla, which typically exhibits a slightly elevated pH relative to other body sites [82].

1.3.2.2   Antimicrobial Lipids (AMLs)

Healthy skin produces a range of antimicrobial free fatty acids and sphingosines displaying natural antimicrobial activity.

Triglycerides produced in the sebaceous glands [13] are hydrolyzed by lipases secreted by the skin microbiome, principally by *Cutibacterium acnes* [11] releasing free fatty acids which then disperse over the surface of skin (Figure 1.6).

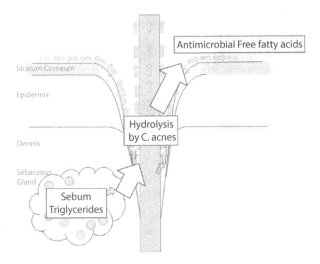

Figure 1.6 The critical role of Cutibacterium acnes in liberating antimicrobial free fatty acids from sebum.

In humans, the major free fatty acid liberated in this way is a mono-unsaturated 16:1 fatty acid called sapienic acid (16:1Δ6) [83], which has been shown to be antimicrobial against the skin pathogen S. *aureus in vitro* [84–87]. Furthermore, levels of this antimicrobial fatty acid are reduced in atopic skin, with levels of sapienic acid *in vivo* negatively correlating with *in-vivo* counts of S. *aureus* [88].

The other major type of antimicrobial fatty acid is sphingosine which is liberated from stratum corneum ceramides by the action of acid and alkaline ceramidases [89]. Like sapienic acid, sphingosine has been shown to have antimicrobial efficacy *in vitro* [87] and to be reduced in atopic skin (150 μM vs 270 μM in healthy skin), with this decline being correlated with decreased acid ceramidase activity [89].

Antimicrobial lipids are discussed in more detail in Chapter 11 of this book.

1.3.2.3 Antimicrobial Peptides (AMPs)

Antimicrobial peptides are a family of small endogenously produced compounds present in the stratum corneum and released through sweat and sebaceous secretions which form a protective layer characterized by direct antimicrobial activity [90, 91], which facilitates the formation of epithelial tight junctions [92] and which may be promoted by the presence of commensal microorganisms [80, 93].

Principle AMPs of human skin include cathelicidins such as LL-37 characterized by an N-terminal signal peptide, dermcidins characterized by a cysteine residue disulfide bridge, the S100 protein, the ribonuclease RNAse7 and defensins, notably human-beta-defensins (hBD) 1, 2 and 3, as well as lysozyme and iron-binding proteins such as lactoferrin [94].

The constitutive expression of several AMPs, including LL-37 and hBD-1, hBD-2 and hBD-3, coupled to their antimicrobial function supports the existence of a functional role in which healthy skin uses AMPs as a means to manage the normal composition of the skin microbiome by deterring pathogens and commensal overgrowth. The intricate relationship with normal healthy skin, evidenced by the reported synergy between microbiome-derived antimicrobial compounds with human LL-37 [95] is also evidenced by both the role of the endogenous multifunctional skin proteases Kallikrein 5 and Kallikrein 7 in the enzymatic release of active LL-37 from its precursor proform hCAP18 [96] and the observed increase in skin AMPs following the topical application of niacinamide [97].

Antimicrobial peptides are discussed in more detail in Chapter 12 of this book.

1.3.3   Nutritional and Microenvironmental Aspects of Skin Impacting the Microbiome

The scope thus far has been focused on the barrier and defensive properties of healthy skin and how those elements can shape the microbiome. However, healthy skin is also a source of nutrients which support the growth of, or in some cases are critical to the survival of, the normal skin microbiome. Despite the expected importance of understanding the nutritional linkages between skin and its microbiome, little systematic work has been undertaken in the area and the sort of detailed food webs needed for a thorough ecological understanding of the skin microbiome are largely absent from the scientific literature.

1.3.3.1   *Amino Acids*

The commensal microbiome, including *Micrococcus, Staphylococcus, Cutibacterium* and *Malassezia* has a requirement for organic nitrogen that can be fulfilled by endogenously produced amino acids [76]. Millimolar concentrations of amino acids are exuded onto skin every day in the form of eccrine sweat (Figure 1.7), providing rich supplies of serine, glycine, alanine and other amino acids [64] and similar amounts provided from

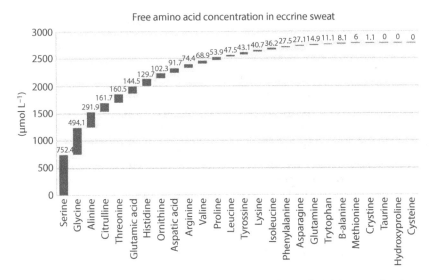

Figure 1.7 Free amino acid composition of eccrine sweat (reproduced from Harker & Harding 2013).

below via the stratum corneum [75], which can provide usable substrates for growth of commensal *Staphylococcus epidermidis* and the skin pathogen *Staphylococcus aureus* [98].

1.3.3.2   Sebaceous Lipids

The levels of lipids in the skin can affect microbiome diversity [48, 50, 99]. Some microbes, such as *Cutibacterium* and *Malassezia*, are particularly dependent on lipids for growth and co-localize with areas of the body where such nutrients are abundant [30, 76]. During puberty, the sebaceous gland becomes activated [100], leading to a shift from a diverse fungal community to one that is dominated by *Malassezia* species [101]. *Cutibacterium acnes* is also notably more abundant in sebaceous regions of skin [76, 102].

1.3.3.3   Organic Acids and Other Materials

Lactate and urea are both abundant on skin, the former from eccrine sweat and the latter as a by-product of lactate/citrulline cycling in the skin surface urea cycle [103] and may support growth of skin bacteria such as *Acinetobacter* [73], which may in part contribute to the above expected presence of urease metabolism pathways in skin bacteria [104].

1.4   A Balanced Skin Microbiome Supports the Normal Functioning of Healthy Skin

Perhaps it should come as no surprise given the millennia over which our skin and skin microbiome have co-evolved, but as our understanding improves it is becoming increasingly apparent that the microbiome of healthy skin is not an inert layer or passenger but is instead an active contributor to the development and maintenance of healthy skin.

This section will explore the role of the microbiome in maintaining healthy skin; from supporting the immune system, to helping maintain skin's normal pH, to the indirect benefits that come from metabolizing various compounds present in the skin.

1.4.1   Pathogen Exclusion

One of the most well-recognized beneficial functions of the commensal skin microbiome is to help prevent colonization of skin by pathogenic microbes [65, 73, 105].

Several different mechanisms contribute to this beneficial effect, in its simplest form this is a question of ecological real estate, whereby the normal skin microbiome, by utilizing resources (nutrients and space) that could otherwise be taken up by pathogens, makes it harder for less desirable microorganisms to gain a foothold on healthy skin [73].

In addition to the sort of passive exclusion described above, the commensal microbiome also plays a direct, active role in dissuading pathogen colonization through the production of bacteriocins and short chain fatty acids (SCFAs) which impede pathogen survival [106, 107]. This is well illustrated by the relationship between *S. epidermidis* and *S. aureus* where competition for nutrients and adhesin receptors [108] can inhibit the formation of, or destroy existing, *S. aureus* biofilms through the production of phenol-soluble modulins [109–111].

Finally, the commensal microbiome may utilize an indirect, skin mediated mechanism to prevent pathogen colonization by amplifying the innate immune response to pathogens [93] or by releasing serine proteases which promote the production of the host endogenous antimicrobial peptides, including human beta defensins 2 and 3, which have been shown to target the skin pathogen *S. aureus* [112, 113].

1.4.2   Contribution to Skin pH

The contribution of cutibacteria and to a lesser extent staphylococci builds on early work demonstrating the role of these organisms in the hydrolytic generation of free fatty acids [11, 13] and later work on the contribution of free fatty acids to the maintenance of skin pH [79]. *In vivo*, these members of the normal skin microbiome produce lipase enzymes that break down sebaceous triglycerides, releasing fatty acids such as sapienic acid and butyric acid [83, 114]. These fatty acids provide important functions in maintaining pH, exerting direct antimicrobial effects and support the function of the skin barrier by contributing to its acidic pH [79].

1.4.3   Microbial Contribution to Skin Barrier Integrity

In addition to their contribution to skin pH and hydration through the hydrolysis of sebaceous triglycerides (described above) and the deterrence of pathogens through the production of short chain fatty acids (SCFAs) [49, 115], the commensal microbiome has been reported to contribute to contribute to skin barrier integrity via a number of different mechanisms.

Human autologous inoculation studies were performed, wherein cultures of the commensal skin microorganisms *S. epidermidis* were recovered from individuals, cultured and applied back to the facial skin of test subjects. These investigations have demonstrated that subjects receiving a topical "top-up" of *S. epidermidis* exhibited a 5–15-fold increase in the number of this organism and also significant improvements in skin condition across a range of skin barrier metrics, including water content, evaporative water loss and lipid content [116].

Separately, investigations into the topical application of *Streptococcus thermophilus* have lent support to the potential role of skin microorganisms in supporting ceramide production via the action of bacterial sphingomyelinase. Through a series of experiments involving application of the organism to *in-vitro* keratinocytes and *in-vivo* healthy and atopic subjects, this work offers an interesting perspective into how the microbiome may play a supportive role in key processes of skin barrier formation [117–119].

An emerging area of research with intriguing potential is the apparent contribution of the commensal skin microbiome to the development of normal skin. Although such work is in its early stages, results such as those of Meisel *et al.* [120] where genes of the epidermal differentiation complex (EDC)—a gene complex enriched in genes encoding for various stages of keratinocyte cornification and which in humans is located on chromosome 1q21—were differentially expressed in a comparison of germ-free and conventionally raised mice, are suggestive of a positive contribution from the commensal microbiome.

In addition, *in-vitro* studies using laboratory grown keratinocytes suggest that skin pathogens actively degrade epidermal tight junctions (an integral part of the living barrier of skin), whereas commensal organisms did not [121], and that in addition, the expression of antimicrobial peptides (see Subsection 1.3.2.3) was also associated with increased tight junctional development [122, 123].

1.5   Conclusion

This is truly an exciting time to be a microbiologist. The sequencing revolution which gave life to the new science of microbiomics also prompted a renaissance in skin microbiology and the opportunity to revisit past insights equipped with new data and the tools of modern science.

In our team's opinion, one of the most profound changes arising from this rejuvenation of interest in the skin microbiome is the shift away from a monolithic view of skin microorganisms as being either negative actors or passive bystanders and towards a holistic perspective embracing the beneficial interplay between skin and skin microbiome in the maintenance of healthy skin (Figure 1.8).

Despite the work of the HMP increasing the number of academic and commercial research projects focused on the skin microbiome, gaps in our understanding remain.

One of these is the ongoing need to ensure we have skin microbiome data which is properly representative of the diversity of skin and which

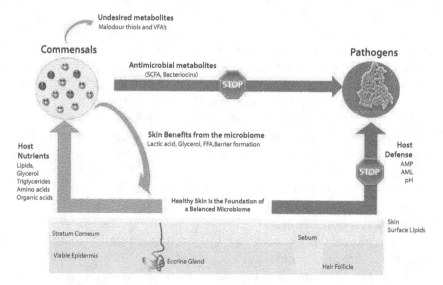

Figure 1.8 Holistic interaction of skin and microbiome.

properly reflects the diversity of human ethnicities, ages, lifestages and climatic conditions. Without a concerted effort in this area we run the risk of overlooking new associations between skin and microbiome.

Another area is the need to build a more complete understanding of skin microbiome function grounded in a more holistic interpretation of "microbiome ecology" that takes new insights such as those emerging from the combined microbiome/metabolome studies of Pieter Dorrestein [30] to build an ecological perspective on human-microbiome and microbe-microbe interactions within the microbiome.

Acknowledgments

The authors would like to express gratitude to the following individuals for their contributions to this chapter and the previously unpublished scientific studies reported therein: Dr. Barry Murphy and Dr. David Arnold (Unilever R&D Port Sunlight); Dr. Gordon James (Unilever R&D Colworth); Drs. Anindya Dasgupta, Amitabha Majumdar and Rupak Mitra (Unilever R&D Bangalore); Dr. Cheri Chi (Unilever R&D Shanghai); and Dr. Stacy Hawkins (Unilever R&D Trumbull).

References

1. Pillsbury, G.M., Rebell, G., The Bacterial Flora of the Skin. *J. Investig. Dermatol.*, 18, 3, 173–86, 1952.
2. Marples, M., *The Ecology of the Human Skin*, Thomas, Springfield, IL 1965.
3. Marples, M., The Normal Flora of Human Skin. British *J. Dermatol.*, 81, 1, 2–13, 1969.
4. Rothman, S. and Lorincz, A., Defense Mechanisms of the Skin. *Annu. Rev. Med.*, 14, 215–242, 1963.
5. Van Abbe, N., The Investigation of Dandruff. *J. Soc. Cosmetic Chem.*, 15, 609–630, 1964.
6. Roia, F. and Vanderwyck, R., Resident Microbial Flora of the Human Scalp and Its Relationship to Dandruff. *J. Soc. Cosmetic Chem.*, 20, 113–134, 1969.
7. Ackerman, A. and Kligman, A., Some Observations on Dandruff. *J. Soc. Cosmetic Chem.*, 20, 81–101, 1969.
8. Strauss, J. and Pochi, P., Effect of Orally Administered Antibacterial Agents on Titratable Acidity of Human Sebum. *J. Investig. Dermatol.*, 47, 577–581, 1966.
9. Kraus, S., Reduction in skin surface free fatty acids with topical tetracycline. *J. Investig. Dermatol.*, 51, 431–434, 1968.

10. Freinkel, R. and Shen, Y., The Origin of Free Fatty Acids in Sebum II: Assay of the lipases of the cutaneous bacteria and effects of pH. *J. Investig. Dermatol.*, 53, 422–427, 1969.

11. Marples, R., Kligman, A., Lantis, L., Downing, D., The Role of the Aerobic Microflora in the Genesis of Fatty Acids in Human Surface Lipids. *J. Investig. Dermatol.*, 55, 173–178, 1970.

12. Nicolaides, N., Skin Lipids: Their Biochemical Uniqueness. *Science*, 186, 19–26, 1974.

13. Stewart, M., Downing, D., Pochi, P., Strauss, J., The Fatty Acids of the Human Sebaceous Gland Phosphotidylcholine. *Biochem. Biophys. Acta*, 529, 380–386, 1978.

14. Montes, L. and Wilborn, W., Location of Bacterial Skin Flora. *British J. Dermatol.*, 81, 23–25, 1969.

15. Jahns, A. and Alexeyev, O., Microbial colonization of normal skin Direct visualization of 194 skin biopsies. *Anaerobe*, 38, 47–49, 2016.

16. Jahns, A., Golovleva, I., Palmer, R., Alexeyev, O., Spatial distribution of bacterial-fungal communities in facial skin. *J. Dermatol. Sci.*, 70, 71–73, 2013.

17. Furzeland, S., Atkins, D., Ferdinando, D., Ginkel, M., Singleton, S., Jones, D., A New Microscopy Ultrastructural Visualisation Method for 3D distribution of microbes in the scalp. *World Congress of Hair Res.*, 2014.

18. Peterson, J., Garges, S., Giovanni, M., McInnes, P., Wang, L., Schloss, J., Bonazzi, V., McEwen, J., Wetterstrand, K., Deal, C., The NIH Human Microbiome Project. *Genome Res.*, 19, 2317–2323, 2009.

19. Lloyd-Price, J., Abu-Ali, G., Huttenhower, C., The healthy human microbiome. *Genome Med.*, 8, 1, 51, 2016.

20. Luzopone, C. and Knight, R., Species Divergence and the Measurement of Microbial Diversity. *FEMS Microbiol. Rev.*, 32, 557–578, 2008.

21. Kong, H., Andersson, B., Clavel, T., Common, J., Jackson, S., Olson, N., Segre, J., Traidl-Hoffmann, C., Performing Skin Microbiome Research: A Method to the Madness. *J. Investig. Dermatol.*, 137, 561–568, 2017.

22. Grice, E. and Segre, J., The Skin Microbiome. *Nat. Rev. Microbiol.*, 9, 244–253, 2011.

23. Byrd, A., Belkaid, Y., Segre, J., The human skin microbiome. *Nat. Rev. Microbiol.*, 16, 143–155, 2018.

24. Proctor, L., LoTempio, J., Marquitz, A. *et al.*, A review of 10 years of human microbiome research activities at the US National Institutes of Health, Fiscal Years 2007-2016. *Microbiome*, 7, 1, 31, 2019.

25. Methé, B., Nelson, K., Pop, M. *et al.*, A Framework for Human Microbiome Research. *Nature*, 486, 215–221, 2012.

26. Llorens-Rico, V.A.R.J., Tracking Humans and Microbes. *Nature*, 569, 632–633, 2019.

27. Proctor, L.M., Creasy, H.H., Fettweis, J.M. *et al.*, The Integrative Human Microbiome Project. *Nature*, 569, 641–648, 2019.

28. Procter, L., Whats Next for the Human Microbiome? *Nature*, 569, 623–625, 2019.

29. Chng, K., Tay, A., Li, C., Ng, A., Wang, J., Suri, B., Matta, S., McGovern, N., Janela, B., Wong, X., Sio, Y., Au, B., Wilm, A., Sessions, P., Lim, T., Tang, M., Ginhoux, F., Connolly, J., Lane, E., Chew, F., Common, J., Nagarajan, N., Whole metagenome profiling reveals skin microbiome-dependent susceptibility to atopic dermatitis flare. *Nat. Microbiol.*, 1, 1–10, 2016.

30. Bousilami, A., Porto, C., Rath, C., Wang, M., Guo, Y., Gonzalez, A., Berg-Lyon, D., Ackermann, G., Christensen, G., Nakatsuji, T., Zhang, L., Borkowski, A., Meehan, M., Dorrestein, K., Gallo, R., Bandeira, N., Knight, R., Alexandrov, T., Dorrestein, P., Molecular cartography of the human skin surface in 3D. *Proc. Natl. Acad. Sci. U S A*, 112, 17, E2120-9, 2015.

31. Gilbert, J. and Lynch, S., Community Ecology as a Framework for Human Microbiome Research. *Nat. Med.*, 25, 884–889, 2019.

32. Perez Perez, G.I., Gao, Z., Jourdain, R., Ramirez, J., Gany, F., Clavaud, C., *et al.* Body Site Is a More Determinant Factor than Human Population Diversity in the Healthy Skin Microbiome. *PLoS ONE* 11, 4, e0151990, 2016.

33. Bibel, D. and Lovell, D., Skin Flora Maps: A Tool in the Study of Cutaneous Ecology. *J. Investig. Dermatol.*, 67, 265–269, 1976.

34. Jo, J., Kennedy, E., Kong, H., Topographical and physiological differences of the skin mycobiome in health and disease. *Virulence*, 8, 324–333, 2019.

35. White, T., Findley, K., Dawson, T.L., Scheynius, A., Boekhout, T., Cuomo, C., Xu, J., Saunders, C., Fungi on the skin: Dermatophytes and Malassezia. *Cold Spring Harbour Perspect. Med.*, 4, a019802, 1–16, 2014.

36. Findley, K., Oh, J., Yang, J., Conlan, S., Deming, C., Meyer, J., Schoenfold, D., Nomicos, E., Park, M., Kong, H., Segre, J., Topographic diversity of fungal and bacterial communities in human skin. *Nat. Int. J. Med.*, 498, 367–370, 2013.

37. Gao, Z., Perez-Perez, G., Chen, Y., Blaser, M., Quantitation of Major Human Cutaneous Bacterial and Fungal Populations. *J. Clin. Microbiol.*, 48, 10, 3575–3581, 2010.

38. Mayser, P. and Gaitanis, G., Physiology and Biochemistry, in: *Malassezia and the skin: Science and Clinical Practice*, pp. 121–137, Springer, Berlin-Heidelberg, 2010.

39. Hay, R. a. M. G., Introduction: Malassezia yeasts from a historical perspective, in: *Malassezia and the skin: science and clinical practice*, 11, pp. 1–16, Springer, Berlin-Heidelberg, 2010.

40. Wu, G., Zhao, H., Li, C., Rakapakse, M., Wong, W., Xu, J., Saunders, C., Reeder, N., Reilman, R., Scheynius, A., Sun, S., Billmyre, B., Li, W., Averette, A., Mieczkowski, P., Heitman, J., Theelen, B., Schroder, M., Sessions, P., Butler, G., Maurer-Stroh, S., Boekhout, T., Genus-Wide Comparative Genomics of Malassezia Delineates Its Phylogeny, Physiology, and Niche Adaptation on Human Skin. *PLoS Genet.* 11, 11, e1005614, 2015.

41. Zhang, E., Tanaka, T.T.R., Makimura, K.N.A., Sugita, T., Characterization of Malassezia microbiota in the human external auditory canal and on the sole of the foot. *Microbiol. Immunol.*, 56, 238–244, 2012.
42. Ashbee, H., Update on the genus Malassezia. *Med. Mycol.*, 45, 287–303, 2007.
43. Clavaud, C., Jourdain, R., Bar-Hen, A., Tichit, M., Bouchier, C., Pouradier, F., El-Rawadi, C., Guillot, J., Menard-Szczebara, F., Breton, L., Latge, J.-P., Mouyna, I., Dandruff Is Associated with Disequilibrium in the Proportion of the Major Bacterial and Fungal Populations Colonizing the Scalp. *PLOS one*, 8, 3, e58203, 2013.
44. Xu, Z., Wang, Z., Yuan, C., Liu, X., Yang, F., Wang, T., Wang, J., Manabe, K., Qin, O., Wang, X., Zhang, Y., Zhang, M., Dandruff is associated with the conjoined interactions between host and microorganisms. *Sci. Rep.*, 6, 24877, 2016.
45. Hannigan, G., Meisel, J., Tyldsley, A., Zheng, Q., Hodkinson, B., SanMiguel, A., Minot, S., Bushman, F., Grice, E., The Human Skin Double-Stranded DNA Virome: Topographical and Temporal Diversity, Genetic Enrichment, and Dynamic Associations with the Host Microbiome. *mbio*, 6, 5, e01578-15, 2015.
46. Tirosh, O., Conlan, S., Deming, C., Lee-Lin, S., Huang, X., Su, H., Freeman, A., Segre, J., Kong, H., Expanded skin virome in DOCK8-deficient patients. *Nat. Med.*, 12, 1815–1821, 2018.
47. Van Zyl, L., Abrahams, Y., Stander, E., Kirby-McCollough, B., Jourdain, R., Clavaud, C., Breton, L., Trindade, M., Novel Phages of Healthy Skin metaviromes from South Africa. *Sci. Rep.*, 8, 1, 12265, 2018.
48. Shibagaki, N., Suda, W., Clavaud, C., Bestian, P., Takayasu, L., Iioka, E., Kurakawa, R., Yamashita, N., Hattori, Y., Yamashita, N., Shindo, C., Breton, L., Hattori, M., Aging-related changes in the diversity of women's skin microbiomes associated with oral bacteria. *Sci. Rep.*, 7, 1–10, 2017.
49. Barnard, E. and Li, H., Shaping of cutaneous function by encounters with commensals. *J. Physiol.*, 595, 437–450, 2017.
50. Mukherjee, S., Mitra, R., Maitra, A., Gupta, S., Kumaran, S., Chakrabortty, A., Majumder, P., Sebum and Hydration Levels in Specific Regions of Human Face Significantly Predict the Nature and Diversity of Facial Skin Microbiome. *Sci. Rep.*, 6, 1–11, 2016.
51. Kong, H., Oh, J., Deming, C., Conlan, S., Grice, E., Beatson, M., Nomicos, E., Polley, E., Komarow, H., Murray, P., Lurner, M.S.J., Temporal shifts in the skin microbiome associated with disease flares and treatment in children with atopic dermatitis. *Genome Res.*, 22, 850–859, 2012.
52. Cawley, A., Arnold, D., Mayes, A., Hoptroff, M., Murphy, B., Grimshaw, S., Gorman, C., MacGuire-Flanagan, A., Tazzioli, J., Paterson, S., Hawkins, S., Qualls, A., Examination of the skin microbiome associated with dry and non-dry skin. *World Congress Dermatol. (Poster 1885)*, 2019.
53. Gilbert, J., Our Unique Microbial Identity. *Genome Biol.*, 16, 97, 2015.

54. Leake, S., Pagni, M., Falquet, L., Taroni, F., Greub, G., The salivary microbiome for differentiating individuals: Proof of principle. *Microbes Infect.*, 18, 6, 399–405, 2016.
55. Meadow, J., Altrichter, A., Bateman, A., Stenson, J., Brown, G., Green, J., Bohannan, B., Humans differ in their personal microbial cloud. *PeerJ*, 3, e1258, 2015.
56. Franzosa, E., Huang, K., Meadow, J., Gevers, D., Lemon, K., Bohannan, B., Huttenhower, C., Identifying personal microbiomes using metagenomic codes. *Proc. Natl. Acad. Sci. U S A*, 112, 22, E2930-8, 2015.
57. Fierer, N., Lauber, C., Zhou, N., McDonald, D., Costello, E., Knight, R., Forensic identification using skin bacterial communities. *Proc. Natl. Acad. Sci. U S A*, 107, 14, 6477–81, 2010.
58. Kuiper, I., Microbial forensics: next-generation sequencing as catalyst. *EMBO Rep.*, 17, 8, 1085–1087, 2016.
59. Hampton-Marcell, J., Lopez, J., Gilbert, J., The human microbiome: An emerging tool in forensics. *Microbiol Biotechnol.*, 10, 2, 228–230, 2017.
60. Kupferschmidt, K., How your microbiome can put you at the scene of the crime. *Science*, 2016.
61. Lee, S., Woo, S., Choi, G., Hong, Y., Eom, Y., Microbial Forensic Analysis of Bacterial Fingerprint by Sequence Comparison of 16S rRNA Gene. *J. Forensic Res.*, 2015.
62. Vogt, A., Hadam, S., Heiderhoff, M., Audring, H., Lademann, J., Sterry, W., Peytavi-Blume, U., Morphometry of human terminal and vellus hair follicles. *Exp. Dermatol.*, 16, 11, 946–950, 2007.
63. Pagnoni, A., Kligman, A., Gammal, S., Stoudemayer, T., Determination of the density of follicles on various regions of the face by cyanoacrylate biopsy: Correlation with sebum output. *British J. Dermatol.*, 131, 6, 862–865, 1994.
64. Harker, M. and Harding, C., Amino acid composition, including key derivatives of eccrine sweat: Potential biomarkers of certain atopic skin conditions. *Int. J. Cosmetic Sci.*, 35, 2, 163–168, 2013.
65. Eyerich, S., Eyerich, K., Traidl-Hoffmann, C., Biedermann, T., Cutaneous Barriers and Skin Immunity: Differentiating A Connected Network. *Trend. Immunol.*, 39, 4, 315–327, 2018.
66. Michaels, A., Chandrasekaren, S., Shaw, J., Drug permeation through human skin: Theory and *in vitro* experimental measurement. *Am. Inst. Chem. Eng.*, 5, 985–996, 1975.
67. Baroni, A., Buomino, E., DeGregorio, V., Roucco, E., Ruocco, V., Wolf, R., Structure and function of the epidermis related to barrier properties. *Clin. Dermatol.*, 30, 3, 257–62, 2012.
68. Elias, P., Stratum Corneum Defensive Functions: An Integrated View. *J. Investig. Dermatol.*, 125, 2, 183–200, 2005.
69. Lee, S., Jeong, S., Ahn, S., An Update of the Defensive Barrier Function of Skin. *Yonsei Med. J.*, 47, 3, 293–306, 2006.

70. Voegali, R. and Rawlings, A., Desquamation: It Is Almost All About Proteases, in: *Treatment of Dry Skin Syndrome*, pp. 150–178, Springer, Berlin-Heidelberg, 2012.

71. Egelrud, T., Desquamation in the Stratum Corneum. *Acta Derm. Venereol. Suppl. (Stockh).*, 208, 44–45, 2000.

72. Ishida-Yamamoto, A. and Kishibe, M., Involvement of corneodesmosome degradation and lamellar granule transportation in the desquamation process. *Med. Mol. Morphol.*, 44, 1, 1–6, 2011.

73. Wilson, M., The Indigenous Microbiota of the Skin, in: *Bacteriology of Humans An Ecological Perpsective*, Blackwell, USA, pp. 56–94, 2008.

74. Bouwstra, J., de Graaf, A., Gooris, G., Nijsse, J., Wiechers, J., v. Aelst and, A.C., Water Distribution and Related Morphology in Human Stratum Corneum at Different Hydration Levels. *J. Investig. Dermatol.*, 120, 5, 750–758, 2003.

75. Sylvestre, J., Couissou, C., Guy, R., Delgado-Charro, M., Extraction and quantification of amino acids in human stratum corneum *in vivo. Br J Dermatol.*, 163, 3, 458–65, 2010.

76. Bojar, R. and Holland, K., Review: The human cutaneous microflora and factors controlling colonisation. *World J. Microbiol. Biotechnol.*, 18, 889–903, 2002.

77. Zapka, C., Leff, J., Henley, J., Tittl, J., De Nardo, E., Butler, M., Griggs, R., Fierer, N., Edmonds-Wilson, S., Comparison of Standard Culture-Based Method to Culture-Independent Method for Evaluation of Hygiene Effects on the Hand Microbiome. *mBio*, 8, 2, e00093–17, 2017.

78. Elias, P., The how, why and clinical importance of stratum corneum acidification. *Exp. Dermatol.*, 26, 11, 999–1003, 2017.

79. Fluhr, J. and Elias, P., Stratum corneum pH: Formation and Function of the 'Acid Mantle'. *Exogenous Dermatol.*, 1, 163–175, 2002.

80. Coates, R., Moran, J., Horsburgh, M., Staphylococci: Colonizers and pathogens of human skin. *Future Microbiol.*, 9, 1, 75–91, 2014.

81. Lambers, H., Piessens, S., Bloem, A., Pronk, H., Finkel, P., Natural skin surface pH is on average below 5, which is beneficial for its resident flora. *Int. J. Cosmetic Sci.*, 28, 5, 359–370, 2006.

82. Kwaszewska, A., Sobiś-Glinkowska, M., Szewczyk, E., Cohabitation–relationships of corynebacteria and staphylococci on human skin, *Folia Microbiol (Praha).* 59, 6, 495–502, 2014.

83. Prouty, S. and Pappas, A., Sapienic Acid: Species-Specific Fatty Acid Metabolism of the Human Sebaceous Gland, in: *Lipids and Skin Health*, pp. 139–157, Springer, New York, USA, 2015.

84. Wille, J. and Kydonieus, A., Palmitoleic Acid Isomer (C16:1Δ6) in Human Skin Sebum Is Effective against Gram-Positive Bacteria. *Skin Pharmacol. Appl. Physiol.*, 16, 3, 176–187, 2003.

85. Cartron, M., England, S., Chiriac, A., Josten, M., Turner, R., Rauter, Y., Hurd, A., Sahl, H., Jones, S., Foster, S., Bactericidal Activity of the Human Skin

Fatty Acid cis-6-Hexadecanoic Acid on *Staphylococcus aureus. Antimicrobial Agents Chemother.*, 58, 7, 3599–3609, 2014.

86. Neumann, Y., Ohlsen, K., Donat, S., Engelmann, S., Kusch, H., Albrecht, D., Cartron, M., Hurd, A., Foster, S., The effect of skin fatty acids on *Staphylococcus aureus. Archives Microbiol.*, 197, 2, 245–267, 2015.

87. Fischer, C., Drake, D., Dawson, D., Blanchette, D., Brogden, K., Wertza, P., Antibacterial Activity of Sphingoid Bases and Fatty Acids against Gram-Positive and Gram-Negative Bacteria. *Antimicrobial Agents Chemother.*, 56, 3, 1157–1161, 2012.

88. Takigawa, H., Nakagawa, H., Kuzukawa, M., Mori, H., Imokawa, G., Deficient Production of Hexadecenoic Acid in the Skin Is Associated in Part with the Vulnerability of Atopic Dermatitis Patients to Colonization by *Staphylococcus aureus. Dermatology*, 211, 3, 240–248, 2005.

89. Arikawa, J., Ishibashi, M., Kawashima, M., Takagi, Y., Ichikawa, Y., Imokawa, G., Decreased Levels of Sphingosine, a Natural Antimicrobial Agent, may be Associated with Vulnerability of the Stratum Corneum from Patients with Atopic Dermatitis to Colonization by *Staphylococcus aureus. J. Investig. Dermatol.*, 119, 2, 433–439, 2002.

90. Rieg, S., Seeber, S., Steffen, H., Humeny, A., Kalbacher, H., Stevanovic, S., Kimura, A., Garbe, C., Schittek, B., Generation of Multiple Stable Dermcidin-Derived Antimicrobial Peptides in Sweat of Different Body Sites. *J. Investig. Dermatol.*, 126, 2, 354–365, 2006.

91. Glaser, R., Harder, J., Lange, H., Bartels, J., Christophers, E., Schroder, J., Antimicrobial psoriasin (S100A7) protects human skin from Escherichia coli infection. *Nat. Immunol.*, 6, 1, 57–64, 2005.

92. Kiatsurayanon, C., Niyonsaba, F., Smithrithee, R., Akiyama, T., Ushio, H., Hara, M., Okumura, K., Ikeda, S., Ogawa, H., Host Defense (Antimicrobial) Peptide, Human b-Defensin-3, Improves the Function of the Epithelial Tight-Junction Barrier in Human Keratinocytes. *J. Investig. Dermatol.*, 134, 8, 2163–2173, 2014.

93. Wanke, I., Steffen, H., Christ, C., Krismer, B., Gotz, F., Peschel, A., Schaller, M., Schittel, B., Skin Commensals Amplify the Innate Immune Response to Pathogens by Activation of Distinct Signaling Pathways. *J. Investig. Dermatol.*, 131, 2, 382–390, 2011.

94. Braff, M., Bardan, A., Nizet, V., Gallo, R., Cutaneous Defense Mechanisms by Antimicrobial Peptides. *J. Investig. Dermatol.*, 125, 1, 9–13, 2005.

95. Nakatsuji, T., Chen, T., Narala, S., Chun, K., Two, A., Yun, T., Shafiq, F., Kotol, P., Bouslimani, A., Melnik, A., Latif, H., Kim, J., Lockhart, A., Artis, K., David, G., Taylor, P., Streib, J., Dorrestein, P., Grier, A., Gill, S., Zengler, K., Hata, T., Leung, D., Gallo, R., Antimicrobials from human skin commensal bacteria protect against *Staphylococcus aureus* and are deficient in atopic dermatitis. *Sci. Transl. Med.*, 9, 378, 22, 9, 2017.

96. Yamasaki, K., Schauber, J., Coda, A., Lin, H., Dorschner, R., Schechter, N., Bonnart, C., Descargues, P., Hovnanian, A., Gallo, R., Kallikrein-mediated

proteolysis regulates the antimicrobial effects of cathelicidins in skin. *FASEB J.*, 20, 12, 2068–2080, 2006.

97. Mathapathi, M., Mallemalla, P., Vora, S., Iyer, V., Tiwari, J., Chakrabortty, A., Majumdar, A., Niacinamide leave-on formulation provides long-lasting protection against bacteria *in vivo*. *Exp. Dermatol.*, 26, 9, 827–829, 2017.

98. Sivakanesan, R. and Dawes, E., Anaerobic Glucose and Serine Metabolism in *Staphylococcus aureus*. *J. Gen. Microbiol.*, 118, 143–157, 1980.

99. Moissl-Eichinger, C., Probst, A., Birarda, G., Auerbach, A., Koskinen, K., Wolf, P., Holman, H., Human age and skin physiology shape diversity and abundance of Archaea on skin. *Sci. Rep.*, 7, 1, 4039, 2017.

100. Tax, G., Urban, E., Palotas, Z., Puskas, R., Konya, Z., Biro, T., Kemeny, L.K., Propionic Acid Produced by Propionibacterium acnes Strains Contributes to their pathoginicity. *Acta Dermato Venereol.*, 96, 1, 43–49, 2016.

101. Jo, J., Deming, C., Kennady, E., Conlan, S., Polley, E., Ng, W., Segre, J., Kong, H., Diverse human skin fungal communities in children converge in adulthood. *J. Investig. Dermatol.*, 136, 12, 2356–2363, 2016.

102. Lee, H., Jeong, S., Lee, S., Kim, S., Han, H., Jeon, C., Effects of cosmetics on the skin microbiome of facial cheeks with different hydration levels. *Microbiologyopen.*, 7, 2, e00557, 2018.

103. Kroll, L., Hoffman, D., Cunningham, C., Koenig, D., Impact of Stratum Corneum Damage on Natural Moisturising Factor (NMF) in the Skin, in: *Treatment of Dry Skin Syndrome*, pp. 441–452, Springer, Berlin-Heidelberg, 2012.

104. Bewick, S., Gurarie, E., Weissman, J., Beattie, J., Davati, C., Flint, R., Thielen, P., Trait-based analysis of the human skin microbiome. *Microbiome*, 7, 1, 101, 2019.

105. Chiller, K., Selkin, B., Murakawi, G., Skin Microflora and Bacterial Infections of the Skin. *J. Investig. Dermatol. Symp. Proc.*, 6, 3, 170–174, 2001.

106. Gallo, R. and Nakatsuji, T., Microbial Symbiosis with the Innate Immune Defense System of the Skin. *J. Investig. Dermatol.*, 131, 10, 1974–1980, 2011,

107. Christensen, G. and Bruggemann, H., Bacterial skin commensals and their role as host guardians. *Beneficial Microbes*, 5, 2, 201–215, 2014.

108. Frank, D., Feazel, L., Bessesen, M., Price, C., Janoff, E., Pace, N., The Human Nasal Microbiota and *Staphylococcus aureus* Carriage. *PLoS One*, 5, 5, e10598, 2010.

109. Cogen, A., Yamasaki, K., Sanchez, K., Dorschner, R., Lai, Y., MacLeod, D., Torpey, J., Otto, M., Nizet, V., Kim, J., Gallo, R., Selective Antimicrobial Action Is Provided by Phenol-Soluble Modulins Derived from *Staphylococcus epidermidis*, a Normal Resident of the Skin. *J. Investig. Dermatol.*, 130, 1, 192–200, 2010.

110. Geohegan, J., Irvine, A., Foster, T., *Staphylococcus aureus* and Atopic Dermatitis: A Complex and Evolving Relationship. *Trends. Microbiol.*, 26, 6, 484–497, 2018.

111. Iwase, T., Uehara, Y., Shinji, H., Tajima, A., Seo, H., Takada, K., Agata, T., Mizune, Y., *Staphylococcus epidermidis* Esp inhibits *Staphylococcus aureus* biofilm formation and nasal colonization. *J. Bacteriol.*, 195, 8, 1645–55, 2013.

112. Lai, Y., Cogen, A., Radek, K., Park, H., MacLeod, D., Leichtle, A., Ryan, A., Nardo, A., Gallo, R., Activation of TLR2 by a Small Molecule Produced by *Staphylococcus epidermidis* Increases Antimicrobial Defense against Bacterial Skin Infections. *J. Investig. Dermatol.*, 130, 9, 2211–2221, 2010.

113. Sugimoto, S., Iwamoto, T., Takada, K., Okuda, K., Tajima, A., Iwase, T., Mizune, Y., *Staphylococcus epidermidis* Esp Degrades Specific Proteins Associated with *Staphylococcus aureus* Biofilm Formation and Host-Pathogen Interaction. *J. Bacteriol.*, 195, 8, 1645–1655, 2013.

114. Wang, Y., Zhang, L., Yu, J., Huang, S., Wang, Z., Chun, K., Lee, T., Chen, Y.-T., Gallo, R., Huang, C.-M., A Co-Drug of Butyric Acid Derived from Fermentation Metabolites of the Human Skin Microbiome Stimulates Adipogenic Differentiation of Adipose-Derived Stem Cells: Implications in Tissue Augmentation. *J. Investig. Dermatol.*, 137, 1, 46–56, 2017.

115. Shu, M., Wang, Y., Yu, J., Kuo, S., Coda, A., Jiang, Y., Gallo, R., Huang, C., Fermentation of Propionibacterium acnes, a commensal bacterium in the human skin microbiome, as skin probiotics against methicillin-resistant *Staphylococcus aureus*. *PLoS One*, 8, 2, e55380, 2013.

116. Nodake, Y., Matsumoto, S., Miura, R., Honda, H., Ishibashi, G., Matsumoto, S., Dekio, I., Sakakibara, R., Pilot study on novel skin care method by augmentation with *Staphylococcus epidermidis*, an autologous skin microbe–A blinded randomized clinical trial. *J. Dermatol. Sci.*, 79, 2, 119–26, 2015.

117. Di Marzio, L., Cinque, B., De Simone, C., and C. M.G, Effect of the lactic acid bacterium Streptococcus thermophilus on ceramide levels in human keratinocytes *in vitro* and stratum corneum *in vivo*. *J. Investig. Dermatol.*, 113, 1, 98–106, 1999.

118. Di Marzio, L., Centi, C., Cinque, B., Masci, S., Giuliani, M., Arcieri, A., Zicari, L., De Simone, C., Cifone, M., Effect of the lactic acid bacterium Streptococcus thermophilus on stratum corneum ceramide levels and signs and symptoms of atopic dermatitis patients. *Exp. Dermatol.*, 12, 5, 615–20, 2003.

119. Di Marzio, L., Cinque, B., Cupelli, F., De Simone, C., Cifone, M., Giuliani, M., Increase of skin-ceramide levels in aged subjects following a short-term topical application of bacterial sphingomyelinase from Streptococcus thermophilus. *Int. J. Immunopathol. Pharmacol.*, 21, 1, 137–43, 2008.

120. Meisel, J., Sfyroera, G., Bartow-McKenney, C., Gimblet, C., Bugayev, J., Horwinski, J., Kim, B., Brestoff, J., Tyldsley, A., Zheng, Q., Hodkinson, B., Artis, D., Grice, E., Commensal microbiota modulate gene expression in the skin. *Microbiome*, 6, 1, 20, 2018.

121. Ohnemus, U., Kohrmeyer, K., Houdek, P., Rohde, H., Wladykowski, E., Vidal, S., Horstkotte, M., Aepfelbacher, M., Kirschner, N., Behne, M., Moll, I., Brandner, J., Regulation of Epidermal Tight-Junctions (TJ) during Infection

with Exfoliative Toxin-Negative *Staphylococcus* Strains. *J. Investig. Dermatol.*, 128, 4, 906–916, 2008.

122. Kiatsurayanon, C., Niyonsaba, F., Smithrithee, R., Akiyama, T., Ushio, H., Hara, M., Okumura, K., Ikeda, S., Ogawa, H., Host Defense (Antimicrobial) Peptide, Human b-Defensin-3, Improves the Function of the Epithelial Tight-Junction Barrier in Human Keratinocytes. *J. Investig. Dermatol.*, 134, 8, 2163–2173, 2014.

123. Hattori, F., Kiatsurayanon, C., Okumura., Ogawa, K.,.H., Ikeda, S., Okamoto, K., Niyonsaba, F., The antimicrobial protein S100A7/psoriasin enhances the expression of keratinocyte differentiation markers and strengthens the skin's tight junction barrier. *British J. Dermatol.*, 171, 4, 742–753, 2014.

2

The Gut Microbiome-Skin Axis: Impact on Skin and Systemic Health

David Drake

Iowa Institute for Oral Health Research, University of Iowa College of Dentistry, Iowa City, Iowa, USA

Abstract

We are in the midst of a revolution of knowledge regarding the human microbiome. The revolution comes from the explosion of knowledge on the role of our microbiomes in systemic disease, overall well-being, behavior, and many other health states that we previously would have never thought of microbiomes driving these complex states. Of all the complex microbiomes across the body, substantial evidence has shown that the gut microbiome appears to be the pivotal microbiome in the body. While there was always some sense of interactions between the microbiomes of the body, only recently has evidence built a fascinating picture of two- and three-way interactions between our microbiomes and organ systems. Now we are obtaining exciting data showing how one microbiome—the gut microbiome—has a definitive effect on the composition and metabolic activity of the skin microbiome. We are in a new era of discovery on how important our microbiomes are to our health and vitality. As we move into a new decade, more interactions and levels of regulation are sure to be discovered.

Keywords: Microbiome, regulatory T cells, dysbiosis, oral microbiome, gut microbiome

Email: david-drake@uiowa.edu

Nava Dayan (ed.) Skin Microbiome Handbook: From Basic Research to Product Development, (33–44) © 2020 Scrivener Publishing LLC

2.1   Introduction

We are in the midst of a revolution of knowledge regarding the human microbiome. We have known for some time that there are more micro-organisms than human cells in our bodies, and we have known that the microbial communities differ across the body, shaped by multiple complex factors. We have progressed from the classical infectious disease paradigm years ago where we relied on Koch's postulates, to early definitive statements outlining how one determines causative agents in infectious diseases. Now we know about the complex interactions within microbial communities that lead to disease [1–5]. The revolution comes from the explosion of knowledge on the role of our microbiomes in systemic disease, overall well-being, behavior, and many other health states that we previously would have never thought of microbiomes driving these complex states.

Of all the complex microbiomes across the body, substantial evidence has shown that the gut microbiome appears to be the pivotal microbiome in the body. An imbalance in the gut microbiota has been strongly associated with obesity and diabetes [6–9]. The scope of the impact the gut microbiome has on organ systems and systemic health is incredible. New evidence now shows that the gut microbiome has significant influence on our body's chrono clocks and circadian rhythms [10]. The consequences of this influence result in considerable impact on our systemic, metabolic homeostasis. There have been multiple other studies showing strong links to systemic diseases and conditions, including obesity, chronic kidney disease, hypertension, and breast cancer [11–20]. Suffice it to say that the gut microbiome appears to be *the* pivotal microbiome in the human body that has far-reaching impact on our overall health.

The skin microbiome is also a fascinating biome that serves many purposes, one of which, and of paramount importance, is a barrier protection against colonization by pathogens [21–25]. There are several skin diseases that have been shown to be associated with shifts in the composition of the skin microbiome and interactions with the host immune system [26–35]. While there was always some sense of interactions between the microbiomes of the body, only recently has evidence built a fascinating picture of two- and three-way interactions between our microbiomes and organ systems. Now we are obtaining exciting data showing how one microbiome—the gut microbiome—has a definitive effect on the composition and metabolic activity of the skin microbiome [36–39].

2.2 The Gut-Skin Microbiome Axis

The gut and skin have several shared characteristics such as having heavy vasculature, nerve innervation, and distinct microbiomes [10, 27, 36, 37, 39–41]. Because these microbiomes interact extensively with the external environment, complex and strongly integrated neuroendocrine and immune system components create biomes that serve as portals to the outside world [29, 37, 38]. Suffice it to say, proper functioning of both the skin and gut are essential for overall body homeostasis and well-being of our bodies—and ultimately survival.

Dysbiosis—taxonomic and functional—of the gut microbiome can have a staggering effect on host overall health. The spectrum of maladies and diseases is impressive, such as Type I and II diabetes, inflammatory bowel disease, colorectal carcinoma, liver cirrhosis, allergies, atherosclerosis, Alzheimer's disease, rheumatoid arthritis, cardiovascular disease, and many others [11–20]. Therefore, it should not be a surprise that dysbiosis of the gut microbiome impacts skin health as well.

It has been shown—and is not terribly surprising—that diet has a profound impact on the gut microbiome [14–16, 20]. It has been known for many years that gastrointestinal (GI) diseases can have manifestations on the skin. These include atopic dermatitis, acne, and psoriasis [37, 38, 40, 42–44]. Many GI diseases that have considerable impact on the gut microbiome in terms of major shifts in microbial composition, community dominance, and metabolic activity, have marked impact on the skin and concomitantly, the skin microbiome [14–16, 20]. In many cases, this can be diagnostic as distinct presentations of skin maladies is indicative of a primary, and in some cases—severe—GI disorders and diseases [36, 37, 40, 45–48]. In the next section, we will investigate this link—the gut-skin microbiome axis.

2.3 The Gut-Skin Microbiome Axis: Principle Pathways

It has been shown that the gut microbiome has a significant effect on the adaptive immune system and involves the induction of immunoglobulin A, exerting a balance/maintenance between effector T cells and regulatory T cells [49–54]. Emerging and exciting new evidence is showing that the gut microbiome exerts a significant effect on skin homeostasis due to its regulatory effect on systemic immunity [29, 37–39]. In addition, studies have also shown that gut microbiome functional dysbiosis—resulting in shifts in metabolites—may influence cutaneous physiology, pathology, and skin site-specific immune responses. Collectively, these data have established the notion that there is a direct link between the well-being, if you will, of the gut microbiome and skin homeostasis [30, 37–39, 41].

It is not all bad; several rodent and human studies have also shown that the gut microbiome can have beneficial effects on the skin [37, 42, 55]. Mice receiving *Lactobacillus reuteri* supplementation experienced significantly increased dermal thickness, enhanced folliculogenesis, and increased sebocyte production, which led to thicker, shinier fur [56]. In another study, oral supplementation of *Lactobacillus brevis* in rats resulted in a significant decrease in transepidermal water loss [57]. This effect has also been shown in humans—after 12 weeks of oral supplementation with *L. brevis*, a significant reduction in transepidermal water loss was also observed as in rats—but a significant increase in corneal hydration was also observed in humans [58]. Similar results were seen in a study with human subjects taking *L. paracasei* supplements for two months, resulting in decreased skin sensitivity and transepidermal water loss [59].

A number of studies have shown that the gut microbiome has a significant effect on allostasis— the recovery of homeostasis after some stressor— and this is mediated by gut microbiome-mediated effects on both the innate and adaptive immune systems [36–38, 60]. There are multiple studies that have shown that probiotics—primarily *Lactobacillus* species—have a marked effect on several clinical responses, including accelerated wound healing, suppression of dermatitis, reduction in hypersensitivity, and skin restoration after ultraviolet (UV) radiation exposure [37, 46, 47, 55–57, 61]. A primary mode of action appears to be through influencing T cell differentiation in response to immune stimuli [62, 63]. Oral administration of *Lactobacillus casei* has been shown to inhibit differentiation of CD+8 T cells into cutaneous hypersensitivity effector cells and concomitantly a decrease in their recruitment to the skin [37, 62]. This particular bacterium increases recruitment of FoxP3+ regulatory T cells to the skin—resulting in decreased apoptosis-mediated skin inflammation [62, 63]. So, the important end result is that skin homeostasis is restored through modulation of the immune system—with the gut microbiome being the primary driver. We will see more later how the gut microbiome plays a pivotal role in multiple skin diseases and conditions.

It is well known that Th17 cells are abundant in both the intestine and the skin, since both organs are an interface to the external environment [64–69]. It is also well known that pro-inflammatory cytokines from these cells appear to contribute significantly to the pathogenesis of several chronic inflammatory dermatoses, which we will cover later. It becomes particularly intriguing when one views the data that the balance between Th17 cells and their counterpart regulatory T cells is strongly influenced by the gut microbiome—establishing this link or triad if you will—between the gut microbiome, the innate and adaptive immune systems, and the skin [53, 54, 69].

2.4   Dysbiosis of the Gut Microbiome and Skin Dyshomeostasis

If the composition and function of the gut microbiome reaches a state of imbalance—and multiple variables can cause this—the impact is far beyond intestinal dysbiosis and disease. There is growing evidence that dysbiosis of the gut microbiome can have a marked impact on the overall homeostasis of the skin [10, 36–38, 40, 55, 60, 70]. Compounds such as phenol and p-cresol aromatic amino acids metabolites, are known as biomarkers of dysbiotic gut microbial communities—this is strongly seen when pathogens like *Clostridium difficile* become more dominant within the gut microbiota [37]. These metabolites enter the circulation and appear to preferentially accumulate in the skin. The result is impairment of epidermal differentiation and skin barrier integrity (Figure 2.1). In addition, an

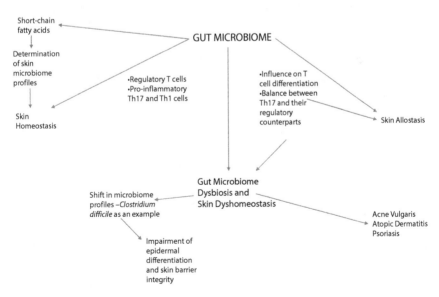

Figure 2.1 Regulation of the gut-skin axis.

increase in epidermal permeability as a result of gut microbiome dysbiosis causes an imbalance between activated effector T cells and their regulatory counterparts [53, 54, 69]. When you then factor in the ensuing production of pro-inflammatory cytokines, one sees a further enhancement of epithelial permeability, resulting in a cascading cycle of systemic inflammation [37, 71]. So, shifts in composition and metabolic function of the gut microbiome has a profound impact on the skin—and potentially the skin microbiome. Although evidence is scant for the latter impact, studies have shown that ingestion of garlic results in bioavailable levels of allyl methyl sulfide in the skin, a breakdown product from garlic. This compound has been shown to be moderately antibacterial [72]. Does this have an impact on the skin microbiome? Clearly, there are likely other compounds that reach the skin from gut metabolism and one wonders if these collectively alter the development and composition of the skin microbiome.

There are three distinct skin disorders that occur that have strong links to intestinal microbiome dysbiosis: Acne Vulgaris, Atopic Dermatitis, and Psoriasis. Each of these is complex and involve metabolic as well as microbial systemic interactions.

2.4.1   Acne Vulgaris

Acne vulgaris is a common chronic skin disease that involves blockage and/or inflammation of the pilosebaceous units. Inflammatory and non-inflammatory lesions result and consist of papules, nodules, and pustules [39, 73]. The pathophysiology of this skin disease is attributed to three primary factors: (1) sebum over-secretion, (2) abnormal keratinocyte desquamation leading to obstruction of the ducts, and (3) inflammation mediated by *Propionibacterium acnes* [43, 74]. It turns out that the regulator of metabolism and cell proliferation, mammalian target of rapamycin complex 1 (mTORC1), is significantly involved through crosstalk between the gut microbiome and the mTOR pathway [75]. Metabolites from the gut microbiota have been shown to not only regulate cell proliferation, but also lipid metabolism and other functions mediated by the mTOR pathway. It also turns out that this relationship is bi-directional: the mTOR pathway can in turn have an impact on the composition of the gut microbiome, thus causing intestinal dysbiosis. So we have a cyclic, bi-directional course between the skin physiology and the gut microbiome, which ultimately has a profound impact on acne pathophysiology [39, 75].

Now add on a third wing—that being psychological stressors and the role of neurotransmitters. It has long been known that there is a connection between acne, gut microbiome dysbiosis, and the brain. And so, it appears as if there is a gut-brain-skin axis in the development and flair-up of this disease. Each one of these wings exerts itself in unique ways, resulting in dysbiosis of the skin inflammatory response, gut microbiome dysbiosis, and perhaps even skin microbiome dysbiosis.

2.4.2   Atopic Dermatitis

Atopic dermatitis or eczema is a chronic disease and an inflammatory dermatosis. Skin barrier dysfunction and altered immune responses appear to be primary players in the development of this condition [31, 32, 34, 35, 39, 41]. One fascinating theory to explain the increased prevalence of this and other allergic diseases is from a less robust state of immune homeostasis versus the more commonly voiced theory of an overresponding immune system to environmental cues [31–35, 39]. This new theory focuses on gut microbiome dysbiosis and the subsequent impact on immune homeostasis—with the microbiome dysbiosis mediated by the typical Western diet. The low fiber and high fat content dramatically change the composition of the gut microbiome, resulting in significantly reduced production of immunomodulatory metabolites. Some key studies suggest that there is a definitive link between dysbiosis of the gut microbiome and atopic skin disease [10, 30, 31, 33, 37, 39, 76, 77]. Similar connections have now been shown between the health and regulation of the gut microbiome and development of the chronic relapsing-remitting inflammatory dermatosis know as Psoriasis [41, 44, 78–81].

2.5   Summary and Future Directions

With the advent of our comprehensive and complex approaches to analyzing the microbiomes of the human body, including not only composition, but also regulation of protein expression and metabolism of whole communities of organisms, we should not be overly surprised to discover that there are connections between multiple organ systems. Our microbiomes do not exist individually on an island; ample evidence over just the past 2–3 years has shown that there are amazing levels of regulation and crosstalk between different microbiomes—like the gut and skin microbiomes discussed here—and systemic organ system regulation and ultimately our overall health. When one adds the brain axis to play in these, one can see that we are on the verge of new and amazing discovery of how our bodies regulate themselves. I believe a key to all of this is the growing understanding of the complex roles our microbiomes have on virtually everything that occurs in human physiology. With future studies dissecting these pathways, we will discover new approaches with prebiotics and probiotics that will help us regulate the homeostasis of our microbiomes. The old saying, "You are what you eat," seems to now have profound implications as a large body of evidence—and still growing at an exponential rate—shows that the pivotal microbiome of the human body is the gut microbiome. We are in a new era of discovery on how important our microbiomes are to our health and vitality. As we move into a new decade, more interactions and levels of regulation are sure to be discovered. How we can manipulate these levels of regulation to improve our overall health I am sure will be an exciting premise.

References

1. Falkow, S., Molecular Koch's postulates applied to microbial pathogenicity. *Rev. Infect. Dis.*, 10, Suppl 2, S274-6, 1988.
2. Fredericks, D. and Relman, D.A., Sequence-based identification of microbial pathogens: A reconsideration of Koch's postulates. *Clin. Microbiol. Rev.*, 9, 1, 18–33, 1996.
3. Byrd, A.L. and Segre, J.A., Adapting Koch's postulates. *Science*, 351, 6270, 224–226, 2016.
4. Ramasamy, S. *et al.*, The role of the skin microbiota in acne pathophysiology. *British J. Dermatol.*, 181, 4, 691–699, 2019.
5. Todd, O.A. and Peters, B.M., Candida albicans and *Staphylococcus aureus* Pathogenicity and Polymicrobial Interactions: Lessons beyond Koch's Postulates. *J. Fungi*, 5, 3, 81, 2019.
6. Cheuk, J., Pender, S., Cagampang, F., PTU-007 The development of obesity and type 2 diabetes harnessing the gut microbiome and host genetics. *Gut*, 68, A114, 2019.
7. Kappel, B. and Lehrke, M., Microbiome, diabetes and heart: A novel link? *Herz*, 44, 3, 223–230, 2019.
8. Sharma, S. and Tripathi, P., Gut microbiome and type 2 diabetes: Where we are and where to go? *J. Nutrition. Biochem.*, 63, 101–108, 2019.
9. Singer-Englar, T., Barlow, G., Mathur, R., Obesity, diabetes, and the gut microbiome: An updated review. *Exp. Rev. Gastroenterol. Hepatol.*, 13, 1, 3–15, 2019.
10. Parkar, S.G., Kalsbeek, A., Cheeseman, J.F., Potential Role for the Gut Microbiota in Modulating Host Circadian Rhythms and Metabolic Health. *Microorganisms*, 7, 2, 41, 2019.
11. BONOMO, R. *et al.*, Gut microbiome and its potential role in obesity-induced neuropathy. *FASEB J.*, 33, 1_supplement, lb624–lb624, 2019.

12. Branchereau, M., Burcelin, R., Heymes, C., The gut microbiome and heart failure: A better gut for a better heart. *Rev. Endocrine Metabol. Disord.*, 20, 407–414, 2019.

13. Chung, S., Barnes, J.L., Astroth, K.S., Gastrointestinal Microbiota in Patients with Chronic Kidney Disease: A Systematic Review. *Adv. Nutrition*, 2019.

14. Dabke, K., Hendrick, G., Devkota, S., The gut microbiome and metabolic syndrome. *J. Clin Investig.*, 129, 10, 4050–4057, 2019.

15. Ding, R.-x. *et al.*, Revisit gut microbiota and its impact on human health and disease. *J. Food Drug Anal.*, 27, 3, 623–361, 2019.

16. Frame, L., Costa, E., Jackson, S., *Current Explorations of Nutrition and the Gut Microbiome: A Systematic Review (P20-032-19)*, Oxford University Press, 2019.

17. Lee, C.J., Sears, C.L., Maruthur, N., Gut microbiome and its role in obesity and insulin resistance. *Ann. N. York Acad. Sci.*, 1461, 1, 37–52, 2020.

18. Rodriguez, D.A. *et al.*, The Gut Microbiota: A Clinically Impactful Factor in Patient Health and Disease. *SN Compr. Clin. Med.*, 1, 3, 188–199, 2019.

19. Tseng, C.-H. and Wu, C.-Y., The gut microbiome in obesity. *J. Formosan Med. Assoc.*, 118, S3–S9, 2019.

20. Vallianou, N. *et al.*, Understanding the Role of the Gut Microbiome and Microbial Metabolites in Obesity and Obesity-Associated Metabolic Disorders: Current Evidence and Perspectives. *Curr. Obesity Rep.*, 8, 3, 317–332, 2019.

21. Kwiecien, K. *et al.*, Architecture of antimicrobial skin defense. *Cytokine Growth Factor Rev.*, 49, 70–84, 2019.

22. Lunjani, N., Hlela, C., O'Mahony, L., Microbiome and skin biology. *Curr Opin. Allerg. Clin. Immunol.*, 19, 4, 328–333, 2019.

23. Parlet, C.P., Brown, M.M., Horswill, A.R., Commensal staphylococci influence *staphylococcus aureus* skin colonization and disease. *Trends Microbiol.*, 27, 6, 497–507, 2019.

24. Polak-Witka, K. *et al.*, The role of the microbiome in scalp hair follicle biology and disease. *Exp. Dermatol.*, 29, 3, 286–294, 2020.

25. Zaher, M.Z., *Investigation of the ability of some commensal members of the nasal and/or skin microbiota to inhibit or eliminate multidrug-resistant Staphylococcus aureus*, CU Theses, 2019.

26. Brandwein, M., Steinberg, D., Meshner, S., Microbial biofilms and the human skin microbiome. *NPJ Biofilms Microbiomes*, 2, 1, 3, 2016.

27. Oh, J. *et al.*, Temporal stability of the human skin microbiome. *Cell*, 165, 4, 854–866, 2016.

28. Meisel, J.S. *et al.*, Commensal microbiota modulate gene expression in the skin. *Microbiome*, 6, 1, 20, 2018.

29. Sherwani, M.A. *et al.*, The skin microbiome and immune system: Potential target for chemoprevention? *PhotoDermatol. Photoimmunol. Photomed.*, 34, 1, 25–34, 2018.

30. Brandwein, M. *et al.*, Beyond the gut: Skin microbiome compositional changes are associated with BMI. *Hum. Microbiome J.*, 13, 100063, 2019.

31. Nakatsuji, T. and Gallo, R.L., The role of the skin microbiome in atopic dermatitis. *Ann. Allergy Asthma Immunol.*, 122, 3, 263–269, 2019.
32. Paller, A.S. *et al.*, The microbiome in patients with atopic dermatitis. *J. Allergy Clin Immunol.*, 143, 1, 26–35, 2019.
33. Pothmann, A. *et al.*, The microbiome and atopic dermatitis: A review. *Am. J. Clin. Dermatol.*, 20, 6, 749–761, 2019.
34. Stalder, J.-F. *et al.*, The emerging role of skin microbiome in atopic dermatitis and its clinical implication. *J. Dermatol. Treatment*, 30, 4, 357–364, 2019.
35. Nibbering, B. and Ubags, N., Microbial interactions in the atopic march. *Clin. Exp. Immunol.*, 199, 1, 12–23, 2020.
36. Lynch, S.V., Gut microbiota and allergic disease. New insights. *Ann. Am. Thoracic Soc.*, 13, Supplement 1, S51–S54, 2016.
37. O'Neill, C.A. *et al.*, The gut-skin axis in health and disease: A paradigm with therapeutic implications. *BioEssays*, 38, 11, 1167–1176, 2016.
38. Vaughn, A.R. *et al.*, Skin-gut axis: The relationship between intestinal bacteria and skin health. *World J. Dermatol.*, 6, 52–58, 2017.
39. Salem, I. *et al.*, The Gut Microbiome as a Major Regulator of the Gut-Skin Axis. *Front Microbiol.*, 9, 1459, 2018.
40. Lee, S.-Y. *et al.*, Microbiome in the gut-skin axis in atopic dermatitis. *Allergy Asthma Immunol. Res.*, 10, 4, 354–362, 2018.
41. Vojvodic, A. *et al.*, Gut Microbiota and the Alteration of Immune Balance in Skin Diseases; From Nutraceuticals to Fecal Transplantation. *Open Access Maced. J. Med. Sci.*, 7, 18, 3034–3038, 2019.
42. Bowe, W., Patel, N.B., Logan, A.C., Acne vulgaris, probiotics and the gut-brain-skin axis: From anecdote to translational medicine. *Benef. Microbes*, 5, 2, 185–99, 2014.
43. Dreno, B. *et al.*, Skin microbiome and acne vulgaris: *Staphylococcus*, a new actor in acne. *Exp. Dermatol.*, 26, 9, 798–803, 2017.
44. Thio, H.B., The microbiome in psoriasis and psoriatic arthritis: The skin perspective. *J. Rheumatol. Suppl.*, 94, 30–31, 2018.
45. Zákostelská, Z. *et al.*, Intestinal microbiota promotes psoriasis-like skin inflammation by enhancing Th17 response. *PloS One*, 11, 7, e0159539, 2016.
46. Beri, K., Perspective: Stabilizing the Microbiome Skin-Gut-Brain Axis with Natural Plant Botanical Ingredients in Cosmetics. *Cosmetics*, 5, 2, 37, 2018.
47. Kim, J.H. *et al.*, Kazachstania turicensis CAU Y1706 ameliorates atopic dermatitis by regulation of the gut-skin axis. *J. Dairy Sci.*, 102, 4, 2854–2862, 2019.
48. Migacz-Gruszka, K. *et al.*, What's new in the pathophysiology of alopecia areata? the possible contribution of skin and gut microbiome in the pathogenesis of alopecia–Big opportunities, big challenges, and novel perspectives. *Int. J. Trichol.*, 11, 5, 185, 2019.
49. Fagarasan, S. *et al.*, Adaptive immune regulation in the gut: T cell–dependent and T cell–independent IgA synthesis. *Annu. Rev. Immunol.*, 28, 243–273, 2009.

50. Alexander, K.L., Targan, S.R., Elson, C.O., III, Microbiota activation and regulation of innate and adaptive immunity. *Immunol. Rev.*, 260, 1, 206–220, 2014.

51. Kato, L.M. *et al.*, The role of the adaptive immune system in regulation of gut microbiota. *Immunol. Rev.*, 260, 1, 67–75, 2014.

52. Thaiss, C.A. *et al.*, The interplay between the innate immune system and the microbiota. *Curr Opin. Immunol.*, 26, 41–48, 2014.

53. Brown, E.M., Kenny, D.J., Xavier, R.J., Gut microbiota regulation of T cells during inflammation and autoimmunity. *Annu. Rev. Immunol.*, 37, 599–624, 2019.

54. Delgobo, M. *et al.*, Gut: Key Element on Immune System Regulation. *Braz. Archives Biol. Technol.*, 62, e19180654, 2019.

55. Szántó, M. *et al.*, Targeting the gut-skin axis—Probiotics as new tools for skin disorder management? *Exp. Dermatol.*, 28, 11, 1210–1218, 2019.

56. Erdman, S. and Poutahidis, T., Probiotic 'glow of health': It's more than skin deep. *Benef. Microbes*, 5, 2, 109–119, 2014.

57. Horii, Y. *et al.*, Effect of heat-killed L actobacillus brevis SBC 8803 on cutaneous arterial sympathetic nerve activity, cutaneous blood flow and transepidermal water loss in rats. *J. Appl. Microbiol.*, 116, 5, 1274–1281, 2014.

58. Ogawa, M. *et al.*, Effects of oral intake of heat-killed Lactobacillus brevis SBC8803 (SBL88™) on dry skin conditions: A randomized, double-blind, placebo-controlled study. *Exp. Ther. Med.*, 12, 6, 3863–3872, 2016.

59. Gueniche, A. *et al.*, Randomised double-blind placebo-controlled study of the effect of Lactobacillus paracasei NCC 2461 on skin reactivity. *Benef. Microbes*, 5, 2, 137–145, 2013.

60. Balato, A. *et al.*, Human Microbiome: Composition and Role in Inflammatory Skin Diseases. *Archivum Immunol. Ther. Exp.*, 67, 1, 1–18, 2019.

61. Fabbrocini, G. *et al.*, Supplementation with Lactobacillus rhamnosus SP1 normalises skin expression of genes implicated in insulin signalling and improves adult acne. *Benef. Microbes*, 7, 5, 625–630, 2016.

62. Chapat, L. *et al.*, Lactobacillus casei reduces CD8+ T cell-mediated skin inflammation. *European J. Immunol.*, 34, 9, 2520–2528, 2004.

63. Hacini-Rachinel, F. *et al.*, Oral probiotic control skin inflammation by acting on both effector and regulatory T cells. *PLoS One*, 4, 3, e4903, 2009.

64. Peiser, M., Role of Th17 cells in skin inflammation of allergic contact dermatitis. *Clin. Dev. Immunol.*, 2013, 2013.

65. Weaver, C.T. *et al.*, The Th17 pathway and inflammatory diseases of the intestines, lungs, and skin. *Annu. Rev. Pathol.: Mechanisms Dis.*, 8, 477–512, 2013.

66. Chen, X. and Oppenheim, J.J., Th17 cells and Tregs: Unlikely allies. *J. Leukocyte Biol.*, 95, 5, 723–731, 2014.

67. Ariotti, S. and Veldhoen, M., Immunology: Skin T Cells Switch Identity to Protect and Heal. *Curr. Biol.*, 29, 6, R220–R223, 2019.

68. Garrett, S.M., Zhao, Q., Feghali-Bostwick, C., Induction of a Th17 Phenotype in Human Skin—A Mimic of Dermal Inflammatory Diseases. *Methods Prot.*, 2, 2, 45, 2019.

69. Powrie, F., Whibley, N., Tucci, A., Regulatory T cell adaptation in the intestine and skin. *Nat. Immunol.*, 2019, 4.

70. Sikora, N., Vargas, F., Dobke, M., Skin Aging and Beauty–Exploring the Gut Microbiota Connection. *J. Aesthet. Reconstr. Surg.*, 5, 1, 1, 2019.

71. Kosiewicz, M.M. *et al.*, Relationship between gut microbiota and development of T cell associated disease. *FEBS Lett.*, 588, 22, 4195–4206, 2014.

72. Chen, C. *et al.*, Broad-spectrum antimicrobial activity, chemical composition and mechanism of action of garlic (Allium sativum) extracts. *Food Control*, 86, 117–125, 2018.

73. Bhate, K. and Williams, H., Epidemiology of acne vulgaris. *British J. Dermatol.*, 168, 3, 474–485, 2013.

74. Rodan, K., Fields, K., Falla, T.J., Efficacy of a twice-daily, 3-step, over-the-counter skincare regimen for the treatment of acne vulgaris. *Clin. Cosmetic Investig. Dermatol.*, 10, 3, 2017.

75. Noureldein, M.H. and Eid, A.A., Gut microbiota and mTOR signaling: Insight on a new pathophysiological interaction. *Microbial Pathog.*, 118, 98–104, 2018.

76. Maarouf, M., Platto, J.F., Shi, V.Y., The role of nutrition in inflammatory pilosebaceous disorders: Implication of the skin-gut axis. *Aust. J. Dermatol.*, 60, 2, e90–e98, 2018.

77. Mahdavinia, M. *et al.*, Effects of diet on the childhood gut microbiome and its implications for atopic dermatitis. *J. Allergy Clin. Immunol.*, 143, 4, 1636, 2019.

78. Tett, A. *et al.*, Unexplored diversity and strain-level structure of the skin microbiome associated with psoriasis. *NPJ Biofilms Microbiomes*, 3, 1, 14, 2017.

79. Yan, D. *et al.*, The role of the skin and gut microbiome in psoriatic disease. *Curr. Dermatol. Rep.*, 6, 2, 94–103, 2017.

80. Codoñer, F.M. *et al.*, Gut microbial composition in patients with psoriasis. *Sci. Rep.*, 8, 1, 3812, 2018.

81. Huang, L. *et al.*, Dysbiosis of gut microbiota was closely associated with psoriasis. *Sci. China Life Sci.*, 62, 6, 807–815, 2019.

3

The Skin and Oral Microbiome: An Examination of Overlap and Potential Interactions between Microbiome Communities

Sandra Buerger

Boston University, College of General Studies, Department of Natural Sciences and Mathematics, Boston, Massachusetts, USA

Abstract

There has been considerable interest in the connection between the gut and brain microbiome, in the form of the gut-brain axis. Considerably less has been said about the connection between the skin microbiome and the oral microbiome, despite the fact that these two microbiomes lie contiguous to each other and have interaction each and every day. This chapter will seek to explore the current research on these connections, limited as it is, and then look towards future directions by exploring the major groups of microbes that have been defined for each group. We will look at the overlap in these microbial groups and explore the potential significance of these interactions.

Keywords: Skin microbiome, oral microbiome, bacterial communication, taxonomy, bacteriome, mycobiome, virome, quorum sensing

3.1 Introduction

3.1.1 Focus of the Chapter

Although scientists have known about the existence of bacteria living on and within the human body since the late 19th century, when Theodor

Email: sbuerger@bu.edu

Nava Dayan (ed.) *Skin Microbiome Handbook: From Basic Research to Product Development*, (45–58) © 2020 Scrivener Publishing LLC

Escherich first recorded the existence of *Escherichia coli* living in the gut of healthy individual [1], the field of microbiology throughout the twentieth century focused more on pathogenic microbes. Sporadic isolation of members of bacteria from the skin, oral cavity and other areas of the body did happen, but it wasn't until the 21st century that we saw an intensive, methodological study of the microbiome [2, 3].

In fact, it was not until 2001 that the term microbiome was commonly used to describe the microbial communities on and within the human body. It was the Nobel Prize winner Joshua Lederberg who brought the term to prominence in 2001 [4]. Lederberg is known for his influence on the field and the ability to bring together different realms of microbiology, pointing the field in new and exciting directions [5]. In his Commentary, written along with Alexa McCray, 'Ome Sweet 'Omics – A Genealogical Treasury of Words, Lederberg described the microbiome as a term used "to signify the ecological community of commensal, symbiotic and pathogenic microorganisms that literally share our body space and have been all but ignored as determinants of human disease."

As the 21st century progressed, the establishment Human Microbiome Project in 2005 and numerous other studies, sought to expand our knowledge of the species that inhabit various hotspots of the microbiome [3]. Initially, the gut was the focus of most studies and to this day still remains the most studied of the microbiomes. Other areas have not had the same intense focus as the gut [6]; however, that does not discount their absolute importance in the role of human health and disease. It was the ease of access to material and established methods to study microbes of the gut, and especially the area of the colon within the wider gut microbiome, that resulted in this lopsided focus. Moreover, many studies have established the vital nature in health of both the skin and the oral microbiome [7].

While initial studies sought to define the "core" microbiome in individuals for each region, understanding a full profile of health will involve establishing not only isolated regions of a healthy microbiome, but the interaction between the different microbiomes. This is a trend that goes beyond the study of the microbiome. Increasingly, scientists have recognized that the future of human health studies must take into account the full body and how systems of the body interact in order to get a realistic understanding of how to treat and deal with various diseases and disorders. Gone are the days where a laser focus on one tissue type is seen as a gold standard. This represents a new direction; as recently as 2018, systems biology was described as having "revolutionized our discovery of biomarkers to prevent, diagnose, and treat disease" [8].

Within the field of microbiome studies, there is a call to adopt this approach. Elodie Ghedin, professor at New York University and director of Center for Genomics and System Biology, said in May 2018 "... it is a third wave of microbiome research, zooming in on the crosstalk among sites, that is helping us truly understand how the different human microbes and their microbial players are interconnected to make a human human" [7]. This represents a new approach, and one with significant challenges. However, there are already some established methodologies that can be applied to interactions between various discrete microbiomes within the human body [8]. In this chapter, we will focus on how these interactions between the skin and oral microbiome, two contiguous areas of the body that have many daily interactions, are being explored and explore the future of studies examining these interactions. We will attempt to synthesize what is known about the "core" composition of the skin and oral microbiome, then examine the promise of studies into quorum sensing (QS) between microbiomes, microbiome-wide association studies (MWAS) and other approaches in elucidating the mysteries behind a healthy skin and oral microbiome.

These approaches give us a wider view of the interactions that are influencing the composition of the microbiome. QS examines bacterial communication through the use of signaling molecules. The distinction between QS and other bacterial signaling is that QS necessitates a specific cell density (a quorum) before the gene activation takes place [9]. Studies that examine the entire microbiome and interactions between these microbiomes and the human body (e.g., QS and MWAS) can serve to give us a better understanding of how the microbiomes affect human health.

3.1.2 Definition of Skin Microbiome

The skin microbiome is recognized as an area with a diverse microbial community (see Table 3.1). Most of these microbes are recognized as commensal, although there are recorded cases where commensal or normal members of the skin microbiome can cause disease. The topography and conditions create a number of unique microenvironments within the skin. This is not surprising considering that the skin is the largest organ of the body and there is substantial heterogeneity from region to region. Generally speaking, we can divide the skin into three regions (1) the sebaceous, (2) moist and (3) dry areas. Each area of the skin has a unique microbial diversity. Bacteria are the most abundant type of microbe found on the skin, while fungi are the least abundant. That holds true even in areas of the skin (such as the feet) where there is a high level of fungal diversity [10–12].

Table 3.1 Summary of conditions on the skin and in the mouth relevant to microbial growth.

Skin	Oral
Multiple regions with different microenvironments	Multiple regions with different microenvironments
(1) Sebaceous	(1) Buccal mucosa, gums and palate
(2) Moist	(2) Saliva, tongue, tonsils, throat
(3) Dry	(3) Plaque
Mainly dry areas	Mainly moist areas
Low pH	Neutral pH
Production of antimicrobial substances	Production of antimicrobial substances

3.1.3   Definition of Oral Microbiome

Similar to the skin microbiome, the oral microbiome is represented by diverse microbial communities [13, 14]. The identification of large numbers of microbial species makes the oral microbiome one of the most diverse sites of the body, exceeded in diversity only by the colon [15].

Once again, closer examination of the oral cavity reveals heterogeneous microenvironments (see Table 3.1). As with the skin microbiome, we can divide the oral microbiome into 3 distinct areas. These areas are based on similarities between the bacterial communities in an individual. In other words, if we were to sample from multiple sites within a single grouping, we would expect to see a consistency in the species level makeup of microbes. The areas include (1) the buccal mucosa, gingiva and hard palate, (2) the saliva, tongue, tonsils and throat and (3) the supra- and subgingival plaque [15].

3.2   Characterization of the Microbiome

3.2.1   Variability and Stability of Skin and Oral Microbiome

There is great variability between individuals in terms of the composition of the microbiomes from all identified sites. Not only in the genetic composition, but also in the density/representation of each group of microbes and even the rate of change.

In fact, even identical twins do not have the same makeups. The variability between identical twins is nearly to the level of non-identical twins, or average variability from person to person. There is an exception of a few taxa that do seem to have a high degree of heritability [16].

However, despite this variability there is stability *within* the individual. In examining similarities between the oral and skin microbiome, we see two areas of the body that are both consistently exposed to new microbes. Yet despite these interactions with environmental microbes, we see the abovementioned stability in the individual microbiome over time. A long-term longitudinal study that examined the skin microbiome showed that all types of microbes (bacteria, fungi and viruses) remained stable over time. Interestingly, the feet showed the most variability [17]. As we shall see below, the feet appear to represent a unique part of the skin microbiome. Correspondingly, the oral microbiome shows individual stability outside of the variation within the three zones discussed above. In fact, with the exception of a high carbohydrate diet, the environment seems to play a relatively minor role in changes that occur within the oral microbiome [15].

Addressing the rate of change, we can once again see a contrast between the skin and oral microbiome. In a study conducted by Flores *et al.*, the skin microbiome changed at the fastest rate, while the oral microbiome, represented by tongue sampling site, changed at the slowest rate out of the three microbiome sites (skin, gut and oral) tested. More diversity appeared to correlate with more individual variance and the degree of variance was found to be very personalized [18]. The variability in the skin microbiome compared to the other two may be the result of the low species abundance as compared to the oral and gut microbiome [16].

3.2.2 Microbial Community

As we continue to consider the microbes that might be detected through any study of the microbiome, we will examine three groupings.

3.2.2.1 *Permeant Mutualistic or Commensal Microbes*

These permeant microbes play important roles in normal physiological tasks, forming an essential part of the healthy body. They are defined as mutualistic and in both the oral mucosa and skin make up parts of the innate immune system. As both the skin and the oral mucosa are potential entry points for pathogens, the presence of these bacteria as competitive antagonistic members of the microbial community can prevent infection or adherence of potential pathogens to either the epidermis or the mucosa [19].

Additionally, we can consider permeant members that do not play any apparent mutualistic role, either in maintenance of normal skin conditions or in the protection against potential pathogens. These commensal organisms exist without causing infection and make up part of the overall microbial community on and within the body.

3.2.2.2   Non-Pathogenic Transient Microbes

Our second category involves transient species that are not part of the permanent microbiome. Because of the nature of the two areas we are exploring and the nature of genetic testing techniques that look at all species present at any given time/space sampling, we are bound to include some microbes that are "just passing through" and don't represent permanent members of the complex community of bacteria.

Studies have shown that colonization of the gut by environmental bacteria is rare. Germ-free mouse studies indicate that these bacteria either fail to establish or are displaced by normal bacteria of the microbiota [16]. Furthermore, a number of studies have shown that the composition of the gut microbiota established in early life plays an important role in lifetime health outcomes [20]. Of course, the environment of the gut has some significant differences that we must consider when comparing the oral mucosa and the skin, but we might suspect that the establishment of transient, non-pathogenic environmental species colonizing the skin or the oral microbiome follows a similar pattern.

As mentioned above, the feet appear to be unique among other sites in the skin microbiome. One possible explanation put forward, is the presence of transient fungal species in the environment [10]. Thus, we cannot discount the presence of transient microbes influencing the makeup of the microbiome; however, we can identify specific situations where the influence has an outsized effect.

3.2.2.3   Pathogenic Microbes

The oral cavity and the skin are constantly exposed to potential pathogens. Many of these are well known and well defined. As historically, microbiology has focused on the pathogenic members as they affect humans, these tend to be the most well defined. While we acknowledge the importance of these microbial interactions, the examination of pathogens of each area is beyond the scope of this chapter.

As much as possible, we will focus in this chapter on the first category, trying to examine the overlap between the microbes that exist in both the oral cavity and skin microbiome as permanent dynamic members. We will also explore the potential influence that permanent members make as they become transient members for each microbiome. Similarly, we will avoid discussing dysbiosis.

3.3   The Core Skin and Oral Microbiomes

3.3.1   Taxonomic Methodology

In the past, reliance on culture techniques has given us a skewed view on the composition of the microbiome. Today, genomic techniques allow us to obtain a more detailed view of the microbes present. Many unculturable representatives have been revealed through shotgun sequencing and genomic analysis tools [10, 16]. Shotgun sequencing has the added benefit of giving information on relative abundance across domains and distinguishing between different strains. Shotgun sequencing looks at fragments from the entire genome as contrasted with 16S rRNA sequencing, which focuses on a single gene. This benefit allows for greater identification of functional genes and, in many cases, identification at a species-specific level [10, 21].

In this section, we will define the most common members and their relative abundance and time/space distribution in the skin and oral microbiomes at the kingdom level for bacteria and fungi, and also examine the acellular representative of the microbiomes' viruses (see Figure 3.1).

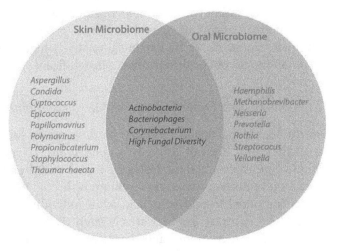

Figure 3.1 Ven Diagram of taxonomic groups and categories of members of the microbiome that are unique to the skin microbiome, unique to the oral microbiome, and shared between the two.

3.3.2   Subgroups of the Microbiome

3.3.2.1   Bacteriome

Within the bacteriome of both the oral and skin microbiome, we see the greatest understanding of the differences and makeup of the microbiome. Bacteria are the best studied members of the microbiomes. There is also some information on the archaeal community within those microbiomes.

Oral Microbiome. Within the oral microbiome, we see a large presence of bacteria from the genus *Streptococcus* (a Firmicutes). These bacteria are found ubiquitously within the oral cavity. Some species have been identified in causing tooth decay, while others have no negative effect on the teeth and tissue of the oral microbiome. *Veillonellaceae* and *Granulicatella* are also represented Firmicutes. Other common taxa include: *Actinomyces, Corynebacterium, Fusobacterium, Haemophilis, Neisseria, Prevotella,* and *Rothia.* In terms of the archaeal members, *Methanobrevibacter* are seen in studies examining the makeup of the oral microbiome [6, 14].

Skin Microbiome. The most common bacteria within the skin microbiome is the *Actinobacteria*. Common, but less prominent taxa include Firmicutes, Proteobacteria, Bacteroidetes, *Staphylococcus, Propionibacterium,* and *Corynebacterium.* Common archaeal taxa include *Thaumarchaeota* [6, 10].

As is evident from the above overview, there is not a very large number of common taxa between the two microbiomes. *Corynebacterium* is an exception to that rule. Additionally, *Actinomyces,* a genus that falls under the broader taxonomic category of Actinobacteria are present in both the skin and oral microbiome. As we are looking at relatively high taxonomic levels, this overlap should not be disregarded as insignificant.

3.3.2.2   Mycobiome (and Other Eukaryotic Microbial Members)

In the skin, the feet in particular have a high diversity of fungal species. These include, but are not limited to, *Aspergillus, Cryptococcus, Rhodotoula* and *Epicoccum.* It should also be noted that prepubescent children have a more diverse fungal representation throughout the skin microbiome as compared to pubescent and adult individuals [10]. The oral microbiome by contrast has a relatively high diversity of fungal species. As in the skin microbiome, age plays a role, with prevalence of *Candida* spp. increasing with age [15]. *Malassezia* is the most common fungi found in the adult skin microbiome, with the exception of the feet [10]. Genetic analysis has shown that healthy individuals have up to 85 genera represented in their oral microbiome. It is important to note that due to a high number of spores in the air, many of these species might be transient spores that were detected and not permeant members of the oral microbiome [15].

3.3.2.3   Virome

Identifying members of a virome in any location represents technical challenges [17, 19, 22]. Differentiating between inclusion of viral DNA in bacterial genomes versus presence of viral DNA from a present virus can be difficult to distinguish. However, a number of researchers have attempted to define both a core virome and differences between different populations for the oral and skin virome.

In both the oral virome and the skin virome, a high prevalence of bacteriophages has been observed [17, 19]. Considering the importance of bacteria in the human microbiome this is not surprising. In the oral microbiome, studies have indicated that there is great variability between individuals, however, a stable oral virome does appear to exist. The most frequent observation is unique viral sequences from individual to individual along with a high prevalence of unique, single appearance viral sequences [17, 22]. Despite this high level of variability, some viruses (notably, human herpesvirus 7 and *Streptococcus* prophage) appear frequently in subjects tested. Observation of distinct differences between sexes is controversial, appearing to exist in some sample groups and not in others [19]. Larger sample sizes will likely be necessary to confirm if a sex-specific difference is observed in the oral virome.

Similar observations have been made for the skin virome. Compared to bacteriome and the mycobiome, the virome of the skin is less consistent over time and space and shows a high degree of individual variation. Studies using different methodologies have failed to discover a core virome for the skin [17, 23]. Much like the oral microbiome, only a few taxonomic groups are identified in multiple subjects. For the skin microbiome, these include polyomavirus and papillomavirus. In both a study by Oh *et al.* and Hannigan *et al.*, papillomaviridae were detected in multiple subjects. However, Oh *et al.* note that the two aforementioned groups were present in only about 50% of their sample.

In both the oral and skin virome, there appears to be less consistency across individuals, indicating that a core virome may not be identifiable. However, it is important to note that small sample sizes and technical limitations exist and that if these limitations are overcome in the future, a clearer view will be achieved.

3.4   Interactions Between Skin and Oral Microbiomes

3.4.1   Potential for Interactions

As we have stressed throughout this chapter, these microbial communities are dynamic and interactions between the microbes are constantly occurring. Interactions between individual members of the skin microbes have been shown [10]. Interactions within the oral microbiome are also the rule. Due to the high rate of exchange and exposure between the oral mucosa and the skin, we would expect similar interactions to occur between the microbes of the oral and skin microbiome. These interactions could fall under the category of antagonistic, commensalistic or mutualistic. Here we are not talking about interactions that benefit the individual human per se, but are viewed from the level of the benefit or cost to the microbial species.

3.4.2   Quorum Sensing

There is ample evidence to show that bacteria are able to communicate in both an interspecies and intraspecies manner. This type of interaction makes use of chemicals and is known as quorum sensing. Quorum sensing (QS) has been established in microbial ecology as a common occurrence in bacterial communities. QS occurs when bacteria reach specific densities and release autoinducer molecules. These chemicals have been shown to induce behaviors in bacteria as diverse as bioluminescence, virulence and biofilm formation. While the expression of bioluminescence likely has no significance to the microbiome, biofilm production and virulence expression certainly could play an important role [9].

3.4.3   Immune System Development

Another area where we might consider the role of crosstalk between the two microbiomes, is that of the development of immunity. The members of the microbiome play a role in the development of effective immunity in that they allow the immune system to differentiate between commensal or mutualistic microbes and pathogenic microbes. This is known as the "old friends" hypothesis. The "old friends" hypothesis postulates that the presence or exposure of varied microbes and antigens, especially in early development, is vital to proper development of the immune system. The high rates of autoimmune disease and hypersensitivities we see today are the result of modern public health measures, including vaccinations and antibiotics [6]. This role must be part of the crosstalk or interactions between the skin and oral microbiome, as both common members of each microbiome would be identified as non-pathogenic by the immune system during an exchange event.

3.4.4   Future Directions

One thing to consider in future studies, is the relative influence of the *composition* versus the gene activity that is taking place [16]. It is perhaps more interesting to look at this gene expression and compare between the oral and skin microbiome, rather than gross composition of family, genera or even species. Furthermore, Gilbert *et al.* suggest that an examination of temporal variability, again in replacement of a single look at the genetic profile, may give us more interesting information and allow for deeper connections between the microbiome and health.

It must also be noted that in the past, due to rapid development of tools to analyze bacteria and a reliance on 16S rRNA sequencing, the focus has been largely bacterial [6, 7]. In the future, researchers need to focus on other microbial members of the microbiome and interactions at the domain level and between acellular microbes and cellular microbes. Fortunately, new genomic techniques have allowed this to become a more realistic possibility [7].

For example, the study of viruses and their contribution, both as bacteriophages and as eukaryotic viruses, is an area that needs to see more development before conclusions can be made about their overall role within the microbiomes [10]. In the oral microbiome, viruses have been well established as pathogenic members of the microbial community [15], however, it seems that a role for bacteriophages may well represent another layer of this dynamic community. A challenge with defining the virome, is that there is no single marker gene—no equivalent of the 16S rRNA gene—that makes bacterial taxonomic studies straightforward [7].

3.5   Conclusion

The skin and oral microbiomes represent an untapped area of research. It can easily be seen that there is much interaction between the two microbial communities. At this juncture, more research needs to be done to define the core microbiome in each location, especially when we consider viruses, which make up important members of each microbiome. Future studies should compare microbiomes in the same individuals. This would necessitate sampling from multiple locations on a single individual. However, the relative ease of getting samples from the skin and oral mucosa make this a reasonable possibility. As we move towards a more comprehensive view of human health, comparing these different microbiomes will be a vital tool in developing a full understanding of a healthy microbiome.

Acknowledgments

Thank you to Michael Huber for his assistance in researching and discussing the topic presented in this chapter.

References

1. Shulman, S.T., Friedmann, H.C., Sims, R.H., Theodor Escherich: The First Pediatric Infectious Disease Physican? *Clin. Infect. Dis.*, 45, 8, 1025–1029, 2007.
2. Blaser, M., The microbiome revolution. *J. Clin. Invest.*, 124, 10, 4162–4165, 2014.
3. NIH HMP Working Group, Peterson, J., Garges, S., Giovanni, M., McInnes, P., Wang, L., Guyer, M., The NIH Human Microbiome Project. *Genome Res.*, 19, 12, 2317–2323, 2009.
4. Lederberg, J. and McCray, A.T., 'Ome Sweet 'Omics—A genealogical treasury of words. *Scientist*, 15, 8, 2001.
5. Oransky, I., Joshua Lederberg. *Lancet*, 371, 2008.
6. Rowan-Nash, A.D., Korry, B.J., Mylonakis, E., Belenky, Cross-Domain and Viral Interactions in the Microbiome. *Microbiol. Mol. Biol. Rev.*, 2019.
7. Taroncher-Oldenburg, G., Jones, S., Blaser, M., Bonneau, R., Christey, P., Clemente, J.C., Elinav, E., Ghedin, E., Huttenhower, C., Kelly, D., Kyle, D., Littman, D., Maiti, A., Maue, A., Olle, B., Segal, L., Vlieg, J.E.T.H., Wang, J., Translating microbiome futures. *Nat. Biotechnol.*, 36, 11, 1037–1042, 2018.
8. Bernabe, B., Cralle, L., Gilbert, J.A., Systems biology of the human microbiome. *Curr. Opin. Biotechnol.*, 51, 146–153, 2018.
9. Eickhoff, M.J. and Bassler, B.L., SnapShot: Bacterial Quorum Sensing. *Cell*, 174, 2018.
10. Byrd, A.L., Belkaid, Y., Segre, J.A., The human skin microbiome. *Nat. Rev. Microbiol.*, 16, 143–155, 2018.
11. Chen, Y.E. and Tsao, H.T., The skin microbiome: Current perspectives and future challenges. *J. Am. Acad. Dermatol.*, 69, 1, 143–155, 2013.
12. Grice, E.A. and Segre, J.A., The skin microbiome. *Nat. Rev. Microbiol.*, 9, 244–253, 2011.
13. Dewhirst, F.E., Chen, T., Izard, J., Paster, B.J., Tanner, A.C.R., Yu, W.H., Lakshmanan, A., Wade, W.G., The Human Oral Microbiome. *J. Bacteriol.*, 192, 19, 5002–5017, 2010.

14. Zaura, E., Keijser, B.J.F., Huse, S.M., Crielaard, W., Defining the health "core microbiome" of oral microbial communities. *BMC Microbiol.*, 9, 259: 259, 2009.

15. Wade, W.G., The oral microbiome in health and disease. *Pharmacol. Res.*, 69, 137–143, 2013.

16. Gilbert, J.A., Blaser, M.J., Caporaso, J.G., Jansson, J.K., Lynch, S.V., Knight, R., Current understanding of the human microbiome. *Nat. Med.*, 24, 4, 392–400, 2018.

17. Oh, J., Byrd, A.L., Park, M., NISC, C.S.P., Kong, H.H., Segre, J.A., Temporal stability of the human skin microbiome. *Cell*, 165, 854–866, 2016.

18. Flores, G.E., Caporaso, J.G., Henley, J.B., Rideout, J.R., Domogala, D., Chase, J., Leff, J.W., Vazquez-Baeza, Y., Gonzalez, A., Knight, R., Dunn, R.R., Fierer, N., Temporal variability is a personalize feature of the human microbiome. *Genome Biol.*, 15, 12, 531, 2014.

19. Perez-Brocal, V. and Moya, A., The analysis of the oral DNA virome reveals which viruses are widespread and rarate among healthy young adults in Valencia (Spain). *PLOS One*, 2018.

20. Tamburini, S., Shen, N., Wu, H.C., Clemente, J.C., The microbiome in early life: implications for health outcomes. *Nat. Med.*, 22, 713–722, 2016.

21. Lee, Y.B., Byun, E.J., Kim, H.S., Potential Role of the Microbiome in Acne: A Comprehensive Review. *J. Clin. Med.*, 8, 7, 987, 2019.

22. Abeles, S.R., Robles-Sikisaka, R., Ly, M., Lum, A.G., Salzman, J., Boehm, T.K., Pride, D.T., Human oral viruses are personal, persistent and gender-consistent. *ISME Journal*, 8, 9, 1753–67, 2014.

23. Hannigan, G.D., Meisel, J.S., Tyldsley, A.D., Zheng, Q., Hodkinson, B.P., SanMiguel, A.J., Minot, S., Bushman, F.D., Grice, E.A., The Human Skin Double-Stranded DNA Virome: Topographical and Temporal Diversity, Genetic Enrichment, and Dynamic Associations with the Host Microbiome. *mBio*, 6, 5, 1578–15, 2015.

Part 2

SKIN MICROBIOME OBSERVATIONAL RESEARCH

4

Skin Microbiome Alterations in Skin Diseases

Travis Whitfill[1,2]*, Gilles R. Dubé[2] and Julia Oh[3]

[1]Yale University School of Medicine, Department of Pediatrics,
New Haven, CT, USA
[2]Azitra, Inc., Farmington, CT, USA
[3]Jackson Laboratory for Genomic Medicine, Farmington, CT, USA

Abstract

A common oversimplification of the skin microbiome is a binary classification of individual microbes as either "beneficial" or "harmful." In reality, however, skin microbes are much more complex and can act as either beneficial or harmful in different scenarios (for example, in altered skin or in healthy skin). In other cases, the ecological dynamics of bacteria interacting in a system add complexities to their characteristics. However, increasing evidence has associated altered microbial communities—or "dysbiosis"–in the skin with unhealthy skin, especially atopic dermatitis, which is highly associated with higher populations of *Staphylococcus aureus*. Here, we review the existing body of evidence around disruptions in the skin microbiome and their associations with skin diseases.

Keywords: Dysbiosis, atopic dermatitis, *S. aureus*, staphylococcal diseases, skin infections

4.1 Introduction and Background

Commensal microorganisms play a crucial role in maintaining human health across a number of organ systems, particularly in the skin [1–7]. Diverse communities of microorganisms populate the skin, and a square centimeter can contain up to a billion microorganisms [8]. These diverse communities of bacteria, fungi, mites and viruses can provide protection

---

**Corresponding author*: travis@azitrainc.com

Nava Dayan (ed.) Skin Microbiome Handbook: From Basic Research to Product Development,
(61–78) © 2020 Scrivener Publishing LLC

against disease and form dynamic, yet distinct niches on the skin [9]. Differences across these distinct niches are driven by topographical and physiological factors including pH, temperature, moisture, sebum and – and these influence the resident fungi [10] and bacteria [11, 12]. Site specificity may also exacerbate skin disorders, which often present in a skin-specific manner (such as atopic dermatitis or psoriasis) [13]. On top of topography and physiology, recent research has also uncovered the role of genetics in driving differences in the virome [14] and other microbiota [15]. Microbial communities are established early in life and play a critical role in establishing immune tolerance to skin microbes [16, 17].

There is a complex but critical role in the interaction between microbes and the cutaneous immune system in homeostasis, and a number of studies have associated altered microbial communities in the skin with cutaneous diseases [8, 18]. The term "dysbiosis" is poorly defined, but generally is described as an alteration of the microbiome away from steady-state conditions and is generally associated with disease states and shifts in microbial communities [19]. Specifically in the context of the skin microbiome, "dysbiosis" can refer to a reduced diversity or hyper-diversified microbial community compared to healthy individuals [20]. Associations between alterations in the skin microbiome and diseases have long been described; however, extensive studies over the past decade have teased out some of the complex relationships between host, environmental, and microbial factors in health and disease states.

In this chapter, we describe microbial and immune interactions, their deviations, and their associations with different skin diseases. We provide a summary of skin conditions associated with dysbiosis (with a focus on atopic dermatitis, acne vulgaris, psoriasis, and skin health) and summarize traditional and newly emerging therapeutic approaches to treating skin diseases by altering the skin microbiome.

4.2 Interactions Between Microbes and Host

Interactions between microbiota and the host both shape the resident microbial community and prevent colonization by pathogenic bacteria in a process termed 'colonization resistance' [21]. A common oversimplification of the skin microbiome is to classify individual microbial species as either "beneficial" or "harmful." In reality, however, skin microbes are much more complex and can act as either beneficial or harmful in different scenarios (for example, in healthy skin or in altered skin). This may be due to individual strain diversity or the microbe's microenvironment. Indeed, ecological dynamics of bacteria interacting in a system add complexities to their impact on the skin. For example, one particular species of bacteria, while on its own may be benign, but in non-intact skin, this same species may increase in its relative abundance to other microbes on the skin and cause a cutaneous response. These relationships are summarized in Figure 4.1.

Cutaneous commensals are essential for the function of the immune system [22, 23]. The immune system has evolved closely with resident microorganisms in the skin to allow the maintenance of commensal partners and the elimination of possible pathogens. To operate optimally, the skin microbiota, epithelial cells and innate and adaptive arms of the immune system need to communicate effectively. Keratinocytes can begin this dialogue by sensing microorganisms, especially pathogen-associated molecular patterns (PAMPs), through pattern recognition receptors (PRRs) [6].

The skin microbiome and immune-microbiome interactions are primarily established early in life [24]. Regulatory T cells are especially important in establishing immune tolerance to commensal microbes, and this process occurs during the neonatal stages of infancy [25, 26]. After the establishment of the skin microbiome during infancy, different microorganisms have been shown to elicit distinct effects on the immune system. For example, skin colonization with *Staphylococcus epidermidis* has been shown to induce increased levels of the cytokine interleukin-1α (IL-1α), which promotes skin-homing T cells to produce cytokines that contribute to host defense and skin inflammation [22, 27]. Notably, under steady-state conditions, induction of effector T cells in response to skin microorganisms occurs in the absence of classical inflammation in a process termed 'homeostatic immunity' [28, 29]. This process represents an essential mechanism

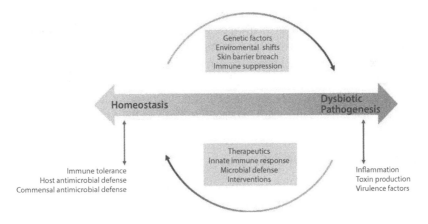

Figure 4.1 Balance between homeostasis and dysbiotic pathogenesis.

whereby different commensals educate distinct aspects of the immune system to respond to future pathogen exposures [22, 27]. This concept was demonstrated by Naik *et al.* when mice given topical *S. epidermidis* were better protected against fungal and parasitic skin infections [22, 27].

4.3   Summary of Known Associations Between Skin Dysbioses and Skin Diseases

A number of studies have observed a lower microbial diversity in damaged skin compared to healthy individuals [20]. There is strong evidence of a microbial component of the pathophysiology of several diseases—such as in atopic dermatitis—but the relationship is less clear in other skin diseases such as psoriasis. Importantly, strain-level genetic diversity has important consequences on virulence and pathogenicity, underscoring the importance of sampling and sequencing methodology in analyzing the skin microbiome. A summary of the associations between altered skin microbiota and skin conditions is presented in Table 4.1.

4.3.1   The Role of *S. Aureus* in Skin Disease

A number of studies have described the mechanisms by which *S. aureus* becomes an opportunistic pathogen and causes skin infections or a cutaneous immune response [30]. *S. aureus* has evolved dozens of pathogenic mechanisms, including: (1) immune evasion by binding to host antibodies (e.g., the Staphylococcal binder of immunoglobulin, Sbi, which helps protect *S. aureus* from innate immune defense and can bind to IgG and complement factor) [31, 32]; (2) resistance to host antimicrobial peptides (AMPs) via expression of proteases [33]; (3) "superantigen" production [34], which prevent chemokine production [35] and inhibit neutrophil chemotaxis in bacterial clearance [36]; (4) toxin production such as staphylococcal exfoliative toxins A and B (ETA/ETB) [37]; and (5) evasion of host proteases [38, 39], among many others. Increased *S. aureus* communities have been associated with psoriasis and especially in atopic dermatitis.

4.3.2   Atopic Dermatitis

Atopic dermatitis (AD), or eczema, is a chronic, pruritic, inflammatory skin disease common in children but also prevalent in many adults. The primary features of the disease are dry, scaly, itchy skin. It has long been known that dysbiosis is a driving feature of AD, with the cutaneous

Table 4.1 Summary of skin diseases and associated skin dysbioses.

Skin condition	Species-level associations	References	Strain-level associations	References
Atopic dermatitis	Increased S. aureus	[43–49]	Increased CC1 S. aureus	[56–58]
Acne vulgaris	Presence of C. acnes	[66, 67]	Increased Type IA C. acnes	[73]
Acneiform rash due to EGFR inhibitors	Increased S. aureus	[89]	Not yet identified	
Body odor	S. hominis, S. haemolyticus, and S. lugdunensis metabolites	[85]	Not yet identified	
Dandruff	Increased Malassezia restricta Filobasidium floriforme	[86]	Not yet identified	
Psoriasis	Increased S. aureus, S. pyogenes, and Malassezia; general community shifts	[78–82]	Not yet identified	

microbiome dominated by *S. aureus* during flares and characterized by a lack of microbial diversity. In addition, disruptions of the skin barrier and subsequent immune dysregulation—driven by a T_H2 response—are hallmarks of the disease concurrent with the *S. aureus* colonization [40–42].

Numerous studies have shown that *S. aureus* is prevalent on the skin of AD patients [43–49]. A recent meta-analysis of 95 observational studies showed the prevalence of *S. aureus* carriers in AD patients was 70% on lesional skin compared to 39% on nonlesional AD skin or healthy control skin [50]. Additionally, the proportion of *S. aureus* colonization on AD flares has been strongly correlated with severity of AD [51]. Metagenomic sequencing analyses have revealed clonal *S. aureus* strains are associated with more severe AD patients [25]. Several studies have defined *S. aureus* population structure based on multilocus sequence typing (MLST), which is a tool that characterizes isolates of bacterial species using the internal fragments of housekeeping genes [52]. These studies have shown that strains from clonal complex 30 (CC30) are most abundant in healthy populations [53–56] but are underrepresented in AD patients while strains from CC1 are over-represented in AD patients compared to healthy controls [56–58]. There tend to be clonal, homogeneous populations of *S. aureus* strains present on AD patients; in contrast, there are heterogenous populations of *S. epidermidis* present in AD patients, with *S. epidermidis* communities in both flares and post-flares composed of strains from diverse clades of the phylogenetic tree [25].

A typical open-ended question in the interplay between dysbioses and skin diseases is whether there is correlative or causal relationship between the two. While this interplay may be indistinct in other diseases, in the case of AD, there is increasing evidence to suggest a causal relationship. Kong, Oh *et al.* observed a temporal relationship between *S. aureus* colonization and AD flares in which *S. aureus* colonization preceded AD flares [51]. Subsequently, Meylan *et al.* showed that, in 36 infants that developed AD in a longitudinal study, there was *S. aureus* colonization before clinical onset of AD [59]. Moreover, a separate longitudinal study in infants showed that colonization with non-*S. aureus* staphylococci (particularly *S. epidermidis*) at two months resulted in a lower risk of atopic dermatitis at one year [60]. These results underscore the importance of the skin microbiome—which is dysregulated in AD—in maintaining immune homeostasis and preventing *S. aureus* growth.

4.3.3   Acne Vulgaris

Acne vulgaris is one of the most common skin disorders and affects up to 85% of adolescents and young adults worldwide [61, 62]. Considered a disease of the pilosebaceous unit, acne may cause scarring, pain, and—in many patients—affect self-esteem and mental health [63–65]. An outdated model of acne pathogenesis is the proposition that increased sebum production promotes broad growth of all *Cutibacterium acnes* species (*C. acnes*, previously *Propionibacterium acnes*) [66,67]. However, this model does not satisfy the evidence that *C. acnes* is equally found in acne prone as well as in healthy skin. Indeed, numerous studies aimed at sequencing *C. acnes* strains have begun to shed light on the strain-specific pathogenicity of *C. acnes*. Initially, *C. acnes* population structure was characterized by two distinct serotypes: types I and II [68]. More recent work with MLST has more comprehensively defined *C. acnes* population structure [69–73] and has identified a new phylogenetically distinct clade, type III [69, 70]. While the total populations of *C. acnes* appear to be similar between acne and normal individuals, specific serotypes of *C. acnes* seem to be differentially abundant: Fitz-Gibbon *et al.* reported that several ribotypes of type IA1 are enriched in acne patients but rarely found in health individuals [73]. Type III and some ribotypes of type II were not detected in acne patients.

Mechanistically, it has been proposed that TLR2 bacterial ligands on *C. acnes* promote inflammation in acne by triggering interleukin-1alpha (IL-1α) granulocyte macrophage-colony stimulating factor (GM-CSF) release [74]. Genetic analyses in the strain-level differences associated with acne have revealed that the clustered regularly interspaced palindromic repeats (CRISPR)/Cas locus in health-associated type II [75] is absent in type I strains [76]. Moreover, a plasmid present in type I strains has been identified that harbors a tight adhesion (tad) locus, that is common among pathogens and essential for biofilm formation and virulence [66].

4.3.4   Psoriasis

Psoriasis is a common inflammatory skin disease and effects around 2-3% of the population worldwide [77]. There is a high physical burden of the disease and the pathophysiology is incompletely understood, but is dominated by inflammation from the IL-23/T_H17 axis.

The role of the skin microbiome in psoriasis is poorly understood, and there does not appear to be a clear role of skin microbiota in the pathogenesis of psoriasis, although several studies have identified differential abundancies in skin microbiota between psoriasis patients and healthy volunteers. For example, several species appear to be associated with greater disease burden, including *S. aureus* [78, 79], *Streptococcus pyogenes* [80] and fungi such as *Malassezia* [81, 82]. However, little is known about the specific role of the microbes in psoriasis pathogenesis, if any.

Recent studies have indicated overall microbiome shifts in psoriasis, but no single biomarker has been identified [83, 84]. More work is needed to more comprehensively understand the relationship between skin or gut microbiome shifts and psoriasis.

4.4   Skin Dysbioses in Skin Health

A number of studies have described associations between skin dysbioses and skin health. Body odor, for example, is highly correlated with the microbiome: it is, to a large extent, caused by the metabolism of sweat and sebaceous excretions by the skin microbiota, and there are associations with certain microbial species and a higher body odor. The association with body odor is largely tied to the ability of microbes on the skin to metabolize dipeptide-conjugated thioalcohols such as S-[1-(2-hydroxyethyl)-1-methylbutyl]-(L)-cysteinylglycine. *S. hominis*, *S. haemolyticus*, and *S. lugdunensis* have been shown to metabolize these compounds and are thus more highly associated with body odor, while *S. epidermidis* and *Corynebacterium tuberculostearicum* have shown little ability to metabolize such compounds and, while present in high numbers in the armpit, are typically not associated with body odor [85]. The Axillary Microbiome and its Relationship with Underarm Odor is described in detail in a separate chapter in this book.

Dandruff, which is characterized by mild seborrheic dermatitis, has been weakly associated with skin microbiome disruptions, particularly *Malassezia restricta* [86], and *Filobasidium floriforme*. Additionally, recent studies have revealed significant changes in the microbiome due to aging. The importance of the establishment of the skin microbiome early in life has been well documented, and there have been efforts to understand changes in the microbiome later in life as well. In general, the microbial diversity of the skin increases with age, but a closer analysis has revealed increases in specific microbial species over time, some of which have been associated with skin conditions [87].

4.5   Other Skin Conditions

Skin microbiome alterations have been found in other skin conditions. Most strikingly, the rising use of epidermal growth factor receptor (EGFR) inhibitors in oncology has created new skin problems: in nearly 100% of patients on EGFR inhibitors, an acneiform rash develops [88]. Interestingly, there is a strong dysbiosis associated with this type of skin disease—*S. aureus* is significantly over-represented in the skin and lesions of EGFR patients compared to controls [89]. EGFR ablation leads to decreased production of antimicrobial peptides and skin barrier proteins [48, 89].

4.6 Therapeutic Approaches to Dysbiosis-Associated Skin Diseases

4.6.1 Traditional Methods of Treating Dysbiosis-Associated Skin Diseases

4.6.1.1 Atopic Dermatitis

Current treatment options primarily address the inflammation or microbial component of AD. For example, bleach baths are an effective option for moderate to severe AD [90, 91] via their anti-staphylococcal activity [92]. Topical corticosteroids are the mainstay treatment option for AD [90], and topical calcineurin inhibitors (e.g., tacrolimus, pimecrolimus) are used as second-line agents [93]. Crisaborole is a recently approved phosphodiesterase-4 (PDE-4) inhibitor for AD with some success in mild-to-moderate AD patents [94]. Other methods include occlusive therapy, although the body of evidence lacks robustness [95]. The most recently approved treatment option is dupilumab, an anti-IL-4Rα monoclonal antibody, and has achieved remarkable success in moderate-to-severe AD patients [96, 97].

4.6.1.2 Acne Vulgaris

Mainstay therapeutics for acne include anti-inflammatory agents, keratolytic agents and antimicrobials. Some include systemic antibiotics and retinoids, or topical agents such as benzoyl peroxide and salicylic acid [98]. Topical or oral antibiotics are used in acne patients to target the underlying microbial etiology. Topical clindamycin or erythromycin is typically used and for the more moderate-to-severe cases of acne, systemic antibiotics may be used such as tetracyclines or trimethoprim [98]. However, systemic antibiotics are typically not preferred due to their effects of the gut and other microbiomes—and especially due to the potential for antibiotic resistance, a growing problem in acne [99].

Systemic isotretinoin, a pro-drug for retinoic acid, is also a common option used for moderate-to-severe acne [100]. The mechanism of action of isotretinoin is incompletely understood [66]; however, it is known that it drastically reduces sebum production and the size of the pilosebaceous duct, thereby altering the duct into less favorable conditions for *C. acnes* colonization [101, 102]. Additionally, it was recently reported that isotretinoin normalizes TLR-2-mediate innate immune responses towards *C. acnes* [103]. A number of newer therapies are in clinical development—including novel antibacterial treatments, anti-inflammatory agents (e.g., anti-IL-17 or IL-1β), and others.

4.6.2 Emerging Therapeutic Approaches to Treating Dysbiosis-Associated Skin Diseases

Newly emerging strategies for treating microbial dysbiosis in skin diseases include the use of live microbes (termed "live biotherapeutic products" when in development for skin diseases). For example, *Lactobacillus* is a common strain that is classified as Generally Regarded as Safe (GRAS) by the FDA, and has been explored for topical use [104]. Other approaches have invoked the topical use of ammonia oxidizing bacteria or topical use of "beneficial" strains of *C. acnes* to treat acne.

Early studies have also shown that topical application of wild-type *S. epidermidis* may offer a viable therapeutic approach to treating skin conditions and skin diseases. In a double-blind, randomized clinical trial at Nagaski University, for example, topical application of autologous *S. epidermidis* in healthy volunteers increased lipid content of the skin, suppressed water evaporation, improved skin moisture retention, and promoted acidification of the skin surface, all without showing undesirable effects [105]. Not only does topical application of *S. epidermidis* appear to have beneficial structural and compositional effects, but also positive cutaneous immune-modulatory effects [106]. Topical application of certain strains of *S. epidermidis* has been shown to enhance innate skin immunity and limit pathogen invasion [27, 106].

In Nakatsuji *et al.*, species of *S. epidermidis* and *S. hominis* were isolated from the skin showed activity against *S. aureus*; topical application of these strains to human subjects with eczema reduced *S. aureus* colonization [107]. It is likely that topical application of *S. epidermidis*, *S. hominis*, and other "beneficial" or benign skin commensals represents a significant opportunity for novel topical therapeutics. While few well-characterized topically applied live bacteria are on the market, many are being characterized and are in development and offer an exciting and viable therapeutic modality in the near future.

4.7   Conclusion and Future Directions

Recently, the microbiome field has rapidly progressed from a collection of inferences and correlates towards a mechanistic understanding of the microbiome's role in disease risk. A number of studies have recently highlighted a better mechanistic understanding of key host-microbe interactions that underlie or drive diseases in the skin. Specifically, the immune interactions between microbes and skin have been of high interest and have shed light on the regulation of homeostasis. Skin microbiota modulate expression of innate factors such as cytokines, chemokines, and antimicrobial peptides and can elicit immune cell responses such as CD8$^+$ T cells or dendritic cells. In addition, skin commensals play a key role in maintaining barrier function and commensal-immune interactions can impact epithelial biology in the skin. Finally, the skin microbiome is established early in life and its priming and education of the immune system are crucial during the neonatal period of early life.

Disruptions in the commensal-immune crosstalk drive disease states and can lead to the introduction of opportunistic pathogens. There is a clear role of *S. aureus* in the disease severity and possible pathogenesis of atopic dermatitis, and there are specific types of *C. acnes* that are associated with acne vulgaris. While previous treatment options have centered around a general antiseptic or anti-inflammatory approach, newer therapeutic options have emerged around using novel approaches such as live microbes or targeted therapy against the microbial factor driving the skin disease. Other novel approaches have leveraged phages for specific antimicrobial activity, and future work may further elucidate the role of other microbial players on the skin including fungi and mites. It is clear that more research is needed in understanding skin-microbe interactions and leveraging this knowledge into more effective therapeutic options for skin diseases.

Acknowledgements

Dr. Oh is on the Scientific Advisory Board of Azitra Inc.

References

1. Structure, function and diversity of the healthy human microbiome. *Nature*, 486, 7402, 207–214, 2012.
2. Wikoff, W.R. *et al.*, Metabolomics analysis reveals large effects of gut microflora on mammalian blood metabolites. *Proc. Natl. Acad. Sci. U. S. A.*, 106, 10, 3698–703, 2009.

3. Salzman, N.H. *et al.*, Enteric defensins are essential regulators of intestinal microbial ecology. *Nat. Immunol.*, 11, 1, 76–82, 2010.

4. Kau, A.L. *et al.*, Human nutrition, the gut microbiome and the immune system. *Nature*, 474, 7351, 327–336, 2011.

5. Ravel, J. *et al.*, Vaginal microbiome of reproductive-age women. *Proc. Natl. Acad. Sci. U. S. A.*, 108 Suppl 1, 4680–7, 2011.

6. Grice, E.A. and Segre, J.A., The skin microbiome. *Nat. Rev. Microbiol.*, 9, 4, 244–53, 2011.

7. Diaz Heijtz, R. *et al.*, Normal gut microbiota modulates brain development and behavior. *Proc. Natl. Acad. Sci. U. S. A.*, 108, 7, 3047–52, 2011.

8. Weyrich, L.S. *et al.*, The skin microbiome: Associations between altered microbial communities and disease. *Aust. J. Dermatol.*, 56, 4, 268–274, 2015.

9. Oh, J. *et al.*, Biogeography and individuality shape function in the human skin metagenome. *Nature*, 514, 7520, 59–64, 2014.

10. Findley, K. *et al.*, Topographic diversity of fungal and bacterial communities in human skin. *Nature*, 498, 7454, 367–70, 2013.

11. Grice, E.A. *et al.*, Topographical and temporal diversity of the human skin microbiome. *Science*, 324, 5931, 1190–2, 2009.

12. Costello, E.K. *et al.*, Bacterial community variation in human body habitats across space and time. *Science*, 326, 5960, 1694–7, 2009.

13. Oh, J. *et al.*, Biogeography and individuality shape function in the human skin metagenome. *Nature*, 514, 59, 2014.

14. Tirosh, O. *et al.*, Expanded skin virome in DOCK8-deficient patients. *Nat. Med.*, 24, 12, 1815–1821, 2018.

15. Picard, C. *et al.*, Primary Immunodeficiency Diseases: An Update on the Classification from the International Union of Immunological Societies Expert Committee for Primary Immunodeficiency 2015. *J. Clin. Immunol.*, 35, 8, 696–726, 2015.

16. Scharschmidt, Tiffany, C. *et al.*, A Wave of Regulatory T Cells into Neonatal Skin Mediates Tolerance to Commensal Microbes. *Immunity*, 43, 5, 1011–1021, 2015.

17. Scharschmidt, T.C. *et al.*, Commensal Microbes and Hair Follicle Morphogenesis Coordinately Drive Treg Migration into Neonatal Skin. *Cell Host Microbe*, 21, 4, 467–477.e5, 2017.

18. Oh, J. *et al.*, The altered landscape of the human skin microbiome in patients with primary immunodeficiencies. *Genome Res.*, 23, 12, 2103–14, 2013.

19. Vandegrift, R. *et al.*, Cleanliness in context: Reconciling hygiene with a modern microbial perspective. *Microbiome*, 5, 1, 76, 2017.

20. Wallen-Russell, C. and Wallen-Russell, S., Meta Analysis of Skin Microbiome: New Link between Skin Microbiota Diversity and Skin Health with Proposal to Use This as a Future Mechanism to Determine Whether Cosmetic Products Damage the Skin. *Cosmetics*, 4, 2, 14, 2017.

21. Buffie, C.G. and Pamer, E.G., Microbiota-mediated colonization resistance against intestinal pathogens. *Nat. Rev. Immunol.*, 13, 11, 790–801, 2013.

22. Naik, S. *et al.*, Compartmentalized control of skin immunity by resident commensals. *Science*, 337, 6098, 1115–9, 2012.
23. Harrison, O.J. *et al.*, Commensal-specific T cell plasticity promotes rapid tissue adaptation to injury. *Science*, 363, 6422, 2019.
24. Scharschmidt, T.C., Establishing Tolerance to Commensal Skin Bacteria: Timing Is Everything. *Dermatol. Clin.*, 35, 1, 1–9, 2017.
25. Byrd, A.L. *et al.*, *Staphylococcus aureus* and *Staphylococcus epidermidis* strain diversity underlying pediatric atopic dermatitis. *Sci. Transl. Med.*, 9, 397, eaal4651, 2017.
26. Scharschmidt, T.C. *et al.*, A Wave of Regulatory T Cells into Neonatal Skin Mediates Tolerance to Commensal Microbes. *Immunity*, 43, 5, 1011–21, 2015.
27. Naik, S. *et al.*, Commensal-dendritic-cell interaction specifies a unique protective skin immune signature. *Nature*, 520, 7545, 104–8, 2015.
28. Belkaid, Y. and Tamoutounour, S., The influence of skin microorganisms on cutaneous immunity. *Nat. Rev. Immunol.*, 16, 6, 353–66, 2016.
29. Belkaid, Y. and Harrison, O.J., Homeostatic Immunity and the Microbiota. *Immunity*, 46, 4, 562–576, 2017.
30. Kord, M. *et al.*, Evaluation of Biofilm Formation and Presence of Ica Genes in *Staphylococcus epidermidis* Clinical Isolates. *Osong Public Health Res. Perspect*, 9, 4, 160–166, 2018.
31. Zhang, L. *et al.*, *Staphylococcus aureus* expresses a cell surface protein that binds both IgG and beta2-glycoprotein I. *Microbiology*, 145, Pt 1, 177–83, 1999.
32. Burman, J.D. *et al.*, Interaction of human complement with Sbi, a staphylococcal immunoglobulin-binding protein: indications of a novel mechanism of complement evasion by *Staphylococcus aureus*. *J. Biol. Chem.*, 283, 25, 17579–93, 2008.
33. Drapeau, G.R., Role of metalloprotease in activation of the precursor of staphylococcal protease. *J. Bacteriol.*, 136, 2, 607–13, 1978.
34. Fitzgerald, J.R. *et al.*, Genome diversification in *Staphylococcus aureus*: Molecular evolution of a highly variable chromosomal region encoding the Staphylococcal exotoxin-like family of proteins. *Infect Immun.*, 71, 5, 2827–38, 2003.
35. Chung, M.C. *et al.*, The crystal structure of staphylococcal superantigen-like protein 11 in complex with sialyl Lewis X reveals the mechanism for cell binding and immune inhibition. *Mol. Microbiol.*, 66, 6, 1342–55, 2007.
36. Koymans, K.J. *et al.*, Staphylococcal Superantigen-Like Protein 1 and 5 (SSL1 & SSL5) Limit Neutrophil Chemotaxis and Migration through MMP-Inhibition. *Int. J. Mol. Sci.*, 17, 7, 2016.
37. Vath, G.M. *et al.*, The crystal structure of exfoliative toxin B: A superantigen with enzymatic activity. *Biochemistry*, 38, 32, 10239–46, 1999.
38. Nagase, H., Visse, R., Murphy, G., Structure and function of matrix metalloproteinases and TIMPs. *Cardiovasc. Res.*, 69, 3, 562–73, 2006.

39. Boden, M.K. and Flock, J.I., Evidence for three different fibrinogen-binding proteins with unique properties from *Staphylococcus aureus* strain Newman. *Microb. Pathog.*, 12, 4, 289–98, 1992.

40. Geoghegan, J.A., Irvine, A.D., Foster, T.J., *Staphylococcus aureus* and Atopic Dermatitis: A Complex and Evolving Relationship. *Trends Microbiol.*, 26, 6, 484–497, 2018.

41. David Boothe, W., Tarbox, J.A., Tarbox, M.B., Atopic Dermatitis: Pathophysiology. *Adv. Exp Med. Biol.*, 1027, 21–37, 2017.

42. Egawa, G. and Kabashima, K., Multifactorial skin barrier deficiency and atopic dermatitis: Essential topics to prevent the atopic march. *J. Allergy Clin. Immunol.*, 138, 2, 350–358, 2016.

43. Higaki, S. *et al.*, Comparative study of staphylococci from the skin of atopic dermatitis patients and from healthy subjects. *Int. J. Dermatol.*, 38, 4, 265–9, 1999.

44. Guzik, T.J. *et al.*, Persistent skin colonization with *Staphylococcus aureus* in atopic dermatitis: Relationship to clinical and immunological parameters. *Clin. Exp. Allergy*, 35, 4, 448–55, 2005.

45. Park, H.-Y. *et al.*, *Staphylococcus aureus* Colonization in Acute and Chronic Skin Lesions of Patients with Atopic Dermatitis. *Ann. Dermatol.*, 25, 4, 410–416, 2013.

46. Tauber, M. *et al.*, *Staphylococcus aureus* density on lesional and nonlesional skin is strongly associated with disease severity in atopic dermatitis. *J. Allergy Clin. Immunol.*, 137, 4, 1272–1274.e3, 2016.

47. Nakatsuji, T. *et al.*, *Staphylococcus aureus* Exploits Epidermal Barrier Defects in Atopic Dermatitis to Trigger Cytokine Expression. *J. Invest. Dermatol.*, 136, 11, 2192–2200, 2016.

48. Kobayashi, T. *et al.*, Dysbiosis and *Staphylococcus aureus* Colonization Drives Inflammation in Atopic Dermatitis. *Immunity*, 42, 4, 756–66, 2015.

49. Seite, S. *et al.*, Microbiome of affected and unaffected skin of patients with atopic dermatitis before and after emollient treatment. *J. Drugs Dermatol.*, 13, 11, 1365–72, 2014.

50. Totte, J.E. *et al.*, Prevalence and odds of *Staphylococcus aureus* carriage in atopic dermatitis: A systematic review and meta-analysis. *Br. J. Dermatol.*, 175, 4, 687–95, 2016.

51. Kong, H.H. *et al.*, Temporal shifts in the skin microbiome associated with disease flares and treatment in children with atopic dermatitis. *Genome Res.*, 22, 5, 850–9, 2012.

52. Larsen, M.V. *et al.*, Multilocus sequence typing of total-genome-sequenced bacteria. *J. Clin. Microbiol.*, 50, 4, 1355–61, 2012.

53. Feil, E.J. *et al.*, How clonal is *Staphylococcus aureus*? *J. Bacteriol.*, 185, 11, 3307–16, 2003.

54. Monecke, S. *et al.*, Molecular epidemiology of *Staphylococcus aureus* in asymptomatic carriers. *Eur. J. Clin. Microbiol. Infect Dis.*, 28, 9, 1159–65, 2009.

55. Melles, D.C. *et al.*, Natural population dynamics and expansion of pathogenic clones of *Staphylococcus aureus*. *J. Clin. Invest.*, 114, 12, 1732–40, 2004.

56. Fleury, O.M. *et al.*, Clumping Factor B Promotes Adherence of *Staphylococcus aureus* to Corneocytes in Atopic Dermatitis. *Infect Immun.*, 85, 6, 2017.

57. Rojo, A. *et al.*, *Staphylococcus aureus* genomic pattern and atopic dermatitis: may factors other than superantigens be involved? *Eur. J. Clin. Microbiol. Infect Dis.*, 33, 4, 651–8, 2014.

58. Yeung, M. *et al.*, Identification of major clonal complexes and toxin producing strains among *Staphylococcus aureus* associated with atopic dermatitis. *Microbes Infect*, 13, 2, 189–97, 2011.

59. Meylan, P. *et al.*, Skin Colonization by *Staphylococcus aureus* Precedes the Clinical Diagnosis of Atopic Dermatitis in Infancy. *J. Invest Dermatol.*, 137, 12, 2497–2504, 2017.

60. Kennedy, E.A. *et al.*, Skin microbiome before development of atopic dermatitis: Early colonization with commensal staphylococci at 2 months is associated with a lower risk of atopic dermatitis at 1 year. *J. Allergy Clin. Immunol.*, 139, 1, 166–172, 2017.

61. Bhate, K. and Williams, H.C., Epidemiology of acne vulgaris. *Br. J. Dermatol.*, 168, 3, 474–85, 2013.

62. White, G.M., Recent findings in the epidemiologic evidence, classification, and subtypes of acne vulgaris. *J. Am. Acad. Dermatol.*, 39, 2 Pt 3, S34–7, 1998.

63. Klassen, A.F., Newton, J.N., Mallon, E., Measuring quality of life in people referred for specialist care of acne: Comparing generic and disease-specific measures. *J. Am. Acad. Dermatol.*, 43, 2 Pt 1, 229–33, 2000.

64. Dalgard, F. *et al.*, Self-esteem and body satisfaction among late adolescents with acne: Results from a population survey. *J. Am. Acad. Dermatol.*, 59, 5, 746–51, 2008.

65. Yazici, K. *et al.*, Disease-specific quality of life is associated with anxiety and depression in patients with acne. *J. Eur. Acad. Dermatol. Venereol.*, 18, 4, 435–9, 2004.

66. O'Neill, A.M. and Gallo, R.L., Host-microbiome interactions and recent progress into understanding the biology of acne vulgaris. *Microbiome*, 6, 1, 177, 2018.

67. Federman, D.G. and Kirsner, R.S., Acne vulgaris: Pathogenesis and therapeutic approach. *Am. J. Manag. Care*, 6, 1, 78–87; quiz 88-9, 2000.

68. Johnson, J.L. and Cummins, C.S., Cell wall composition and deoxyribonucleic acid similarities among the anaerobic coryneforms, classical propionibacteria, and strains of Arachnia propionica. *J. Bacteriol.*, 109, 3, 1047–1066, 1972.

69. McDowell, A. *et al.*, Propionibacterium acnes types I and II represent phylogenetically distinct groups. *J. Clin. Microbiol.*, 43, 1, 326–34, 2005.

70. McDowell, A. *et al.*, A new phylogenetic group of Propionibacterium acnes. *J. Med. Microbiol.*, 57, Pt 2, 218–24, 2008.

71. Lomholt, H.B. and Kilian, M., Population genetic analysis of Propionibacterium acnes identifies a subpopulation and epidemic clones associated with acne. *PLoS One*, 5, 8, e12277, 2010.

72. McDowell, A. *et al.*, An expanded multilocus sequence typing scheme for propionibacterium acnes: Investigation of 'pathogenic', 'commensal' and antibiotic resistant strains. *PLoS One*, 7, 7, e41480, 2012.

73. Fitz-Gibbon, S. *et al.*, Propionibacterium acnes strain populations in the human skin microbiome associated with acne. *J. Invest Dermatol.*, 133, 9, 2152–60, 2013.

74. Graham, G.M. *et al.*, Proinflammatory cytokine production by human keratinocytes stimulated with Propionibacterium acnes and P. acnes GroEL. *Br. J. Dermatol.*, 150, 3, 421–8, 2004.

75. Brüggemann, H. *et al.*, CRISPR/cas loci of type II Propionibacterium acnes confer immunity against acquisition of mobile elements present in type I P. acnes. *PloS One*, 7, 3, e34171–e34171, 2012.

76. Scholz, C.F. *et al.*, Genome stability of Propionibacterium acnes: a comprehensive study of indels and homopolymeric tracts. *Sci. Rep.*, 6, 20662, 2016.

77. Boehncke, W.H. and Schon, M.P., Psoriasis. *Lancet*, 386, 9997, 983–94, 2015.

78. Tomi, N.S., Kranke, B., Aberer, E., Staphylococcal toxins in patients with psoriasis, atopic dermatitis, and erythroderma, and in healthy control subjects. *J. Am. Acad. Dermatol.*, 53, 1, 67–72, 2005.

79. Chang, H.-W. *et al.*, Alteration of the cutaneous microbiome in psoriasis and potential role in Th17 polarization. *Microbiome*, 6, 1, 154–154, 2018.

80. Raza, N., Usman, M., Hameed, A., Chronic plaque psoriasis: Streptococcus pyogenes throat carriage rate and therapeutic response to oral antibiotics in comparison with oral methotrexate. *J. Coll. Physicians Surg. Pak.*, 17, 12, 717–20, 2007.

81. Rudramurthy, S.M. *et al.*, Association of Malassezia species with psoriatic lesions. *Mycoses*, 57, 8, 483–8, 2014.

82. Prohic, A., Identification of Malassezia species isolated from scalp skin of patients with psoriasis and healthy subjects. *Acta Dermatovenerol. Croat*, 11, 1, 10–6, 2003.

83. Tett, A. *et al.*, Unexplored diversity and strain-level structure of the skin microbiome associated with psoriasis. *NPJ Biofilms Microbiomes*, 3, 1, 14, 2017.

84. Visser, M.J.E., Kell, D.B., Pretorius, E., Bacterial Dysbiosis and Translocation in Psoriasis Vulgaris. *Front. Cell. Infect. Microbiol.*, 9, 7–7, 2019.

85. Bawdon, D. *et al.*, Identification of axillary Staphylococcus sp. involved in the production of the malodorous thioalcohol 3-methyl-3-sufanylhexan-1-ol. *FEMS Microbiol. Lett.*, 362, 16, 2015.

86. Morand, S.C. *et al.*, Complete Genome Sequence of Malassezia restricta CBS 7877, an Opportunist Pathogen Involved in Dandruff and Seborrheic Dermatitis. *Microbiol. Resour. Announc.*, 8, 6, 2019.

87. Shibagaki, N. *et al.*, Aging-related changes in the diversity of women's skin microbiomes associated with oral bacteria. *Sci. Rep.*, 7, 1, 10567, 2017.

88. Fabbrocini, G. *et al.*, Acneiform Rash Induced by EGFR Inhibitors: Review of the Literature and New Insights. *Skin Appendage Disord.*, 1, 1, 31–37, 2015.

89. Lichtenberger, B.M. *et al.*, Epidermal EGFR controls cutaneous host defense and prevents inflammation. *Sci. Transl. Med.*, 5, 199, 199ra111, 2013.

90. Mayba, J.N. and Gooderham, M.J., Review of Atopic Dermatitis and Topical Therapies. *J. Cutan Med. Surg.*, 21, 3, 227–236, 2017.

91. Eichenfield, L.F. *et al.*, Guidelines of care for the management of atopic dermatitis: Section 2. Management and treatment of atopic dermatitis with topical therapies. *J. Am. Acad. Dermatol.*, 71, 1, 116–32, 2014.

92. Lee, M. and Van Bever, H., The role of antiseptic agents in atopic dermatitis. *Asia Pac. Allergy*, 4, 4, 230–40, 2014.

93. Lebwohl, M.G. *et al.*, Pathways to managing atopic dermatitis: Consensus from the experts. *J. Clin. Aesthet. Dermatol.*, 6, 7 Suppl, S2–s18, 2013.

94. Zane, L.T. *et al.*, Crisaborole and its potential role in treating atopic dermatitis: Overview of early clinical studies. *Immunotherapy*, 8, 8, 853–66, 2016.

95. Braham, S.J. *et al.*, Occlusive therapy in atopic dermatitis: Overview. *J. Dermatolog. Treat*, 21, 2, 62–72, 2010.

96. Beck, L.A. *et al.*, Dupilumab treatment in adults with moderate-to-severe atopic dermatitis. *N. Engl. J. Med.*, 371, 2, 130–9, 2014.

97. Simpson, E.L. *et al.*, Two Phase 3 Trials of Dupilumab versus Placebo in Atopic Dermatitis. *N. Engl. J. Med.*, 375, 24, 2335–2348, 2016.

98. Zaenglein, A.L. *et al.*, Guidelines of care for the management of acne vulgaris. *J. Am. Acad. Dermatol.*, 74, 5, 945–73.e33, 2016.

99. Walsh, T.R., Efthimiou, J., Dreno, B., Systematic review of antibiotic resistance in acne: An increasing topical and oral threat. *Lancet Infect. Dis.*, 16, 3, e23–33, 2016.

100. Layton, A., The use of isotretinoin in acne. *Dermato-endocrinology*, 1, 3, 162–169, 2009.

101. King, K. *et al.*, A double-blind study of the effects of 13-cis-retinoic acid on acne, sebum excretion rate and microbial population. *Br. J. Dermatol.*, 107, 5, 583–90, 1982.

102. Leyden, J.J. and McGinley, K.J., Effect of 13-cis-retinoic acid on sebum production and Propionibacterium acnes in severe nodulocystic acne. *Arch. Dermatol. Res.*, 272, 3-4, 331–7, 1982.

103. Dispenza, M.C. *et al.*, Systemic isotretinoin therapy normalizes exaggerated TLR-2-mediated innate immune responses in acne patients. *J. Invest Dermatol.*, 132, 9, 2198–205, 2012.

104. Maekawa, T. and Hajishengallis, G., Topical treatment with probiotic Lactobacillus brevis CD2 inhibits experimental periodontal inflammation and bone loss. *J. Periodontal Res.*, 49, 6, 785–91, 2014.

105. Nodake, Y. *et al.*, Pilot study on novel skin care method by augmentation with *Staphylococcus epidermidis*, an autologous skin microbe - A blinded randomized clinical trial. *J. Dermatol. Sci.*, 79, 2, 119–26, 2015.

106. Linehan, J.L. *et al.*, Non-classical Immunity Controls Microbiota Impact on Skin Immunity and Tissue Repair. *Cell*, 172, 4, 784–796.e18, 2018.

107. Nakatsuji, T. *et al.*, Antimicrobials from human skin commensal bacteria protect against *Staphylococcus aureus* and are deficient in atopic dermatitis. *Sci. Transl. Med.*, 9, 378, 2017.

5

The Axillary Microbiome and its Relationship with Underarm Odor

Alexander Gordon James

*Unilever Beauty & Personal Care (Deodorants), Colworth Science Park,
Bedford, UK*

Abstract

The generation of malodour on the skin surface of modern humans is caused by the biotransformation of naturally secreted non-odorous precursor molecules into volatile odorants by members of the commensal microbiome. Specifically in the axilla (underarm), malodour is mediated mainly by the bacterial metabolism of amino acid- and dipeptide-conjugated substrates originating from the apocrine gland. Of particular relevance are the conversion of S-hydroxyalkyl-L-cysteinylglycine precursors into thioalcohols such as 3-methyl-3-sulfanylhexan-1-ol, and the conversion of N^{α}-acyl-L-glutamine precursors into volatile fatty acids such as 3-hydroxy-3-methylhexanoic acid and 3-methyl-2-hexenoic acid. Historically, culture-based microbiological studies revealed that the axillary microbiota consists primarily of Gram-positive bacteria of the genera *Staphylococcus*, *Corynebacterium* and *Cutibacterium* (formerly *Propionibacterium*). While this has been confirmed by culture-independent metataxonomics studies, it is now clear that Gram-positive anaerobic cocci such as *Anaerococcus* and *Peptoniphilus* species should also be considered as key components of the commensal microbiome. In this chapter, I will examine in detail the composition of the commensal axillary microbiome and its relationship with underarm odor, focusing on precursor-product relationships, odor-forming metabolic pathways and causal organisms, as well as the effects of microbiome perturbations, including product interventions.

Keywords: *Corynebacterium*, *Staphylococcus*, *Staphylococcus hominis*, Gram-positive anaerobic cocci, volatile fatty acid, thioalcohol, N^{α}-acylglutamine aminoacylase, carbon-sulphur β-lyase

Email: Gordon.James@unilever.com

Nava Dayan (ed.) *Skin Microbiome Handbook: From Basic Research to Product Development*,
(79–130) © 2020 Scrivener Publishing LLC

5.1   Introduction

The generation of malodour on the skin surface of *Homo sapiens* (modern humans) is caused by the biotransformation of naturally secreted non-odorous precursor molecules into volatile odorants by members of the commensal microbiota, also known as the skin microbiome. This is most notably manifested in the axilla (underarm), where a large and permanent population of microorganisms thrives on the various exocrine gland secretions present therein, namely sebum, eccrine sweat and apocrine sweat. Sebum is primarily a complex mixture of lipids secreted by the sebaceous gland into the hair follicle, the function of which is not fully understood [1]. In the context of axillary malodour, often referred to as body odor (BO), it contains many structurally-unusual (*e.g.* methyl-branched) long-chain fatty acids [2], which can be converted into volatile fatty acids (VFAs) by some axillary bacteria [3] although, as discussed in the sections below, this is now believed to be only a minor contributory route to BO [4]. The eccrine sweat gland is the most prevalent exocrine organ and produces an aqueous solution mainly in response to heat and exercise, as well as emotional stimuli, which is secreted directly onto the skin surface [5]. Its main function is thermoregulation, as the principal component, water, evaporates from the skin surface, cooling the body; however, in the occluded environment of the axilla, this process is impeded, resulting in a high level of hydration that supports the existence of a dense skin microbiota. Eccrine sweat is a dilute solution similar in composition to plasma, with the inorganic electrolytes sodium, chloride and potassium being the major solutes [5]. It also contains significant levels of lactate, as well as other organic solutes, notably amino acids, and can thus support microbial growth. Interestingly, the amino acid composition of eccrine sweat bears an extraordinary similarity to that of the epidermal protein profilaggrin [6] (rather than blood plasma, as previously thought) which, when hydrolysed, forms a major part of the natural moisturizing factor within the stratum corneum that maintains the barrier integrity of human skin. In the context of BO, as discussed in the sections below, some of these amino acids, specifically branched aliphatic species such as L-leucine, can be metabolised by axillary bacteria to short-chain, methyl-branched VFAs, such as isovaleric acid [7], which have been long-associated with the acidic note of axillary malodour [8]; however, its main role is probably the aforementioned elevated skin hydration, supporting naturally high numbers of commensal microbes. Another interesting aspect of eccrine sweat, however, is the presence of antimicrobial peptides (AMPs), in particular dermcidin [9], suggesting a role in innate immunity and the regulation of the skin microbiota, a feature we will revisit in a later section. The apocrine gland is similar to the sebaceous gland in that it secretes into the hair follicle, but differs from both the sebaceous and eccrine glands in being unique to a few bodily locations including the areolae, genitalia and external auditory meatus (ear canal), as well as the axilla [10]. Apocrine sweat is a lipid-rich viscous fluid, which in its native form is odorless; its chemical composition is poorly defined, although a high level of cholesterol has been reported [11], and it is also likely to contain the antimicrobial enzyme lysozyme [12], another component of the skin's innate immune system. Most notably in relation to BO, however, were pioneering studies undertaken in the 1950s which demonstrated that the generation of malodour on underarm skin is due mainly to the action of the resident microbiota on secretions from the axillary apocrine gland [13]. The discovery of an odor-generating process linked to apocrine glands in the human axilla immediately raised interest both in its current relevance and its evolutionary origin. In other mammalian species, apocrine glands located in specialised sites, *e.g.* the perianal and inguinal regions, are regarded as scent glands, which become active with phases of the sexual cycle [10]. Furthermore, human apocrine glands do not have a thermoregulatory function, do not develop fully until puberty and, in females, go into atrophy after the menopause. Speculation was further fueled in the 1970s when 16-androstene steroids, and in particular the porcine pheromone 5α-androstenone, were detected in the human axilla [14]. For many years, these 16-androstenes were heavily implicated in BO as well as being labelled as human pheromones, even if now vestigial [15]; however, as discussed in the sections below, their contribution to axillary odor is now believed to be minor [4]. Nevertheless, the evolutionary link between what we currently perceive as BO and a vestigial human chemical signaling mechanism involving the axillary apocrine gland remains a subject of some intrigue, though not one examined in detail in this review.

Since the breakthrough work of Shelley and colleagues on bacterial metabolism of apocrine sweat [13], extensive studies on the axillary microbiota and its relationship with underarm odor have been reported, notably by Leyden *et al.* in the early 1980s [8] and Taylor *et al.* in the early 2000s [16], in each case highlighting the high bacterial density on underarm skin, typically averaging ~10^6 colony-forming units per cm^2 of skin (CFU/cm^2). These studies used traditional culture methods to quantitatively determine the axillary microbial ecology of multiple subjects and correlated the results with subjectively determined odor quality and intensity, respectively. Overlaying modern taxonomic terminology [4] established that the microbiota consists mainly of representatives of the Gram-positive bacterial genera *Staphylococcus, Corynebacterium* and *Cutibacterium* (formerly *Propionibacterium* [17]). Leyden and colleagues showed that significantly higher numbers of both total bacteria, and in particular corynebacteria, were associated with a "pungent, apocrine" odor quality [8], while Taylor and colleagues found highly significant associations between both total aerobic bacteria, and in particular corynebacteria, and malodour intensity [16]. These studies formed much of the microbiological evidence in support of the widely accepted view that members of the *Corynebacterium* genus are the primary causal agents of BO.

Until relatively recently, our understanding of the microbial communities on human skin sites was based wholly on traditional culture methods, which rely on the cultivability of genera of interest in specific selective growth media, and cannot normally identify individual species without further biochemical or genetic tests. As discussed in the sections below, however, over the past decade or so, we have witnessed a revolution in microbiology, manifested in the adoption of culture-independent metataxonomic approaches [18], especially 16S rRNA gene profiling, to probe the skin microbiome. Several such studies have been carried out in the axilla, and with the advent of 2nd and 3rd generation high-throughput DNA sequencing technologies, the breadth and depth of data generated has increased massively. Specifically in relation to the axillary microbiome, metataxonomic studies confirm it is dominated by members of the *Staphylococcus, Cutibacterium* (formerly *Propionibacterium* [17]) and *Corynebacterium* genera [19], although the presence of taxa not previously indicated by culture-based methods is also evident, most notably Gram-positive anaerobic cocci (GPAC) belonging to the *Anaerococcus* and *Peptoniphilus* genera [20, 21].

The currently accepted view is that VFAs and thioalcohols (sulfanylalkanols) are the primary causal molecules of axillary malodour. The unsaturated aldehyde 2-nonenal has also been implicated, but specifically in older (40+) subjects [22]; moreover, the formation of this odorant is believed to be chemical (oxidative degradation of unsaturated fatty acids) rather than biochemical, and thus does not involve a contribution from the microbiome. In the past, 16-androstene steroids were heavily touted as causal molecules of BO [15] but, as highlighted in the sections below, on the basis of various strands of evidence [23–25], their contribution is now believed to be minor [4]. The involvement of short-chain ($C_2 - C_5$) VFAs has long been acknowledged, and various metabolic routes to these acids have been elucidated [3, 7]. However, in the early 1990s, it was established that a group of structurally-unusual medium-chain ($C_6 - C_{10}$) acids, in particular the *trans* (*E*) isomer of 3-methyl-2-hexenoic acid (3M2H), is the main aspect of VFA-based underarm odor [24]. It was initially thought that these acids were carried to the skin surface non-covalently bound to two "apocrine secretion odor-binding proteins" (ASOBs) [26]. However, Natsch *et al.* [27] later showed that 3M2H, and the structurally related 3-hydroxy-3-methylhexanoic acid (3H3MH), are covalently bound to L-glutamine residues in axillary sweat, and released by the bacterial enzyme N^α-acylglutamine aminoacylase, the encoding gene for which was cloned and heterologously expressed from an axillary *Corynebacterium* strain. The same group later reported that a wide range of medium-chain VFAs are present in axillary sweat as L-glutamine N^α-conjugates, with 3H3MH and 3M2H being the dominant species [28]. While the studies of Natsch and colleagues [27, 28] support the microbiological evidence that corynebacteria are the primary BO-causing microbes, more recent evidence has challenged this view, as will be discussed in the sections below. In the context of VFA-based malodour, Fujii *et al.* described an axillary *Anaerococcus* strain capable of efficiently releasing 3H3MH from its L-glutamine N^α-conjugated precursor [29].

Thioalcohols are an important aspect of human BO that were first reported in three simultaneous publications in 2004 [30–32]. They possess a particularly pungent odor, and can be detected at the pg/L level, an order of magnitude lower than many other volatile aroma-bearing chemicals emanating from skin [31]. The most abundant of these thioalcohols is 3-methyl-3-sulfanylhexan-1-ol (3M3SH), which was described by Troccaz *et al.* [30] as having a "sweat and onion-like" smell, and by Hasegawa *et al.* [32] as possessing a "strong meaty, fruity note.....reminiscent of axillary odor". The microbially-transformed precursors to these malodorants were initially believed to be *S*-hydroxyalkyl-L-cysteine conjugates [31], but are now acknowledged to be structurally related dipeptide-conjugated *S*-hydroxyalkyl-L-cysteinylglycine species [33]. The biosynthetic origin of these precursors in the human host is not fully understood, but they are believed to be secreted onto axillary skin via the ATP-binding cassette (ABC) transporter ABCC11 as odorless glutathione (GSH) conjugates [34]. As discussed in the sections below, this transporter has also been linked genetically to BO as humans of East Asian origin in particular are often homozygous for a single nucleotide polymorphism (SNP) in the *ABCC11* allele (538G→A) that leads to loss of transporter function [35, 36], resulting in a reduction in malodour intensity as well as a change in quality [37]. The GSH conjugate of 3M3SH (*S*-G-3M3SH) has never been detected in the axilla; however, the L-cysteinylglycine dipeptide conjugated form, *S*-Cys-Gly-3M3SH, is readily detectable [33] and, consistent with this observation, a human γ-glutamyl transferase (GGT1) was recently demon-strated to localise to the apocrine sweat gland and convert S-G-3M3SH to S-Cys-Gly-3M3SH [34].

As the importance of sulfanylalkanols in BO emerged in the mid-2000s, it was quickly evident that 3M3SH is the prominent thioalcohol-based mal-odorant [30–32]; however, one of these published studies identified three additional thioalcohols, including 3-sulfanylhexan-1-ol and 2-methyl-3-sulfanylbutan-1-ol [31], validating work carried out by ourselves using a combined analytical and organoleptic approach [4]. Based on the premise that the direct precursors to these malodorants would be S-hydroxyalkyl-L-cysteine conjugates, carbon-sulphur (C-S) β-lyase genes were identified, cloned, sequenced and heterologously expressed from two separate axil-lary *Corynebacterium* strains [4, 31]. In each case, the expressed protein was shown to be a MalY-type cystathionine β-lyase (EC 4.4.1.8) [4] capable of efficiently lysing L-cysteine S-conjugated thioalcohols [31]. In contrast, staphylococcal cystathionine β-lyases, such as that cloned and expressed from *Staphylococcus haemolyticus* by Troccaz *et al.* [38], are of the MetC-type, and show poor conversion of S-hydroxyalkyl-L-cysteine conjugates into thioalcohols. However, an alternative postulate by Starkenmann *et al.* [33] stated that the true thioalcohol precursors are S-hydroxyalkyl-L-cysteinylglycine conjugates, which are enzymatically cleaved by *S. haemo-lyticus*, presumably mediated by an alternative lytic enzyme to cystathionine β-lyase. In support of this, Troccaz *et al.* [39] measured significant (μg/L – mg/L) levels of S-Cys-Gly-3M3SH in the axillary sweat of 49 volunteers over 3 years, and it is now accepted that S-hydroxyalkyl-L-cysteinylglycine conjugates are the physiological precursors of thioalcohols present in apo-crine sweat. However, while accepting this paradigm, Emter & Natsch [40] used both native cellular extracts and purified recombinant enzymes to show that the sequential action of a dipeptidase and C-S (cystathionine) β-lyase mediates release of 3M3SH from its dipeptide precursor in an axil-lary *Corynebacterium* strain, and argued that this was representative of the physiological route to the thioalcohol aspect of BO.

As discussed in the sections below, in conjunction with academic groups at the universities of York and Oxford, we have now elucidated the pathway by which S-Cys-Gly-3M3SH is taken up and metabolised by a limited range of staphylococcal species present in the axilla, namely *Staphylococcus homi-nis*, *S. haemolyticus* and *Staphylococcus lugdunensis*, producing and secret-ing the pivotal thioalcohol malodorant 3M3SH [41]. Of these, the most abundant species typically present on axillary skin is *S. hominis* [42], and the biological significance of this taxon in BO has recently been confirmed using both metataxonomics [43] and real-time (quantitative) polymerase chain reaction (qPCR) assays [44], with each of these studies showing a strong correlation between *S. hominis* and malodour intensity. This appears to contradict earlier work using culture-based studies at the genus level that had either discounted the contribution of staphylococci [16] or linked them only to the "faint acid, non-apocrine" note of BO [8]; however, both these observations are likely due to the dominance of the non-thioalcohol producing species *Staphylococcus epidermidis* on axillary skin [41, 42]. We recently showed that S-Cys-Gly-3M3SH is actively taken up by *S. hominis* via a specific secondary active transporter, $PepT_{Sh}$, a member of the proton-coupled oligopeptide transporter (POT) family [45]. A combination of structural, biochemical and cell-based assays revealed how this di- and tri-peptide transporter can recognise thioalcohol-conjugated peptides, and also demonstrated that transport is coupled to the inwardly directed proton electrochemical gradient. Further to this, in conjunction with the University of York, we have now identified and characterised a novel C-S β-lyase enzyme found only in a small monophyletic group of human-associated staphylococci (including *S. hominis, S. haemolyticus* and *S. lugdunensis*) that is able to catalyse the lysis of L-cysteine S-conjugated 3M3SH (S-Cys-3M3SH) with greater efficiency than a wide range of other related C-S β-lyase enzymes [46].

In this chapter, I will utilise published work by ourselves and others to examine in detail the composition of the commensal axillary microbiome and its relationship with underarm odor, focusing on precursor-product relationships, odor-forming metabolic pathways and causal organisms. As well as reviewing the existing literature, some relevant new data is presented, including material recently submitted for publication, and considered alongside that already available in the public domain to reach an informed view on the current state-of-the-art, as well as future perspectives. While the area has been reviewed quite recently by experienced practitioners in the field [47, 48], neither publication does full justice to the significant recent advances made in our understanding of the axillary microbiome and its association with, in particular, thioalcohol-based malodor – in no small part due to developments since their publication. The former is concise in nature, focusing mainly on the influence of metataxonomics (16S rRNA gene profiling) to probe the axillary microbiome, and speculating on the future potential of metatransciptomics (analysis of meta-mRNAs via sequencing of corresponding meta-cDNAs [18]) as a route to understanding its metabolic activity [47]. In reality, the years since have seen precious little movement in the application of metagenomics (analysis of shotgun-sequenced DNA recovered from a microbiota sample [18]), let alone metatransciptomics, to the skin microbiome, mainly due to the difficulties in sampling sufficient DNA or mRNA, respectively. The review by Natsch [48] is an informative, entertaining and in-part personal account of the author's experiences as a BO practitioner, but with a focus mainly on the future design of more specific deodorant-active materials. We last reviewed the area ourselves in 2012 (published in-print in 2013) in what was a comprehensive appraisal of the state-of-the-art at the time [4]. However, the aforementioned developments since then in our understanding of the axillary microbiome and its association with thioalcohol-based malodour in particular have necessitated an update and reassessment of the field. In the main, this chapter is designed to serve exactly this purpose, with additional consideration of the influence of perturbations such as product interventions on the axillary microbiome and consequences for malodour control, both currently and in the future.

5.2   Composition of the Axillary Microbiome

Prior to discussing in detail the microorganisms that inhabit axillary skin, it is worth considering the two words already being interchangeably used in this chapter to define them – microbiota and microbiome. At this stage, it is standard practice to cite a short article co-authored by Nobel-laureate Joshua Lederberg in 2001 [49] although, in reality, both terms, especially microbiota, were in use prior to then. To the purist, these two words are not synonymous – microbiota typically denotes the collection of microorganisms located within a specific environment, while microbiome usually refers to the collection of genomes from all the microorganisms found in a particular environment. However, as their popularity grows in both technical and non-technical literature, it is evident that they are increasingly being treated as synonyms and, as already stated, they are used interchangeably in this chapter.

Pioneering studies carried out in the early 1950s demonstrated that BO is mainly a consequence of the action of the resident microbiome on odorless natural secretions from the apocrine gland [13], an exocrine organ unique to a few bodily locations, specifically the areolae, genitalia, ear canal and axilla [10]. Multiple studies on the axillary microbiota and its relationship with underarm odor have been reported in the years since with much of the early work reviewed by Jackman in 1982 [50]. However, the widest ranging studies with most significance to our current understanding of the problem up to decades later were those described by Leyden *et al.* in 1981 [8] and Taylor *et al.* in 2003 [16]. The earlier publication appears quirkily old-fashioned, in particular with its reference to defunct taxonomic terms such as "diphtheroid"; however, it warrants re-examination in light of what we know now. Traditional culture methods were used to classify and quantify the axillary microbiota of over 200 subjects and correlate the results with subjectively determined odor quality descriptors [8]. It was established that the microbiota consists mainly of "*Micrococcaceae*" (predominantly *Staphylococcus* species, but historically misclassified within this family), "lipohilic and large-colony aerobic diphtheroids" (predominantly *Corynebacterium* species) and *Propionibacterium* (now *Cutibacterium* [17]) species. Significantly higher numbers of corynebacteria in particular were associated with a "pungent, apocrine" odor quality, while high numbers of staphylococci correlated with a "faint acid, non-apocrine" odor quality. In support of this, *in vivo* experiments involving the co-incubation of cultured bacteria with apocrine sweat (both sampled from the axilla) on the volar forearm showed that only corynebacteria generated "apocrine odor" while staphylococci produced an "acid odor" attributed to the VFA isovaleric acid. In our previous review of the area [4], we were keen to translate the findings of Leyden *et al.* [8] in the context of our then-understanding of underarm odor – specifically, that they were indicative of causal links between (a) corynebacteria and thioalcohol and/or medium chain ($C_6 - C_{10}$) VFA malodorants, and (b) staphylococci and short chain ($C_2 - C_5$) VFAs. However, given developments since, implicating a monophyletic group of staphylococci, especially *S. hominis*, in thioalcohol-based malodour [41, 46], this interpretation can now be seen as erroneous, at least in part. In this respect, it is likely that the results from the Leyden *et al.* study [8] were confounded by the dominance on axillary skin of the non-thioalcohol producing species *S. epidermidis* [41, 42].

The later study reported by Taylor *et al.* [16] determined the microbial ecology of axillary skin using a range of selective and non-selective culture media, and was broadly supportive of the earlier findings [8]. In total, 36 subjects were sampled, and high variability was observed in colonisation dynamics, as summarised in Table 5.1. Generally, however, axillae carried a high-density microbiome, typically averaging ~10^6 CFU/cm^2, and were dominated by *Staphylococcus* species or "aerobic coryneforms" (essentially *Corynebacterium* species), although in a few individuals, the dominant colonisers were *Propionibacterium* (now *Cutibacterium* [17]) species. When microbial counts were compared with subjectively determined malodour intensities for individual axillae at the time of sampling, highly significant

Table 5.1 Culture-based baseline profile of the axillary microbiota and its relationship to malodour intensity (adapted from Taylor et al. [16] and James et al. [4]).

Genus	Prevalence (%)	Density range (log$_{10}$ CFU/cm^2)	Mean density (log$_{10}$ CFU/cm^2)	Correlation with malodour
Staphylococcus	98.4	1.72 – 7.00	5.76	ns
Corynebacterium	93.4	0.72 – 7.51	6.07	$p < 0.0001$
Micrococcus	45.0	0.72 – 4.72	3.19	$p < 0.05$
Cutibacterium	87.5	0.72 – 7.07	5.36	ns
Malassezia	21.7	0.72 – 2.67	1.20	ns

ns, not statistically-significant.

associations (p < 0.0001) were found for total aerobes and corynebacteria. A significant association was also found between *Micrococcus* species and malodor intensity (p < 0.05), but the low prevalence and density of this genus on underarm skin (Table 5.1) precludes it from a contributory role, as outlined previously [4]. No correlations were observed for staphylococci, cutibacteria or *Malassezia* fungi [16]. In the case of the staphylococci, and what we know now about *S. hominis* and others, and thioalcohols [41, 45, 46], this is probably another example of historical data confounded by the dominance on axillary skin of the non-thioalcohol producing species *S. epidermidis* [41, 42].

With the culture-based data appearing to support the pivotal role of corynebacteria in BO, Taylor *et al.* [16] undertook a further characterisation of these organisms, using 16S rRNA gene sequencing to analyse isolates from colonies sampled from aerobic coryneform-selective plates. The 16S rRNA gene sequence was obtained for 74 of these isolates, and directly compared to sequences lodged on the ribosomal database project (RDP) website (http://rdp.cme.msu.edu/). The highest similarity match for a large majority (n = 50) of these was *Corynebacterium* sp. G-2, while the next most dominant species match was *Corynebacterium mucifaciens* (n = 8), and instances were also found of *Corynebacterium afermentans*, *Corynebacterium amycolatum*, *Corynebacterium genitalium*, *Corynebacterium riegelii* and *Corynebacterium striatum* [16]. We later showed that *Corynebacterium* sp. G-2 is synonymous with *Corynebacterium tuberculostearicum* [4] suggesting this may represent the dominant *Corynebacterium* species on axillary skin, a postulate later supported by a metataxonomics study [43]. A proportion of the organisms identified by rRNA gene sequence analysis as *C. tuberculostearicum* (n = 9) or *C. mucifaciens* (n = 4) were also analysed biochemically for their ability to metabolise fatty acids, this being the basis of the A/B phenotyping of corynebacteria that we previously linked to BO [3]. All were negative and thus members of the *Corynebacterium* (B) sub-group; however, in a separate study, most fatty acid-catabolising *Corynebacterium* (A) strains isolated from the axillae of two subjects were identified by rRNA gene sequence analysis as *C. amycolatum* [4]. We tentatively inferred from these results that *C. tuberculostearicum* represents the dominant *Corynebacterium* (B) species on axillary skin, as well as being the main representative of the genus overall, with *C. amycolatum* as the principal representative of sub-group (A). As highlighted above, the former interpretation has been confirmed by a metataxonomics study [43], but the latter remains unvalidated. However, as discussed in the sections below, we anyway now believe that the A/B phenotyping of axillary corynebacteria is much less important in the context of malodour than we previously felt [4].

While the above studies employed a genetic approach, 16S rRNA sequencing, to probe the *Corynebacterium* population of axillary skin, organisms subjected to this had previously been isolated by culturing on a selective medium [4, 16]. However, starting in the mid-2000s, we have witnessed a revolution in microbiology, manifested in the adoption of completely culture-independent methods to probe the taxonomic and genomic composition of microbial communities, approaches now termed as metataxonomics and metagenomics, respectively [18]. Due to the inherent difficulties in sampling sufficient DNA for metagenomic studies, recent advances in our understanding of the skin microbiome have mainly been driven by metataxonomics, especially via amplification, sequencing and profiling of the bacterial (and archaeal) 16S rRNA marker gene; this being complemented by whole-genome sequencing of relevant organisms. Published metataxonomic studies on the human skin microbiota that include the axilla as a sampling site began to appear in the late 2000s [19, 20], and with the advent of a wave of 2nd and then 3rd generation high-throughput DNA sequencing platforms, the breadth and depth of data generated has increased massively. At this point, however, it is worth highlighting that, despite the advantages of metataxonomics and indeed all the aforementioned molecular approaches, none can efficiently differentiate between live and dead microbes (unlike culture-based methods), as they rely on the analysis of DNA extracted from a microorganism, rather than its viability.

Molecular analysis of the human microbiome, including that of skin, exploded in the mid-late 2000s, driven mainly by the following two events:

1. The 2005 launch, by 454 Life Sciences, of the first of the 2nd generation DNA sequencing platforms based on sequencing-by-synthesis technology [51]. This large-scale parallel pyrosequencing system [52] massively increased throughput compared to traditional Sanger sequencing, achieving ~500 Mbp per run with ~500 bp read lengths, at significantly lower cost.

2. The 2007 launch, by the US National Institutes of Health (NIH), of the Human Microbiome Project (HMP), with the aim of increasing our understanding of the microbiota involved in human health and disease, and including the skin as a target site [53].

In relation to the skin microbiome, the first of these occurrences gave rise to a wealth of metataxonomics data on various skin sites, including the axilla, while both events in tandem were responsible for exponentially increasing the number of relevant genome sequences accessible to the skin microbiology community. NIH support for the HMP ceased at the end of 2016, and the website was archived the following year, although all its datasets remain available via a central repository (https://portal.hmpdacc.org/). Its legacy included the Integrated Microbial Genomes (IMG) database and comparative analysis system [54], which has since evolved into the IMG & Microbiomes (IMG/M) platform (https://img.jgi.doe.gov/), under the auspices of the Joint Genome Institute (JGI), to support the annotation, analysis and distribution of microbial genome and microbiome datasets [55]. IMG/M continues to provide open access to hundreds of skin-relevant bacterial genomes, each processed through the IMG annotation pipeline, with a variety of analytical and visualisation tools also available.

In 2007, 454 Life Sciences was acquired by Roche Diagnostics, although it continued to exist as a separate business unit until 2013, at which point it was shut down by Roche, who subsequently ceased to support the platform in 2016. The principal reason for its demise was simply that of being superseded by a new wave of high-throughput sequencing-by-synthesis platforms such as that developed by Solexa [56] prior to their acquisition by Illumina (https://www.illumina.com/systems/sequencing-platforms.html), aswell as non-optical ion semiconductor sequencing [57], developed and commercialised by Ion Torrent, now a subsidiary of ThermoFisher (https://www.thermofisher.com/uk/en/home/brands/ion-torrent.html); these provided similar read lengths, but with increased throughput, greater accuracy and lower cost, and remain the bedrock of microbial genome, metagenome and metataxonome sequencing projects to the present day. However, even these are now being rivalled by a 3rd generation of DNA sequencing platforms, based on single molecule, real-time, long-read sequencing [58], such as that developed and commercialised by Pacific Biosciences (https://www.pacb.com/), as well as Oxford Nanopore Technologies' MinION (https://nanoporetech.com/products/minion), the first portable real-time device for nucleic acid sequencing that connects directly to a computer via a USB cable. In contrast to the 2nd generation platforms, these techniques include the option of omitting any amplification steps during library preparation, therefore enabling single molecule sequencing with much higher read lengths [58]. The approach is inherently prone to high error rates, but much effort has been invested to minimise this issue.

The first published culture-independent metataxonomic studies on the bacterial microbiota of human skin appeared in the late 2000s and, in the main, confirmed the culture-based view that the dominant genera on most surface sites are *Propionibacterium* (now *Cutibacterium* [17]), *Staphylococcus* and *Corynebacterium* [19, 20]. It was evident, however, that other taxa are present and, at species-level in particular, even within these established genera, the diversity is much greater than previously revealed by culture-based methods [19]. Specifically in relation to the axillary microbiome, early metataxonomic studies suggest it is dominated by members of the *Staphylococcus* genus (*Firmicutes* phylum) and *Propionibacterineae* (probably *Cutibacterium* (formerly *Propionibacterium* [17]) species) and *Corynebacterineae* (probably *Corynebacterium* species) suborders (*Actinobacteria* phylum), as well as members of the *Micrococcineae* suborder (probably *Micrococcus* species), although the presence of taxa not previously indicated by culture-based methods is also evident, particularly additional members of the *Firmicutes* and *Actinobacteria* phyla [20, 21]. Of particular note among the *Firmicutes* are representatives of a heterogeneous group of organisms traditionally classified as GPAC, notably members of the *Anaerococcus* and *Peptoniphilus* genera, which were identified on multiple skin sites [20] and were subsequently confirmed as significant components of the resident axillary microbiome [21]. Historically, these obligate anaerobes had been commonly isolated from clinical specimens [59], but were not universally considered as human skin commensals. More recently published studies on the composition of the axillary microbiome, including our own [37], have confirmed the dominance by some or all of the genera *Staphylococcus, Corynebacterium, Cutibacterium* (formerly *Propionibacterium* [17]), *Anaerococcus* and *Peptoniphilus* [43, 60–63]. In the main, these later studies have continued to rely on the metataxonomics approach, but there is also evidence of alternative approaches being adopted, as well as a move away from western (US or European) subjects. For example, our own published study was conducted on Filipino subjects as part of a wider investigation into the effect on BO of the 538G→A SNP in the *ABCC11* allele [37], as discussed below. The study by Okamoto *et al.* [61] was conducted on Japanese male subjects as part of an investigation into the relationship between the microbiota and two different axillary odor quality descriptors, "cumin-like, spicy BO" (C-type) and "weak, milk-like BO" (M-type). It is unclear to what extent these descriptors relate to specific VFA or thioalcohol malodorants, or variances in *ABCC11* genotype, and anyway, no differences in microbiome profile between the C-type and M-type subjects were detected by metataxonomics. The notable aspect of this study was the additional use of genus-level qPCR assays to determine corynebacterial and staphylococcal levels (as well as total bacteria), showing an increased density of each in the C-type subjects. These findings highlight the key distinction between these two approaches – while metataxonomics provides a high-resolution profile of a microbial community, it can only reliably determine *relative* abundance of each taxon; qPCR can provide an indication of *absolute* abundance of specific taxa, or indeed all bacteria present, dependent on the selection of primer and probe. The latter approach is one also being adopted by ourselves, especially at species-level to quantitatively differentiate between the dominant axillary *Staphylococcus* species, *S. epidermidis*, and the key odor-forming species, *S. hominis* [44]. The study by Lam *et al.* [62] was conducted on Filipino subjects, but specifically focusing on pre-pubescent children and teenagers, with sampling undertaken on several skin sites including the axilla. The notable aspect of this study was its use of metagenomics, an approach usually constrained by difficulties in sampling sufficient DNA from skin for shotgun sequencing; this method allowed analysis of both the profile of the microbiome, and its metabolic capability in relation to odor. Similar to the findings of metataxonomic studies on adult subjects, the axillary bacterial profile of children and teenagers, at both genus- and species-level, was dominated by staphylococci, cutibacteria and corynebacteria; GPAC were not detected (mean relative abundance (MRA) cut-off, 0.1%), though this may be an artefact of the metagenomics approach, rather than reflective of a key age-related difference. *Staphylococcus* species were found to strongly correlate with odor intensity in children and teenagers, with isovaleric acid (from L-leucine) and acetic acid (from L-lactic acid and glycerol, via pyruvate) production being identified as likely metabolic routes to BO [62], consistent with previous findings by ourselves, as discussed below [7]. The study by Li *et al.* [63] was conducted on a large number of US-based subjects (n = 169) who were sub-divided according to their age, gender and ethnic origin, this therefore representing the first such study to include all these variables. Another notable aspect was the novel metataxonomics approach employed, namely intergenic spacer profiling (IS-pro), developed and commercialised by IS-Diagnostics (http://isdiagnostics.nl/); this provides species-level differentiation of bacteria according to the length of their 16S-23S rDNA intergenic spacer region. The technique is reliant on a database of >500 identifiable species which covers most members of the axillary microbiota; however, there are notable exceptions, namely *Anaerococcus* (apart from *Anaerococcus prevotii*) and *Peptoniphilus* species, which explains their absence from the study results. Among the study's main findings were that older subjects (55+) had the highest number of total bacteria (based on IS-pro peak intensities), while the diversity of *Corynebacterium* species also increased with age [63]. Gender appeared to have little effect on microbiome abundance or diversity, but ethnic differences were apparent, notably the significantly higher levels of *S. hominis* observed in East Asian subjects. Although not highlighted in the paper, this observation is surprising, given the pivotal role of this bacterium in thioalcohol-based malodour [41, 44], and the fact that most humans of

East Asian origin are homozygous for a loss-of-function SNP in the gene encoding the apocrine ABCC11 transporter responsible for mediating the secretion of thioalcohol precursors onto axillary skin [34].

Figure 5.1 shows the results of a recent metataxonomics study undertaken by ourselves on female subjects in the UK (n = 50), applying our current protocol based on 16S rRNA gene amplification, sequencing and profiling, using the Illumina sequencing-by-synthesis platform (https://www.illumina.com/systems/sequencing-platforms.html). Illustrated are

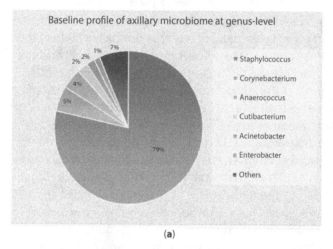

(a)

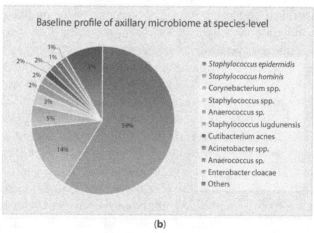

(b)

Figure 5.1 Metataxonomic baseline profile of the axillary microbiome at genus-level (a) and species-level (b) based on 16S rRNA gene amplification and sequencing, using the Illumina sequencing-by-synthesis platform (https://www.illumina.com/systems/sequencing-platforms.html). In each case, all taxa with a mean relative abundance of >1% are indicated.

baseline profiles of the axillary microbiome at genus-level (a) and species-level (b), showing all taxa with an MRA of >1%. The results are broadly consistent with relevant published studies [20, 21, 37, 43, 60, 61] although, for this panel at least, *Peptoniphilus* levels fell below the MRA cut-off.

5.3   16-Androstene Steroids and Axillary Malodour

Paradoxically, given their low volatility, some steroids have an odor perceivable by at least a proportion of the human population. In particular, this relates to the 16-androstene steroid 5α-androstenone, as well as the structurally related 5α-androstenol, which are known to be present in apocrine sweat [14, 15], are perceived by some as having a sweaty and urinous or musk-like smell, respectively, and were previously heavily implicated in axillary malodour [15]. Interestingly, the ability to smell 5α-androstenone is determined by two non-synonymous SNPs in the *OR7D4* allele encoding human olfactory receptor 7D4, that alter the phenotype such that subjects are less sensitive to this 16-androstene, and perceive it as less unpleasant [64] – this being consistent with Amoore's earlier observation of some individuals' inability to perceive specific odorants including 5α-androstenone, a concept termed specific anosmia [23]. With the role of 5α-androstenone, in particular, as a porcine pheromone being well established, these 16-androstenes were also heavily touted as being the basis of a chemical signalling mechanism in humans connected to the axillary apocrine gland, albeit now probably vestigial in evolutionary terms [15]. In relation to their putative contribution to BO, a detailed investigation on the biochemical origins of 16-androstenes on axillary skin was conducted in our laboratories and published in 2003 [25]. This was focussed entirely on corynebacteria, earlier studies having established that other members of the axillary microbiota are incapable of metabolising steroids, apart from non-odor forming *Micrococcus* species [65]. Our study demonstrated that axillary corynebacteria can only produce 16-androstenes from precursor steroids where the C16 double bond is already present (*i.e.* structurally related 16-androstenes), confirming earlier work on a smaller number of test bacteria [15]. In incubations with one such substrate, 5,16-androstadien-3-ol, some mixed populations of axillary corynebacteria generated many different steroid metabolites identifiable by gas chromatography/mass spectrometry (GC/MS), including 5α-androstenol and 5α-androstenone, which were assembled into a proposed metabolic map of 16-androstene microbial biotransformations [25]. When individual *Corynebacterium* strains were isolated and individually incubated with 5,16-androstadien-3-ol, a few were capable of efficient, rapid reactions, but no single isolate could carry out the full complement of biotransformations observed with the mixed populations. A key observation was the small proportion of 16-androstene transforming bacteria isolated from axillary skin – from a panel of 21 individuals, only 4 of 18 mixed corynebacterial populations, and 4 of 45 individual *Corynebacterium* isolates could metabolise 5,16-androstadien-3-ol. It is of course possible that both this study and others before it [15] have failed to isolate the most active bacteria or identify the true substrate; however, even the strongest advocates of 16-androstenes as causal molecules of axillary malodour have failed to produce any direct evidence connecting them to the condition at the low levels (pmol/cm^2) present physiologically. The association between these steroids and BO originates from studies in the 1970s highlighting the presence of the porcine pheromone 5α-androstenone in the human axilla [14], the fact that it possesses a urine-like smell characteristic of axillary odor, and the belief that the levels present would exceed its low olfactory threshold [15]. However, there are no reports in the literature where GC or GC/MS studies incorporating organoleptic assessments have been used to directly link 16-androstenes to underarm odor; in fact Zeng *et al.* [24], who used exactly this approach to implicate 3M2H and other medium-chain VFAs in BO, stated explicitly that this wasn't true of the 16-androstenes. As we surmised in a previous review [4], in light of this evidence and the biotransformation data published by ourselves [25], as well as the high levels of specific anosmia reported for 16-androstenes [23], a phenomenon since characterised genetically [64], it is likely that the contribution of these steroids to axillary malodour is much less significant than previously thought. References to 5α-androstenone and/or 5α-androstenol in the context of BO have become increasingly rare in the literature in recent years, although they did figure prominently in a 2011 review otherwise focussed on treatments for axillary malodour [66]. The only citation of note since then revived a historical hypothesis on the putative apocrine precursor of 5α-androstenol being a β-glucuronide conjugate [67]; this publication came from an unexpected source, the group concerned being responsible for many of the key recent developments in our understanding of the origins of thioalcohol-based malodour [30, 33, 39].

5.4 The Axillary Microbiome, VFAs and Malodour

It is widely acknowledged that short-chain (C_2 – C_5) and medium-chain (C_6 – C_{10}) VFAs are among the causal molecules of axillary malodour. The involvement of the short-chain acids in BO has long been recognised, and various metabolic routes to these, as well as some medium-chain VFAs, from substrates readily available on axillary skin, have been previously outlined by ourselves [3, 7]. Propionibacteria (now cutibacteria [17]) and staphylococci were shown to ferment glycerol, from triacylglycerol hydrolysis, and L-lactic acid, naturally abundantly present on skin, to acetic and propionic acid. Although this pathway in staphylococci was also later identified during a metagenomics study by Lam *et al.* [62] as a metabolic route to BO, there is in fact little evidence that either of these VFAs is a major axillary malodorant. More importantly, staphylococci are capable of converting branched aliphatic amino acids, such as L-leucine, to the highly odorous short-chain (C_4 – C_5) methyl-branched VFAs, such as isovaleric acid, which are historically associated with the acidic note of axillary malodor [8]. L-Leucine and its methyl-branched counterparts L-valine and L-isoleucine are present at significant levels in eccrine sweat, where the free amino acid content is now known to closely match the amino acid composition of the epidermal protein profilaggrin [6]. At the time, however, we proposed that the major metabolic route to short-chain VFAs in the axilla was the partial degradation (via β-oxidation) of structurally-unusual long-chain fatty acids present in sebum, particularly methyl-branched species [2]; this pathway is mediated by a sub-group (A) of the *Corynebacterium* genus, while the other sub-group, corynebacteria (B), are incapable of growth on fatty acids [3]. This belief was based primarily on *in vitro* kinetic data showing higher rates of VFA generation by corynebacteria (A) than staphylococci [7], as well as the significant *in-vivo* association found at genus level between total *Corynebacterium* (A + B), but not *Staphylococcus* density, and malodour intensity [16] (Table 5.1). However, this position was revised during our last review of the area in 2012-13, partly on the realisation that, although corynebacteria (A) metabolise fatty acids at a faster rate than staphylococci do branched aliphatic amino acids, culture-based ecology studies show that, on average, <10% of axillary *Corynebacterium* isolates are members of the (A) sub-group [4], while the prevalence and density of the *Staphylococcus* genus is universally high across test populations [8, 16]. Furthermore, a reevaluation of Nicolaides' seminal 1974 publication on the structural features of skin lipids revealed that sebum does not contain significant quantities of any *iso*-methyl-branched, odd carbon number long-chain fatty acids which could act as substrates for isovaleric acid, the most prominent of the short-chain VFA malodorants, through β-oxidation by corynebacteria (A) [2]; meanwhile, L-leucine, the precursor for this VFA via staphylococcal amino acid metabolism, is plentiful on axillary skin [6]. Similar to our recent identification of *S. hominis* as the key driver of thioalcohol-based malodour [41, 44], there is a paradox here, given there is no direct association between staphylococcal numbers and malodour intensity in the axilla [16]. While the former can be explained by the dominance of the non-thioalcohol producing species *S. epidermidis* on axillary skin [41, 42], the latter is a more challenging discrepancy, given that essentially all human-associated *Staphylococcus* species, including *S. epidermidis*, can generate VFAs via this route [7]. This apparent paradox can probably be explained by the observations of Leyden and colleagues in their 1981 publication [8], where they concluded that staphylococci were responsible for the "faint acid, non-apocrine" note of BO. Our current position thus remains that the major metabolic route to short-chain VFAs in the axilla is the biotransformation of branched aliphatic amino acids by *Staphylococcus* species, with the conversion of L-leucine to isovaleric acid being the most important example.

While the biotransformation of branched aliphatic amino acids and methyl-branched long-chain fatty acids can explain the origins of short-chain VFA malodorants on axillary skin, as well as a few medium-chain acids, these pathways cannot account for the highly structurally-unusual medium-chain VFAs, such as 3M2H, described originally by Zeng *et al.* [24], and later by Natsch *et al.* [27, 28]. Initially, it was proposed that these were transported to the skin surface non-covalently bound to two apocrine secretion odor-binding proteins, ASOB1 and ASOB2, and released onto axillary skin following interaction with the microbiota, perhaps via the action of bacterial proteases on the ASOBs [26]. ASOB2 was subsequently shown to be identical to apolipoprotein D, a member of the lipocalin family of carrier proteins which typically transport small hydrophobic ligands [68]. Given the putative evolutionary link between BO and a vestigial human chemical signaling mechanism involving the axillary apocrine gland, this observation raised the intriguing possibility that human odorants could, like some non-human mammalian pheromones, be transported by lipocalins, akin to the role of major urinary proteins in rodents [69]. Subsequently, however, Natsch and colleagues established that 3M2H and its even more abundant structural counterpart 3H3MH, as well as lower levels of a variety of other structurally-unusual medium-chain VFAs, are actually present in axillary sweat as covalently-bound conjugates of L-glutamine, and released on the skin surface by the bacterial enzyme N^α-acylglutamine aminoacylase [27, 28]. These studies were a landmark, providing the first published example of an axillary odor-forming enzyme being purified and characterised, and its encoding gene cloned (from an axillary *Corynebacterium* isolate), sequenced and heterologously expressed [27]. In support of the L-glutamine conjugates hypothesis, Troccaz and colleagues later measured significant (mg/L) levels of N^α-3-hydroxy-3-methylhexanoyl-L-glutamine (Gln-3H3MH) in the axillary sweat of 49 volunteers over 3 years, cementing its role as a key malodour precursor [39]. Proponents of the lipocalins hypothesis persist, but it is difficult to rationalise against the backdrop of the high levels of Gln-3H3MH present on axillary skin [4]. Akiba *et al.* [70] attempted to combine the L-glutamine conjugates and lipocalins hypotheses on the origins of medium-chain VFAs in the axilla by proposing that 3H3MH was covalently bound to the N-terminal L-glutamine residue of apolipoprotein D, which was then proteolytically cleaved as Gln-3H3MH. It is true that this residue is predicted to be L-glutamine, after cleavage of the putative signal peptide at residues 1-20 of the apolipoprotein D precursor (http://www.ncbi.nlm.nih.gov/protein/NP_001638.1), but this means one complete VFA-conjugated protein would be required per molecule of Gln-3H3MH produced. Given the levels of Gln-3H3MH reported by Troccaz *et al.* [39], a 1:1 ratio of apolipoprotein D to 3H3MH would require unrealistically high levels of this protein (g/L) in axillary sweat, which would seem to rule out this hybrid hypothesis as a viable physiological mechanism [4].

As reported previously, our internal studies provide a modicum of support to the L-glutamine conjugates hypothesis, in that we were able to isolate axillary bacteria, mainly *Corynebacterium* species, with the ability to hydrolyse both the model substrate carbobenzyloxy-L-glutamine (Z-Gln) to benzyl alcohol, and the putative physiological precursor N^α-3-methyl-2-hexenyl-L-glutamine (Gln-3M2H) to 3M2H [4]. However, the N^α-acylglutamine aminoacylase activity of these bacteria was insufficient to explain the high levels of 3M2H we have detected in axillary samples by GC-MS, the only exception being *Corynebacterium* sp. Ax20, an axillary isolate described by Natsch *et al.* [27, 28], which efficiently hydrolysed both substrates. In a follow up study, various medium manipulations were undertaken in an attempt to increase yields of benzyl alcohol from Z-Gln in incubations with axillary *Corynebacterium* strains. However, despite testing a multitude of media ranging from simple buffer to complex broth, N^α-acylglutamine aminoacylase activities remained stubbornly low [4]. At this stage, it was unclear whether our internal studies had failed either to isolate the most active bacteria, or to identify the optimum physiological conditions *in vitro* for expression of the enzyme, although the results of the medium manipulation study appeared to favour the former. Furthermore, genetic analysis of *Corynebacterium* sp. Ax20 in our laboratory failed to find an exact match for its 16S rRNA sequence, although it was more similar to *Corynebacterium glaucum* than *C. striatum*, the speciation initially attributed by Natsch and colleagues to Ax20 [27, 31], though omitted in later publications [40, 48]. As was highlighted at the time, none of the genetically analysed axillary *Corynebacterium* isolates described by Taylor *et al.* [16] matched *C. glaucum*, while only one matched *C. striatum*, supporting the notion that we'd failed to isolate the most aminoacylase-active bacteria by traditional culture methods [4]. However, more recent metaxonomics data from our own internal studies [unpublished data], aswell as the literature [43] indicates that these two species are indeed present on axillary skin at low abundance, suggesting that, even if the causal bacteria for this route to BO have yet to be isolated, it is not *C. glaucum* and/or *C. striatum* we should be pursuing. An intriguing new insight emerged in a 2014 publication from Fujii and colleagues [29]; this proposed that a previously uncharacterised *Anaerococcus* strain (sp. A20) was responsible for the release of 3H3MH from its L-glutamine-conjugated precursor Gln-3H3MH on axillary skin, with this activity being unique to this strain, and not exhibited by any of the other tested *Anaerococcus* species, including the type species *Anaerococcus prevotii* commonly found on human skin. While the speciation of GPAC in the axilla remains poorly defined, strain A20 is now known to represent the species *Anaerococcus nagyae* [71]. The implication of *A. nagyae* in VFA-based malodour remains unvalidated since Fujii and colleagues' 2014 publication, and the causal bacteria for this important route to BO thus remains one of the key gaps in our understanding of the aetiology of the condition; however, should the involvement of *A. nagyae* be confirmed, it raises a fascinating question over the role of *Corynebacterium* species in axillary malodour. Conventionally, members of this genus have been heavily implicated as causal agents, initially by association in microbial ecology studies [8, 16], and subsequently through *in-vitro* precursor-product relationship studies [4, 27, 31]. However, as discussed below, we have recently identified a monophyletic group of human-associated staphylococci (including *S. hominis*) as being responsible for thioalcohol-based malodour [41, 46], while accepting that the major route to short-chain VFAs is via amino acid biotransformations by *Staphylococcus* species [4]. If *A. nagyae* is confirmed as being responsible for the production of medium-chain VFAs on axillary skin, it would leave an unanswered question as to why corynebacteria have historically been shown to correlate with malodour intensity in the underarm [16] and, in particular, the "pungent, apocrine" note of BO [8].

5.5   The Axillary Microbiome, Thioalcohols and Malodour

The presence of sulfanylalkanols on axillary skin, and their prominent role in underarm odor, was first reported in simultaneous publications by

Troccaz *et al.* [30], Natsch *et al.* [31] and Hasegawa *et al.* [32], who each identified 3M3SH as the primary causal molecule of thioalcohol-based malodour, based on its abundance and odor quality, with descriptors ranging from "sweat and onion-like" to "strong meaty, fruity note......reminiscent of axillary odor". Natsch and colleagues further identified a series of additional thioalcohols associated with BO, namely 3-sulfanylhexan-1-ol, 2-methyl-3-sulfanylbutan-1-ol and 3-sulfanylpentan-1-ol [31]. There was an interesting parallel here to work carried out by ourselves using a combination of analytical and organoleptic methods [4]; this identified a series of four thioalcohols involved in underarm odor, specifically two sets of isomers, of molecular weight 120 Da and 134 Da respectively, with, in each case, one isomer possessing a meaty, onion-like smell, characteristic of axillary odor, and the other a less objectionable, occasionally fruity odor. The less unpleasant 134 Da isomer was identified as 3-sulfanylhexan-1-ol, while the meaty, onion-like 120 Da species was confirmed as 2-methyl-3-sulfanylbutan-1-ol, each consistent with Natsch and colleagues' observations [31]. In a similar vein, while we failed at the time to identify our less objectionable 120 Da isomer, it can perhaps be assumed to be 3-sulfanylpentan-1-ol; however, the reasons why we failed to identify a 148 Da thioalcohol equivalent to 3M3SH remain unclear.

Natsch *et al.* also proposed that the substrates for sulfanylalkanols on axillary skin were S-hydroxyalkyl-L-cysteine conjugates [31] and, in a repeat of their pioneering work on N^α-acylglutamine aminoacylase [27], cloned, sequenced and heterologously expressed the gene encoding cystathionine β-lyase (EC 4.4.1.8) from *Corynebacterium* sp. Ax20. Additionally, this recombinant C-S β-lyase was shown to be active against the L-cysteine S-conjugates of various thioalcohols, and was further demonstrated to release these odorants from axillary sweat extracts. We arrived at an identical conclusion on the nature of the thioalcohol precursors, based on the same premise that similar substrate-product relationships exist in other biological environments, such as the aroma of wines fermented from some *Vitis vinifera* (grape vine) varieties [72]. In support of this, we identified the L-cysteine S-conjugate of 2-methyl-3-sulfanylbutan-1-ol in axillary samples using GC/MS and developed an *in-vitro* biotransformation assay to screen axillary bacteria for their ability to cleave mainly a model substrate, S-benzyl-L-cysteine, but also a chemically-synthesised equivalent of the putative physiological 2-methyl-3-sulfanylbutan-1-ol precursor [4]. The results showed that some corynebacteria and staphylococci possess C-S β-lyase activity against both substrates, though in the case of the *Corynebacterium* isolates, there were a greater proportion of positive strains, and the activities tended to be higher. It had previously been reported that, within the axillary microbiome, only members of the *Corynebacterium* genus can cleave *S*-hydroxyalkyl-L-cysteines [31], but clearly this wasn't the case, at least for a minority of *Staphylococcus* isolates. Indeed, a gene encoding cystathionine β-lyase was later cloned and heterologously expressed from an axillary *S. haemolyticus* isolate [38]; however, the recombinant enzyme showed only very low activity against the L-cysteine *S*-conjugate of 3M3SH, and no odor was generated on incubation with sterile axillary sweat. The plot thickened when Starkenmann and colleagues proposed an alternative hypothesis for thioalcohol production on axillary skin based on the human glutathione (GSH) detoxification pathway [33], and provided evidence that the direct precursors are *S*-hydroxyalkyl-L-cysteinylglycines, derived from GSH *S*-conjugates originating from the axillary apocrine gland. In support of this, Troccaz *et al.* [39] measured significant (μg/L – mg/L) levels of *S*-Cys-Gly-3M3SH in the axillary sweat of 49 subjects over a period of 3 years. While GSH-conjugated 3M3SH (*S*-G-3M3SH) has never been detected in the axilla, and its metabolic origin and fate are not fully resolved, the key steps are now believed to be its transport by ABCC11 and conversion to *S*-Cys-Gly-3M3SH by γ-glutamyl transferase (GGT1), both of which have been shown to localise to the axillary apocrine gland [34].

Starkenmann *et al.* [33] showed that a strain of *S. haemolyticus* isolated from axillary skin was more efficient at cleaving *S*-Cys-Gly-3M3SH than either *S. epidermidis* or *Corynebacterium xerosis*. It was hinted that lysis was mediated by a single enzymic step rather than via a combination of a dipeptidase and C-S β-lyase, though clearly not by the *S. haemolyticus* cystathionine β-lyase later described by Troccaz *et al.* [38]. Meanwhile, Emter & Natsch [40], while accepting that L-cysteinylglycine *S*-conjugates were the apocrine-secreted thioalcohol precursors, provided evidence that the sequential action of a corynebacterial dipeptidase and cystathionine β-lyase is required for release of 3M3SH from its dipeptide *S*-conjugated precursor. Again, this group strengthened their case by cloning and heterologously expressing a gene encoding, in this case, a novel metallo-dipeptidase from *Corynebacterium* sp. Ax20 [40]. As discussed below, history would show that Starkenmann and Troccaz were correct in identifying *S. haemolyticus* as a causal organism of thioalcohol-based malodour, and suspecting that an alternative lytic enzyme to cystathionine β-lyase was involved – while Natsch and colleagues were correct in their assertion that the metabolic route to thioalcohol release involved two enzymic steps, a dipeptidase and C-S β-lyase.

Of the bacteria tested in our *in-vitro* biotransformation assay, the highest levels of C-S β-lyase activity were exhibited by *Corynebacterium jeikeium* NCIMB 40928 and 3 strains of *Corynebacterium tuberculostea-ricum*, including the type strain CIP 107291 and two axillary isolates [4]. *C. jeikeium* NCIMB 40928 was selected for a study aimed at cloning and expressing the gene responsible for this activity and, in the absence at the time of N-terminal sequence data, a bioinformatics approach was used to group enzymes with potential C-S β-lyase activity, and enable the design of degenerate primers. Of these, two phylogenetically distinct protein groups, categorised as the MetC- and MalY-type β-lyases, were identified as the most likely homologues of *C. jeikeium* C-S β-lyase. The MetC/MalY classification originated from *Escherichia coli*, which possesses two cys-tathionine β-lyases, one encoded by the ubiquitous *metC* gene, and the other by *malY*, encoding a bifunctional protein (in *E. coli*) also involved in regulating the uptake and metabolism of maltose [73]. The *C. jeikeium* cystathionine β-lyase gene was indeed cloned following amplification with a *malY* primer, while sequence analysis of *Corynebacterium* sp. Ax20 cys-tathionine β-lyase [31] confirmed that this too is a member of the MalY group, as are the putative cystathionine β-lyases of all genome-sequenced *Corynebacterium* strains [4]. Meanwhile, *S. haemolyticus* cystathionine β-lyase [38] is a member of the MetC group, along with the corresponding predicted enzymes of all genome-sequenced *Staphylococcus* strains [4]. By an interest-ing coincidence, we later showed that *C. jeikeium* NCIMB 40928 C-S β-lyase was 100% identical, at both the nucleotide and amino acid level, to the puta-tive cystathionine β-lyase gene and protein of *C. jeikeium* K411 (http://www.uniprot.org/uniprot/Q4JWQ6), the first axilla-relevant *Corynebacterium* species to be genome-sequenced [74]. In a follow-up publication in collab-oration with ourselves, this group further showed that the repressor protein McbR acts as a transcriptional regulator of *malY* and other genes involved in sulphur-containing amino acid biosynthesis in *C. jeikeium* K411 [75].

Following our last review of the axillary microbiome and BO in 2012-13, our position was clearly that of implicating *Corynebacterium* species as the primary causal organisms of thioalcohol-based BO [4]. However, things then moved very quickly in an unexpectedly different direction, driven by our collaboration with the Thomas lab at University of York (http://thomaslabyork.weebly.com/). Our 2015 publication demonstrated that *S*-Cys-Gly-3M3SH is imported and metabolised by a limited range of human-associated staphylococci in the axilla, specifically the species *S. hominis, S. haemolyticus* and *S. lugdunensis*, resulting in the formation and release of the primary thioalcohol malodorant 3M3SH [41]. Furthermore, most members of the *Corynebacterium* genus, including the dominant axil-lary species *C. tuberculostearicum* [4, 43], as well as *S. epidermidis*, the most widespread of the skin-associated staphylococci [42], and indeed the overall dominant member of the axillary microbiome (Figure 5.1b), were shown to be essentially incapable of converting S-Cys-Gly-3M3SH to 3M3SH. Of the thioalcohol-producing *Staphylococcus* species, *S. hominis* is historically recognised as the most prevalent on axillary skin [42], second only in abundance to *S. epidermidis*, an observation validated in a recent metaxonomics study on female subjects in the UK (Figure 5.1b). Furthermore, two recent and independent studies have each shown a strong correlation between *S. hominis* and malodour intensity using both metataxonomics [43] and qPCR [44]. Based on this combined evidence, we would now argue that *S. hominis* is the primary causal organism of thioalcohol-based malodour, although our identification of *S. haemolyticus* as one of the other odor-forming species is notable in confirming previous work by Starkenmann and colleagues [33]. Implicating a major axillary *Staphylococcus* species in BO appears to contradict earlier genus-level studies using traditional culture methods [8, 16]; however, in each case, the conclusions reached by the authors can be attributed to the dominance of the non-thioalcohol producing species *S. epidermidis* on axillary skin [41, 42].

The key feature behind the above breakthrough was the use of the physiological malodour precursor S-Cys-Gly-3M3SH in our published study, in addition to the model substrate S-benzyl-L-cysteinylglycine [41]. In incubations with the latter substrate, most axilla-relevant *Corynebacterium* strains efficiently metabolised S-benzyl-L-cysteinylglycine to benzyl mercaptan, while the two tested *S. epidermidis* isolates showed essentially no activity compared to the negative controls (Figure 5.2a). These results were consistent with those previously reported by ourselves, using the related model substrate S-benzyl-L-cysteine [4] although, interestingly, the benzyl mercaptan yield from a *S. haemolyticus* strain was comparable that of most of the tested corynebacteria. However, in incubations with the physiological malodour precursor S-Cys-Gly-3M3SH, the situation changed dramatically, with all tested corynebacteria showing low or no biotransformation of this substrate (Figure 5.2b), although moderate yields of 3M3SH were subsequently observed for several *C. amycolatum* isolates but, in agreement with the observations of Starkenmann *et al.* [33], a high yield of 3M3SH was observed with *S. haemolyticus*. These results explain why we incorrectly implicated corynebacteria as the primary causal organisms of thioalcohol-based BO [4], but fail to account for previous observations that *Corynebacterium* MalY-type cystathionine β-lyases show high activity against the L-cysteine S-conjugates of thioalcohols involved in BO [4, 31]. Clearly, the inability of axillary corynebacteria (apart from *C. amycolatum*) to convert S-hydroxyalkyl-L-cysteinylglycines

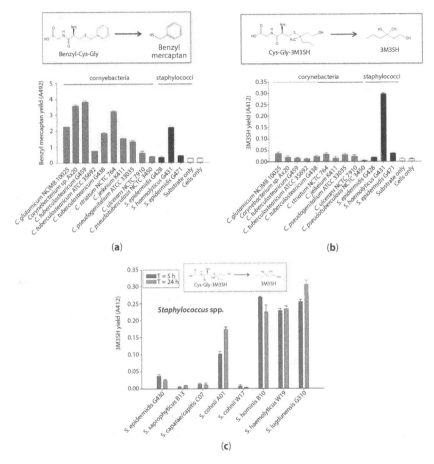

Figure 5.2 Metabolism of the model substrate S-benzyl-L-cysteinylglycine (Benzyl-Cys-Gly) and the physiological malodour precursor S-Cys-Gly-3M3SH to benzyl mercaptan and 3M3SH, respectively, by axilla-relevant *Corynebacterium* and *Staphylococcus* strains (adapted from Bawdon *et al.* [41]). (a) Biotransformation of S-benzyl-L-cysteinylglycine by corynebacteria and staphylococci (24 h incubation); (b) biotransformation of S-Cys-Gly-3M3SH by corynebacteria and staphylococci (24 h incubation); (c) biotransformation of S-Cys-Gly-3M3SH by speciated axillary *Staphylococcus* isolates (5 h & 24 h incubations).

and S-hydroxyalkyl-L-cysteines to thioalcohols is due to a separate metabolic deficiency, possibly the lack of a homologue to the PepT$_{Sh}$ transporter described below [45]. When representative strains of various axilla-relevant *Staphylococcus* species were incubated with S-Cys-Gly-3M3SH, efficient biotransformation to the corresponding thioalcohol was observed for *S. hominis*, *S. haemolyticus* and *S. lugdunensis* (Figure 5.2c). A moderate 3M3SH yield was observed for one *Staphylococcus cohnii* strain, while the other tested isolate of this species showed essentially no activity, a result replicated by *Staphylococcus caprae/capitis* and *Staphylococcus saprophyticus*, with a negligible 3M3SH yield only exhibited by *S. epidermidis*. It was further demonstrated that S-Cys-Gly-3M3SH is actively transported into *S. hominis*, rather than passively diffusing across the cell membrane [41], and also that the intracellular metabolic route to thioalcohol release involves two enzymic steps, requiring both a dipeptidase and a C-S β-lyase [76], as previously shown in *Corynebacterium* sp. Ax20 [40].

In collaboration with both the Thomas lab at University of York and the Newstead group at University of Oxford (https://newsteadgroup.org/lab-members/about/), we went on to show that the active transport of S-Cys-Gly-3M3SH across the *S. hominis* cell membrane is mediated by the secondary transporter $PepT_{Sh}$, a member of the POT family and major facilitator superfamily (MFS) of membrane transporters that facilitate movement of peptides across membranes in response to chemiosmotic gradients [45]. The gene encoding $PepT_{Sh}$ was cloned and overexpressed in *E. coli*, following which the purified protein was reconstituted into liposomes, which established that transport of S-Cys-Gly-3M3SH is coupled to the inwardly directed proton electrochemical gradient. Furthermore, a high-resolution co-crystal structure of $PepT_{Sh}$ bound to S-Cys-Gly-3M3SH was obtained, allowing further insight into the mechanism of ligand recognition and binding. Site-directed mutagenesis of the $PepT_{Sh}$ gene was undertaken, focussing on the substrate binding site, and a series of structural, biochemical and cell-based studies were carried out on the mutated proteins compared to the wildtype. These showed that, while the preferred substrates for $PepT_{Sh}$ are L-alanyl di- and tripeptides, recognition and transport of S-Cys-Gly-3M3SH is enabled by the presence of an extended hydrophobic pocket that accommodates the acyl chain of the S-hydroxyalkyl moiety [45]. Taking things a stage further, in conjunction with the University of York, we have now identified and characterised a novel staphylococcal C-S β-lyase enzyme, termed PatB, that mediates the lysis of S-Cys-3M3SH with greater efficiency and selectivity than a wide range of related C-S β-lyases [46]. Intriguingly, while a PepT-encoding orthologue exists in genome-sequenced representatives of all *Staphylococcus* species, the PatB-type C-S β-lyase is present only in a small monophyletic group of human-associated staphylococci (including *S. hominis*, *S. haemolyticus* and *S. lugdunensis*). Crucially, this enzyme, termed ShPatB in *S. hominis*, is part of the MalY group of C-S β-lyases, and thus distinct from the MetC-type cystathionine β-lyase ubiquitous in all staphylococci, and previously shown in *S. haemolyticus* to be essentially inactive against S-Cys-3M3SH [38].

The gene encoding ShPatB was cloned and overexpressed in *E. coli*, and high-resolution crystal structures obtained of the enzyme both native and bound to the active site ligand and inhibitor L-cycloserine. Through a series of structural and biochemical studies, it was established that ShPatB has evolved to selectively lyse *S*-hydroxyalkyl-L-cysteines via adaptation of the binding site to create a constrained hydrophobic pocket that accommodates the aliphatic *S*-hydroxyalkyl moiety. In common with other C-S β-lyases, ShPatB exists as a homodimer with each subunit covalently bound to a pyridoxal phosphate moiety, this coenzyme being a prerequisite for the deaminating aspect of the catalytic mechanism. However, on account of its unique presence in a monophyletic group of human-associated staphylo-cocci, it is possible to calculate that the PatB-encoding gene was acquired tens of millions of years ago, implying that, in primate evolution, thioal-cohol-based BO (or a vestigial chemical signalling mechanism based on thioalcohols) is an ancient process that long predates the emergence of *H. sapiens* as a species [46]. An overview of the transport and metabolism of *S*-Cys-Gly-3M3SH in *S. hominis* is schematically illustrated in Figure 5.3. The first intracellular step, the removal of L-glycine to produce *S*-Cys-3M3SH, is postulated to be catalysed by aminopeptidase PepA, though the

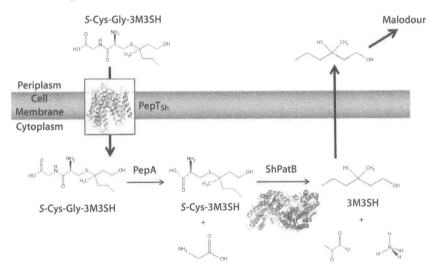

Figure 5.3 Schematic of the transport and intracellular metabolism of *S*-Cys-Gly-3M3SH by *S. hominis* (adapted from Minhas *et al.* [45] and Rudden *et al.* [46]). Passage across the cell membrane is mediated by the POT transporter PepT$_{Sh}$, while removal of L-glycine to generate *S*-Cys-3M3SH is postulated to be catalysed by aminopeptidase PepA. Lysis to 3M3SH, pyruvate and ammonium is mediated by the C-S β-lyase ShPatB, while export of 3M3SH is assumed to be via diffusion across the cell membrane.

identification of the specific peptidase responsible for this reaction remains unconfirmed [46]. Likewise, the route of export of 3M3SH is unknown, but currently assumed to be via diffusion across the cell membrane [45].

5.6   Perturbation of the Axillary Microbiome

Before reflecting on the susceptibility of the axillary microbiome to external perturbations, it is necessary to consider its baseline stability. The permanency of the axillary microbiota has frequently been commented on, notably by ourselves [3, 4, 7, 16], hinting at a significant level of stability which, if true, must be underpinned by probably multiple regulatory mechanisms involving both microbiome and host. Indeed, activities such as the lipase-mediated hydrolysis of (antimicrobial) free fatty acids from sebaceous triacylglycerols and the secretion of bacteriocins have long been postulated to represent mechanisms by which the skin microbiota self-regulates in the axilla and elsewhere [77]. These properties can be seen as an extension of the mechanisms by which the commensal microbiome inhibits the colonisation of skin by opportunistic, potentially-pathogenic microbes [78]. Similarly, host control measures such as AMP production can regulate the commensal microbiota as well as protecting the skin from invasive opportunists, as discussed below. An additional feature that undoubtedly influences axillary microbiome stability is compartmentation, although our understanding here is influenced mainly by well-established insights from other skin sites, for example the colonisation of the hair follicle by *Cutibacterium* (formerly *Propionibacterium* [17]) species, especially *Cutibacterium acnes*. Nakatsuji *et al.* [79] proposed a fundamental change in our understanding of skin microbiome compartmentation, presenting data to support the existence of bacteria in the living epidermis (below the stratum corneum), the dermis and even the subcutaneous adipose tissue, as well as the hair follicle. This radical proposal, which was based mainly on a metataxonomics and total bacteria qPCR study of microdissected skin sections, provides a real challenge to established principles on the transport of particles through skin aswell as the innate immune system. However, Jahns & Alexeyev [80] used fluorescence assays to directly visualise microbes in 194 skin biopsies, and found that stratum corneum and hair follicles were the only compartments showing microbial colonisation. It was also pointed out that while molecular studies detect the genetic fingerprints of microorganisms, both live and dead, visualisation studies provide unequivocal evidence of anatomically intact microbial cells. Our limited internal studies (unpublished) on microbiota location on skin using scanning electron microscopy are supportive of the observations of Jahns & Alexeyev [80]. Given the existence of micro-biota- and host-derived regulatory mechanisms, and the influence of compartmentation, it seems likely that stability is indeed a feature of the axillary microbiota, although individual variability in density and profile is undoubtedly high, even among populations of the same ethnicity and geographic location [16]. As discussed above, age and ethnicity can also have an influence, although gender appeared have little effect on microbiome abundance or diversity [63]; in contrast, a study by Callewaert *et al.* [60] showed that most female axillae are *Staphylococcus*-dominated, while males have a higher tendency to be *Corynebacterium*-dominated. Additionally, as discussed below, *ABCC11* genotype has an influence on the axillary micro-biome, with a shift in profile evident between AA homozygotes and those carrying the G-allele [37]. Notwithstanding this variability, there is as out-lined circumstantial evidence for the stability of the axillary microbiome at an individual level; however, is there any hard evidence? For this, we must initially turn to a culture-based study reported by Hopwood and colleagues [81]; this investigated the microbial colonisation dynamics of the axillae of a single male individual over a period of nearly one year, focussing on staph-ylococci, corynebacteria and propionibacteria (now cutibacteria [17]), with samples taken on a fortnightly basis. The results were interpreted as indi-cating that the axillary microbiota is relatively unstable, although on closer examination, most of the variability is due to fluctuations in the population density of *Corynebacterium* species, while staphylococcal and propionibac-terial/cutibacterial numbers remained fairly constant [81]. Furthermore, the degree of temporal variability recorded in this study is less than the levels of interpersonal variability typically observed in population studies, even among individuals of the same ethnicity and geographic location [16]. A later multi-site metataxonomics study on the topographical and temporal diversity of the skin microbiome similarly showed that the axilla was one of those locations where the microbiota retained significant community struc-ture over time, compared to the level of interpersonal variation recorded at the same site [19].

It is thus reasonable to assume, on the basis of both direct and circum-stantial evidence that, on an individual basis, the axillary microbiome is relatively stable; this takes us back to our original question as to how sus-ceptible it is to external perturbations. Actually, however, there is a paucity of published literature on the effect of either environmental agitations or product interventions on the population density or profile of the microbi-ota at this site; in fact, there is essentially nothing on environmental per-turbations. In terms of product interventions, Callewaert *et al.* [82] used denaturing gradient gel electrophoresis (DGGE) of amplified 16S rRNA genes, a metataxonomics-type method, to study the effect of deodorants and antiperspirants on the bacterial community structure in the axilla. Neither the compositions nor the active ingredients of the formulations used in the study were disclosed but, as they were commercial products, it is likely that most of the deodorants would have contained ethanol and/or another broad-spectrum antimicrobial agent plus fragrance, while most of the antiperspirants would have contained an aluminium salt such as aluminium chlorohydrate, again with fragrance. Leaving aside the influence of fragrance, deodorants are designed to control malodour and usually act by reducing microbiota density or activity through the inclusion of antibacterial ingredients such as those mentioned above, while antiperspirants are designed primarily to reduce sweating via the inclusion of admissible aluminium or aluminium/zirconium complexes [83]; however, aluminium-based antiperspirant salts are also highly effective deodorant ingredients due to their inherent antimicrobial properties. The small-scale study by Callewaert *et al.* [82] showed that, especially with antiperspirant use, there was an increase in overall microbiome diversity, plus an increased MRA of the *Actinobacteria* phylum (probably *Corynebacterium* species), coupled with a reduced MRA of *Firmicutes* (probably *Staphylococcus* species). Based on the traditional link between corynebacteria and BO, this result was interpreted as indicating that use of antiperspirants can reprofile the axillary microbiome to a more malodorous phenotype. However, given the aforementioned antimicrobial properties of aluminium-based antiperspirant salts, and the fact that DGGE measures relative rather than absolute abundance, a more likely explanation is that the numbers of both staphylococci and corynebacteria were reduced, but the former to a greater extent than the latter. Indeed, our internal larger-scale human studies (unpublished), conducted according to the ASTM standard guides for sensory evaluation of axillary deodorancy and recovery of microorganisms from skin [84, 85], show that antiperspirants consistently provide significantly lower expert-assessed malodour intensity scores, and typically reduce bacterial numbers on axillary skin by at least a factor of ten. Furthermore, it is usual for the reduction in staphylococci to be greater than that of corynebacteria, leading inevitably to an apparent change in profile. Similar results were obtained by Urban *et al.* [86] who used both a culture-based and metataxonomics approach to investigate the effect of antiperspirant and deodorant use on the axillary microbiota; this small-scale study showed an increase in species richness with antiperspirant use, but aligned to a reduction in bacterial density. The most recently published report on the influence of antiperspirant use on axillary bacteria was part of a wider study on the impact of cosmetic products on the skin metabolome and microbiome [87].

Using a metatoxonomics approach, this showed that the MRA of both *Staphylococcus* and *Corynebacterium* species decreased with product use, while overall diversity increased, and the MRA of GPAC (*Anaerococcus* and *Peptoniphilus* species) also went up significantly. Absolute abundances were not determined, but the likelihood is that GPAC were less effected than staphylococci and corynebacteria by the antibacterial action of the aluminium-based antiperspirant salt, perhaps due to their anaerobic nature requiring a specific compartment on axillary skin; this would in fact be consistent with culture-based data from our internal human deodorancy studies (unpublished).

A more subtle and targeted route to axillary malodour control was recently reported by ourselves, based on intervention with the cosmetic ingredient niacinamide, the amide form of vitamin B_3 [44]. This approach exploited the skin's innate immune system, in particular the contribution of AMPs, known to be present in both keratinocytes and eccrine sweat [9]. Niacinamide has been shown to stimulate the synthesis and secretion of some AMPs on skin, both *in-vitro* and *in-vivo*, and this has been demonstrated to translate into a hygiene benefit *in-vivo*, reducing levels of both *E. coli* and *Staphylococcus aureus* on human volar forearms [88]. Using a combination of enzyme-linked immunosorbent assays (ELISA) and liquid chromatography / mass spectrometry (LC/MS), we initially showed that high-odor individuals have lower levels of some AMPs (Psoriasin, RNase7, FLG2, S100A8, S100A9) in their axillae, as well as higher densities of *S. hominis*, as determined by qPCR [44]. A human deodorancy study, conducted according to the aforementioned ASTM standard guides [84, 85], was then carried out on an unfragranced niacinamide-containing deodorant roll-on product, compared to a vehicle control. The test product provided both an odor-control benefit at 5 h and 24 h, along with a small, but significant decrease (<0.5 $\log_{10}$) in staphylococcal numbers at 24 h, which was shown by species-level qPCR assays to be driven primarily by a reduction in *S. hominis* (Figure 5.4). It was concluded that niacinamide boosts AMP production on axillary skin, disproportionately targeting the thioalcohol-producing bacterium *S. hominis*, resulting in malodour reduction. These results also suggest that the synthesis and secretion of AMPs is a mechanism by which the human host regulates the commensal microbiota, as well as protecting the skin from opportunistic, potentially-pathogenic microbes. This niacinamide initiative represents a significant shift from the traditional use of broad-spectrum antimicrobial agents; however, an even more radical approach to axillary malodour control has been proposed and piloted by Callewaert and colleagues [89, 90]. Inspired by the success of fecal transplantation as a treatment for some gut disorders such

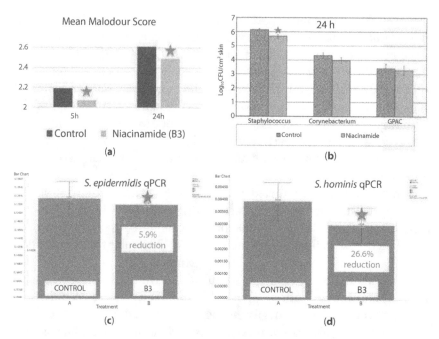

Figure 5.4 Results of a human deodorancy study on a prototype roll-on product containing niacinamide (B3) versus a vehicle control. (a) Mean malodour scores at 5 h and 24 h; (b) culture-based microbiology data at 24 h; (c) *S. epidermidis* qPCR data at 24 h; (d) *S. hominis* qPCR data at 24 h. Red asterisks indicate statistical significance.

as *Clostridium difficile* infection, this proposes the replacement of commensal high-odor microbiomes with low-odor bacteriotherapeutics, either obtained directly from a donor axilla, or by the use of cultured bacterial isolates. Promising results, in terms of both expert-assessed malodour scores and microbiota profiles, were reported from a pilot study on a pair of non-cohabiting monozygotic twins, who acted as donor and recipient, and two additional subjects who were treated with a pure *Staphylococcus* strain [89]. Publication of the results of a larger-scale follow-up study, as reported in a recent press article (https://www.thetimes.co.uk/article/is-this-the-end-of-body-odor-x6zm9twlt), is eagerly anticipated.

5.7 Human Genetics – Influence on Malodour and the Axillary Microbiome

In humans, the axillary apocrine gland is not involved in thermoregulation, does not fully develop until puberty and, in females, goes into atrophy post-menopause. Given that, in other mammals, apocrine glands situated in specialised sites such as the groin are regarded as scent glands [10], the discovery that the main process leading to malodour in humans initiates in the axillary apocrine gland [13] has long raised interest in the evolutionary origin of this exocrine unit, resulting in speculation on the possible existence of a genetic factor to BO. This was investigated by Kuhn & Natsch [91], building on their previous observation that the N^α-acyl-L-glutamine precursors to a wide variety of medium-chain (C_6 - C_{10}) VFAs are present in apocrine sweat [28]. It was proposed that common patterns of these VFAs might contribute to inherited individual-specific BO types, and indeed a study conducted on 12 pairs of monozygotic human twins supported this hypothesis. An attempt was subsequently made to link this genetically determined pattern of N^α-acyl-L-glutamines to polymorphic genes residing in the human leukocyte antigen complex, which is responsible for the regulation of the acquired immune system in *H. sapiens*; however, the evidence here suggested that this wasn't the case [92]. A genetic influence on human axillary odor that has been heavily characterised is a SNP (538G→A) in the *ABCC11* gene, resulting in an L-glycine to L-arginine substitution (G180R) in the corresponding protein, rendering it dysfunctional and subject to proteasomal degradation [35, 93]. Originally, this was shown to be the determinant of human earwax type, with the AA genotype resulting in dry earwax, in contrast to GG and the heterozygote GA which give rise to a wet earwax phenotype [94]; this landmark discovery was the first example of a DNA polymorphism determining a visible human phenotypic trait. Martin and colleagues showed that the *ABCC11* gene product, an ABC transporter and apical efflux pump, is also responsible for the secretion of the L-glutamine N^α-conjugates of 3M2H and 3H3MH, as well as the L-cysteinylglycine S-conjugate of 3M3SH, from the axillary apocrine gland [93]. While the GG and GA genotypes correspond to high levels of these odorants and their precursors in axillary extracts, the AA genotype results in a near-complete absence of N^α-acyl-L-glutamines and S-hydroxyalkyl-L-cysteinylglycines in the underarm due to loss of transporter function [35, 36]. The biosynthetic origin of these precursors in the human host is not fully understood although, in the case of the S-hydroxyalkyl-L-cysteinylglycines, Baumann *et al.* [34] validated Starkenmann and colleagues' earlier hypothesis that these derive from GSH S-conjugates [33], which act as substrates for two key proteins expressed in the axillary apocrine gland, the ABCC11 transporter and GGT1 enzyme, the latter responsible for the deglutamylation of S-G-3M3SH to S-Cys-Gly-3M3SH. In terms of frequency, it was quickly realised that the dominant G-allele prevails in populations of European and African origin, while the

A-allele is most prevalent among East Asians, notably in China and Korea [94]. This pattern has since been validated courtesy of the output from the 2008-2015 '1000 Genomes Project', an international research initiative to establish a detailed catalogue of human genetic variation (https://www.internationalgenome.org/). The frequency of the R180 SNP variant in different geographies and populations is accessible via the Ensembl genome browser (rs17822931), highlighting that intermediate frequencies are evident elsewhere globally, particularly in other parts of Asia; however, the selective pressures underlying this geographical distribution are unknown.

Until the publication of our Philippines-based study [37], there existed only circumstantial evidence on the effect of the *ABCC11* AA genotype on malodour intensity and quality, and no information whatsoever on potential effects on the axillary microbiota. Anecdotally, it was reported that Caucasians and Africans generated a more intense malodour than Asians, especially East Asians who seemingly produce only a faint, acidic underarm odor [93]. Harker and colleagues showed that the intensity of axillary odor was significantly lower in AA homozygotes, compared to individuals with the GA and GG *ABCC11* genotypes [37]. However, AA subjects still exhibited appreciable levels of malodour, although GC/MS analysis of volatile odorants in the axillary headspace showed the absence of both thioalcohols, including 3M3SH, and the medium-chain VFA, 3M2H; short-chain VFAs, including isovaleric acid, were however ubiquitous across all the genotype groups. Likewise, significantly lower levels of the malodour precursors S-Cys-Gly-3M3SH, Gln-3H3MH and Gln-3M2H were detected in the axillae of AA subjects, compared to individuals with the GA and GG genotypes; in fact, S-Cys-Gly-3M3SH was not detected in any AA individuals, while the levels of the N^α-acyl-L-glutamines were negligible. In summary, the results show that AA homozygotes have lower malodour intensity and different odor quality than those carrying the dominant G-allele, with the quality being defined by short-chain VFAs, rather than medium-chain VFAs and thioalcohols. The influence of *ABCC11* genotype on the axillary microbiome composition at genus-level was investigated using the metataxonomics approach, with the results showing a shift in the microbiota profile between AA homozygotes and those carrying the G-allele [37]. While all the genotype groups were dominated by the genera *Staphylococcus*, *Corynebacterium* and *Anaerococcus*, AA subjects had significantly lower MRA of staphylococci and corresponding higher abundance of corynebacteria than the GA and GG groups. It is tempting to retrospectively interpret this as being indicative of higher levels of *S. hominis* in individuals carrying the G-allele, and thus possessing an active ABCC11 transporter, but in the absence of species-level definition, and absolute abundance data, this is highly speculative. Nevertheless, the shift in the microbiota profile in a direction opposite to that expected at the time (based on historical culture-based data [8, 16]) is intriguing; however, given that the main role of the axillary apocrine gland is probably the secretion of malodour precursors rather than nutrients for bacterial growth, the *ABCC11* AA genotype is likely to have a greater effect on odor intensity and quality than microbiome composition. That said, if AA homozygotes possess a defective apocrine sweating process in addition to a near-absence of N^α-acyl-L-glutamines and S-hydroxyalkyl-L-cysteinylglycines in the secretion (as might be expected on the basis of the earwax phenotypic change [94]), another component of the microbiome that one might expect to be affected is the *Micrococcus* genus. The antimicrobial enzyme lysozyme, a component of the skin's innate immune system, has been shown to localise to the axillary apocrine gland, while being absent from sebaceous and eccrine glands [12]. Lysozyme mediates the hydrolysis of glycosidic linkages in peptidoglycan, the major component of Gram-positive bacterial cell walls and, ever since its discovery (by none other than Alexander Fleming, who would later discover penicillin, the world's first antibiotic), the high susceptibility of micrococci to this enzyme has been known [95]. However, while micrococci were detected in the metataxonomics aspect of our Philippines-based study, there was no evidence of an increased MRA in the AA group [37]. A later study investigated the effect of ethnicity on odorant production in the axilla [96]; specifically, this involved the GC/MS analysis of volatile odorants in axillary extracts sampled from 30 *ABCC11* genotyped males of Caucasian (n = 10), East Asian (n = 10) and African-American (n = 10) descent. As expected, the East Asian subjects, nine of whom were AA homozygotes (plus one GA heterozygote), had significantly lower levels of 3M2H and another medium-chain VFA, 7-octenoic acid, than the Caucasian and African-American subjects, all of whom were GG homozygotes. Interestingly, however, the African-American group had significantly higher levels of both VFAs than the Caucasian group, a difference that can't be explained by *ABCC11* genotype and is suggestive of another, as yet uncharacterised genetic influence on human axillary odor.

5.8   Conclusions and Future Perspectives

In this chapter, I have reviewed, in detail, the composition of the commensal axillary microbiome and its relationship with underarm odor, as well as the effects of microbiota perturbations, including product interventions;

I have based this on existing publications from ourselves and others, as well as including some relevant new data in the form of recently published and as-yet unpublished scientific studies. Traditional culture-based studies indicated that the axillary microbiome is dominated by Gram-positive bacteria of the genera *Staphylococcus*, *Corynebacterium* and *Cutibacterium* (formerly *Propionibacterium* [17]), of which historically the corynebacteria show the strongest association with malodour intensity [8, 16]. Based on 16S rRNA gene sequencing, the most abundant *Corynebacterium* species isolated from axillary skin was *C. tuberculostearicum*, a member of subgroup (B), while *C. amycolatum* was the principal representative of the fatty acid-catabolising (A) subgroup, with the former observation subsequently validated in a metataxonomics study [43], although the latter remains unverified. However, our current view anyway is that this A/B phenotyping of axillary *Corynebacterium* species is of much less relevance to axillary odor generation than previously thought [4], although questionmarks remain over the possible role of *C. amycolatum*, as highlighted below. Culture-independent studies on the axillary microbiota, mainly conducted via the metataxonomics approach, have confirmed the dominance of the *Staphylococcus*, *Corynebacterium* and *Cutibacterium* genera (Figure 5.1), but also revealed the presence of taxa not hitherto indicated by culture-based methods, notably *Anaerococcus* and *Peptoniphilus* species [21]. The involvement of these GPAC in axillary malodour remains unresolved, although a significant role has been proposed for *A. nagyae* [29], as highlighted below. Age, ethnicity and gender have each been demonstrated to influence microbiome abundance and/or diversity in the axilla [60, 63], while individual variability in density and profile is high, even among populations of the same ethnicity and geography [16]. A well-characterised SNP (538G→A) in the *ABCC11* gene has also been shown to cause a shift in the axillary microbiota profile for AA homozygotes [37], although it is likely that this genotype has a more pronounced effect on odor intensity and quality than microbiome composition. Notwithstanding this interpersonal variability, there is both direct and circumstantial evidence to suggest that, at an individual level, the axillary microbiome is relatively stable. The susceptibility of this microbiota to environmental perturbations is unknown, although there is some published data on product interventions; in the main, this shows that aluminium-based antiperspirants cause large reductions in microbiome density, with some taxa being more affected than others, leading to apparent changes in profile [82, 86, 87].

There is a growing acceptance that short-chain (C_4 – C_5) and medium-chain (C_6 – C_{10}) VFAs, along with sulfanylalkanols, are the causal molecules of axillary malodour, and although 16-androstene steroids were heavily touted in the recent past, their contribution is now believed to be minor [4]. Our present view on the origins of short-chain VFAs such as iso-valeric acid remains that adopted in 2012-13, namely that the major route is the metabolism of branched aliphatic amino acids by *Staphylococcus* species, rather than the partial degradation of long-chain methyl-branched fatty acids by corynebacteria (A), as previously believed [3, 4]. Meanwhile, the medium-chain VFAs most heavily implicated in malodour, such as 3M2H and 3H3MH, originate from N^{α}-acyl-L-glutamine precursors in axillary sweat [27, 28]; however, a significant challenge remains to identify the causal bacteria for this primary route to BO. The key enzyme mediating release of these VFAs, N^{α}-acylglutamine aminoacylase, was identified in an unspeciated axillary *Corynebacterium* strain whose closest taxonomic matches are *C. striatum* and *C. glaucum* [4, 27]; however, these species are only low-abundance components of the axillary microbiome [4, 43]. More recently, the GPAC species *A. nagyae* was isolated from axillary skin and shown to efficiently convert Gln-3H3MH to 3H3MH [29], a potentially significant insight that, if verified, raises a fascinating question over the role of *Corynebacterium* species in axillary malodour, as outlined below. This work also highlights the lack of species-level diversity data for GPAC on human skin (*e.g.*, see Figure 5.1b); it remains to be established, for example, how abundant *A. nagyae* is in the axilla compared to other *Anaerococcus* species, and whether it is indeed the only species with N^{α}-acylglutamine aminoacylase activity against Gln-3H3MH, as indicated by Fujii *et al.* [29]. Along with structurally-unusual medium-chain VFAs, thioalcohols and in particular 3M3SH have emerged as primary causal molecules of underarm odor [30–32]. It was initially believed that the precursors to these sulfanylalkanols were S-hydroxyalkyl-L-cysteines, and a MalY-type cystathionine (C-S) β-lyase capable of efficiently lysing these substrates was identified in two separate axillary *Corynebacterium* strains [4, 31]; in contrast, staphylococcal cystathionine β-lyases are of the MetC-type, and show poor conversion of S-hydroxyalkyl-L-cysteines into thioalcohols [38]. However, it is now accepted that these L-cysteine S-conjugates are intermediates in the metabolic pathway to thioalcohols in the axilla, with the true precursors, as secreted by the apocrine gland, being S-hydroxyalkyl-L-cysteinylglycines [33, 39]. The pathway by which S-Cys-Gly-3M3SH is taken up and metabolised by the axillary microbiota has recently been elucidated and shown to exist, in full, within only a small monophyletic group of staphylococci, including *S. haemolyticus*, *S. lugdunensis* and especially *S. hominis*, the most abundant of the group on axillary skin, and thus touted as the primary causal bacterium of |thioalcohol-based BO [41]. The key steps in *S. hominis* are mediated by a membrane transporter, $PepT_{Sh}$, responsible for uptake of S-Cys-Gly-3M3SH, an aminopeptidase (putatively PepA) which removes L-glycine to generate S-Cys-3M3SH, and a unique C-S β-lyase, ShPatB, which lyses the L-cysteine S-conjugate to release 3M3SH that is then believed to passively diffuse out the cell [45, 46] (Figure 5.3). Importantly, ShPatB is part of the MalY group of C-S β-lyases, and thus distinct from the MetC-type type cystathionine β-lyase present in all staphylococci, and known to be essentially inactive against S-Cys-3M3SH [38]. The main representatives from each of the principal structural groups of axillary malodorants are displayed in Table 5.2, alongside their corresponding precursor molecules, biochemical routes of formation and causal bacteria.

Our recent breakthrough in implicating a major axillary *Staphylococcus* species in malodour formation appears to contradict historical culture-based genus-level studies that had either discounted the contribution of this genus [16] or linked it only to the "faint acid, non-apocrine" note of BO [8]; however, in each case, the authors' conclusions can be explained by the dominance of the non-thioalcohol producing species *S. epidermidis* on axillary skin [41, 42]. More difficult to explain in light of this and other recent advances, notably our realisation that staphylococci are mainly responsible for the production of short-chain VFAs [4], as well as the unverified link between *A. nagyae* and medium-chain VFAs [29], is why the *Corynebacterium* genus has historically been shown to correlate with malodour intensity in the underarm [16] and, in particular, the "pungent, apocrine" note of BO [8]? While recognising the statistician's mantra that "correlation does not imply causation", this apparent paradox will require explanation, particularly if the *A. nagyae* insight is validated. Possibly, an answer lies in the role of *C. amycolatum*, which is capable of both converting long-chain methyl-branched fatty acids to short-chain VFAs [4] and metabolising S-Cys-Gly-3M3SH to 3M3SH [41], but has not thus far been recognised as a high-abundance component of the axillary microbiome, possibly due to weaknesses in the species-level definition of corynebacteria on human skin (*e.g.*, see Figure 5.1b).

The last *c*15 years have seen a step-change in our understanding of the axillary microbiome and its relationship with underarm odor, as detailed in the sections above and illustrated schematically in Figure 5.5. There are few, if any other parts of the human body where there exists such a high degree of understanding not just of the commensal microbiome, but of its causal links to a cosmetically-relevant phenotype, namely BO. This has been achieved thanks to the efforts not just of ourselves, but numerous other practitioners in the field, including the likes of Andreas Natsch, Myriam Troccaz, Christian Starkenmann and Chris Callewaert, to name

Table 5.2 Key representatives of the major structural classes of axillary malodorants and their precursors, with metabolic routes and causal bacteria indicated. Adapted from Natsch et al. [27, 28], James et al. [4, 7], Starkenmann et al. [33], Fujii et al. [29], Bawdon et al. [41], Minhas et al. [45] and Rudden et al. [46].

Precursor	Malodorant	Metabolic route	Causal bacteria
L-Leucine	Isovaleric acid	Branched aliphatic amino acid metabolism	Staphylococcus species
Nα-E-3-Methyl-2-hexenoyl-L-glutamine (Gln-3M2H)	E-3-Methyl-2-hexenoic acid (3M2H)	Nα-Acylglutamine aminoacylase	Corynebacterium sp. Ax20

(Continued)

Table 5.2 Key representatives of the major structural classes of axillary malodorants and their precursors, with metabolic routes and causal bacteria indicated. Adapted from Natsch et al. [27, 28], James et al. [4, 7], Starkenmann et al. [33], Fujii et al. [29], Bawdon et al. [41], Minhas et al. [45] and Rudden et al. [46]. (*Continued*)

Precursor	Malodorant	Metabolic route	Causal bacteria
N^α-3-Hydroxy-3-methylhexanoyl-L-glutamine (Gln-3H3MH)	3-Hydroxy-3-methylhexanoic acid (3H3MH)	N^α-Acylglutamine aminoacylase	*Corynebacterium* sp. Ax20 *A. nagyae*
S-[1-(2-Hydroxyethyl)-1-methylbutyl]-(L)-cysteinylglycine (S-Cys-Gly-3M3SH)	3-Methyl-3-sulfanylhexan-1-ol (3M3SH)	PepT transporter; PatB C-S β-lyase	*S. hominis* *S. haemolyticus* *S. lugdunensis*

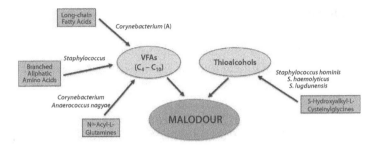

Figure 5.5 Schematic of the microbiological and biochemical origins of axillary malodour, adapted from Natsch *et al.* [27, 28], James *et al.* [3, 4, 7], Starkenmann *et al.* [33], Fujii *et al.* [29], Bawdon *et al.* [41] and Rudden *et al.* [46]. The major routes are the hydrolysis of N$^\alpha$-acyl-L-glutamines to medium-chain (C$_6$ – C$_{10}$) VFAs by corynebacteria and/or *A. nagyae*, and the formation of thioalcohols from S-hydroxyalkyl-L-cysteinylglycines by a monophyletic group of staphylococci (*S. hominis*, *S. haemolyticus* and *S. lugdunensis*).

but a notable few. As detailed above, a few outstanding knowledge gaps remain – how susceptible is the microbiome to environmental perturbations? – and to product interventions beyond aluminium-based antiperspirants? – an improved species-level definition of corynebacteria and in particular GPAC is required, not least to determine the respective roles of *C. amycolatum* and *A. nagyae* – which bacteria are mainly responsible for (medium-chain) VFA-based malodour? – can it really be true that corynebacteria are not one of the main contributors to BO? – and, if so, why do they consistently display such a strong association with malodour intensity? Finally, the biggest future challenge we face is how to exploit all this knowledge to develop a new generation of deodorant systems based on targeting specific bacteria, metabolic pathways or key enzymes, a significant shift from the current reliance on fragrances and broad-spectrum antimicrobial agents. There are encouraging signs that things are already moving in this direction; for example, our niacinamide-based intervention [46] and the bacteriotherapeutic approach proposed and piloted by Callewaert *et al.* [89, 90], both described above. Additional examples include published reports on the screening of plant-derived compounds for their ability to inhibit C-S β-lyase activity in a *Staphylococcus* cell lysate [97], and the identification of a material capable of inhibiting the conversion of Gln-3H3MH to 3H3MH by an *A. nagyae* cell lysate [29].

Acknowledgements

I would like to express my gratitude to the following individuals for their contributions to this document and the recently published, as well as previously unpublished scientific studies reported therein:

- Diana Cox (Unilever R&D Colworth, UK)
- Dr. Robert Cornmell, Sally Grimshaw, Ann-Marie Carvell and Dr. Barry Murphy (Unilever R&D Port Sunlight, UK)
- Dr. Amitabha Majumdar (Unilever R&D Bangalore, India)
- Professor Gavin Thomas and past & current colleagues (University of York, UK)
- Professor Simon Newstead and Dr. Gurdeep Minhas (University of Oxford, UK)

References

1. Picardo, M., Ottaviani, M., Camera, E., Mastrofrancesco, A., Sebaceous gland lipids. *Dermato-Endocrinology*, 1, 68, 2009.
2. Nicolaides, N., Skin lipids: their biochemical uniqueness. *Science*, 186, 19, 1974.
3. James, A.G., Casey, J., Hylians, D., Mycock, G., Fatty acid metabolism by cutaneous bacteria and its role in axillary malodour. *World J. Microbiol. Biotechnol.*, 20, 787, 2004.
4. James, A.G., Austin, C.J., Cox, D.S., Taylor, D., Calvert, R., Microbiological and biochemical origins of human axillary odor. *FEMS Microbiol. Ecol.*, 83, 527, 2013.
5. Bovell, D., The human eccrine sweat gland: Structure, function and disorders. *J. Local Global Health Sci.*, 5, 2015, http://dx.doi.org/10.5339/jlghs.2015.5.
6. Harker, M. and Harding, C.R., Amino acid composition, including key derivatives of eccrine sweat: potential biomarkers of certain atopic skin conditions. *Int. J. Cosmet. Sci.*, 35, 163, 2013.
7. James, A.G., Hylians, D., Johnston, H., Generation of volatile fatty acids by axillary bacteria. *Int. J. Cosmet. Sci.*, 26, 149, 2004.
8. Leyden, J.J., McGinley, K.J., Holzle, E., Labows, J.N., Kligman, A.M., The microbiology of the human axilla and its relationship to axillary odor. *J. Invest. Dermatol.*, 77, 413, 1981.
9. Schittek, B., Hipfel, R., Sauer, B., Bauer, J., Kalbacher, H., Stevanovic, S., Schirle, M., Schroeder, K., Blin, N., Meier, F., Rassner, G., Garbe, C.,

Dermcidin: A novel human antibiotic peptide secreted by sweat glands. *Nat. Immunol.*, 2, 1133, 2001.

10. Collins, P.J., Sweat Glands: Eccrine and Apocrine, in: *Pharmacology of the Skin I*, M.W. Greaves and S. Shuster (Eds.), pp. 193–212, Springer-Verlag, Berlin, Heidelberg, 1989.

11. Labows, J.N., McGinley, K.J., Kligman, A.M., Perspectives on axillary odor. *J. Soc. Cosmet. Chem.*, 34, 193, 1982.

12. Campbell, G.A., Burgdorf, W.H., Everett, M.A., The immunohistochemical localization of lysozyme in human axillary apocrine glands. *J. Invest. Dermatol.*, 79, 351, 1982.

13. Shelley, W.B., Hurley, H.J., Nichols, A.C., Axillary odor – experimental study of the role of bacteria, apocrine sweat, and deodorants. *AMA Arch. Derm. Syphilol.*, 68, 430, 1953.

14. Claus, R. and Alsing, W., Occurrence of 5α-androst-16-en-3-one, a boar pheromone, in man and its relationship to testosterone. *J. Endrocrinol.*, 68, 483, 1976.

15. Gower, D.B., Holland, K.T., Mallet, A.I., Rennie, P.J., Watkins, W.J., Comparison of 16-androstene steroid concentrations in sterile apocrine sweat and axillary secretions: interconversions of 16-androstenes by the axillary microflora – a mechanism for axillary odor production in man? *J. Steroid Biochem. Mol. Biol.*, 48, 409, 1994.

16. Taylor, D., Daulby, A., Grimshaw, S., James, G., Mercer, J., Vaziri, S., Characterization of the microflora of the human axilla. *Int. J. Cosmet. Sci.*, 25, 137, 2003.

17. Scholz, C.F.P. and Kilian, M., The natural history of cutaneous propionibacteria, and reclassification of selected species within the genus *Propionibacterium* to the proposed novel genera *Acidipropionibacterium* gen. nov., *Cutibacterium* gen. nov. and *Pseudopropionibacterium* gen. nov. *Int. J. Syst. Evol. Microbiol.*, 66, 4422, 2016.

18. Marchesi, J.R. and Ravel, J., The vocabulary of microbiome research: a proposal. *Microbiome*, 3, 31, 2015.

19. Grice, E.A., Kong, H.H., Conlan, S., Deming, C.B., Davis, J., Young, A.C., Bouffard, G.G., Blakesley, R.W., Murray, P.R., Green, E.D., Turner, M.L., Segre, J.A., Topographical and temporal diversity of the human skin microbiome. *Science*, 324, 1190, 2009.

20. Costello, E.K., Lauber, C.L., Hamady, M., Fierer, N., Gordon, J.I., Knight, R., Bacterial community variation in human body habitats across space and time. *Science*, 326, 1694, 2009.

21. Egert, M., Schmidt, I., Hohne, H.M., Lachnit, T., Schmitz, R.A., Breves, R., rRNA-based profiling of bacteria in the axilla of healthy males suggests right-left asymmetry in bacterial activity. *FEMS Microbiol. Ecol.*, 77, 146, 2011.

22. Haze, S., Gozu, Y., Nakamura, S., Kohno, Y., Sawano, K., Ohta, H., Yamazaki, K., 2-Nonenal newly found in human body odor tends to increase with aging. *J. Invest. Dermatol.*, 116, 520, 2001.

23. Amoore, J.E., Specific anosmia and the concept of primary odors. *Chem. Senses*, 2, 267, 1977.

24. Zeng, X.-N., Leyden, J.J., Lawley, H.J., Sawano, K., Nohara, I., Preti, G., Analysis of characteristic odors from human male axillae. *J. Chem. Ecol.*, 17, 1469, 1991.

25. Austin, C. and Ellis, J., Microbial pathways leading to steroidal malodour in the axilla. *J. Steroid Biochem. Mol. Biol.*, 87, 105, 2003.

26. Spielman, A.I., Zeng, X.-N., Leyden, J.J., Preti, G., Proteinaceous precursors of human axillary odor: isolation of two novel odor-binding proteins. *Experientia*, 51, 40, 1995.

27. Natsch, A., Gfeller, H., Gygax, P., Schmid, J., Acuna, G., A specific bacterial aminoacylase cleaves odorant precursors secreted in the human axilla. *J. Biol. Chem.*, 278, 5718, 2003.

28. Natsch, A., Derrer, S., Flachsmann, F., Schmid, J., A broad diversity of volatile carboxylic acids, released by a bacterial aminoacylase from axilla secretions, as candidate molecules for the determination of human-body odor type. *Chem. Biodivers.*, 3, 1, 2006.

29. Fujii, T., Shinozaki, J., Kajiura, T., Iwasaki, K., Fudou, R., A newly discovered *Anaerococcus* strain responsible for axillary odor and a new axillary odor inhibitor, pentagalloyl glucose. *FEMS Microbiol. Ecol.*, 89, 198, 2014.

30. Troccaz, M., Starkenmann, C., Niclass, Y., van de Waal, M., Clark, A.J., 3-Methyl-3-Sulfanylhexan-1-ol as a major descriptor for the human axilla-sweat odor profile. *Chem. Biodivers.*, 1, 1022, 2004.

31. Natsch, A., Schmid, J., Flachsmann, F., Identification of odoriferous sulfanylalkanols in human axilla secretions and their formation through cleavage of cysteine precursors by a C-S lyase isolated from axilla bacteria. *Chem. Biodivers.*, 1, 1058, 2004.

32. Hasegawa, Y., Yabuki, M., Matsukane, M., Identification of new odoriferous compounds in human axillary sweat. *Chem. Biodivers.*, 1, 2042, 2004.

33. Starkenmann, C., Niclass, Y., Troccaz, M., Clark, A.J., Identification of the precursor of (S)-3-methyl-3-sulfanylhexan-1-ol, the sulfury malodour of human axilla sweat. *Chem. Biodivers.*, 2, 705, 2005.

34. Baumann, T., Bergmann, S., Schmidt-Rose, T., Max, H., Martin, A., Enthaler, B., Terstegen, L.G., Schweiger, D., Kalbacher, H., Wenck, H., Jedlitschky, G., Jovanović, Z., Glutathione-conjugated sulfanylalkanols are substrates for ABCC11 and γ-glutamyl transferase 1: a potential new pathway for the formation of odorant precursors in the apocrine sweat gland. *Exp. Dermatol.*, 23, 247, 2014.

35. Nakano, M., Miwa, N., Hirano, A., Yoshiura, K.-I., Niikawa, N., A strong association of axillary osmidrosis with the wet earwax type determined by genotyping of the ABCC11 gene. *BMC Genet.*, 10, 42, 2009.

36. Hamada, K., Haruyama, S., Yamaguchi, T., Yamamoto, K., Hiromasa, K., Yoshioka, M., Nishio, D., Nakamura, M., What determines human body odor? *Exp. Dermatol.*, 23, 316, 2014.

37. Harker, M., Carvell, A.-M., Marti, V.P.J., Riazanskaia, S., Kelso, H., Taylor, D., Grimshaw, S., Arnold, D.S., Zillmer, R., Shaw, J., Kirk, J.M., Alcasid, Z.M., Gonzales-Tanon, S., Chan, G.P., Rosing, E.A.E., Smith, A.M., Functional characterisation of a SNP in the ABCC11 allele – Effects on axillary skin metabolism, odor generation and associated behaviours. *J. Dermatol. Sci.*, 73, 23, 2014.

38. Troccaz, M., Benattia, F., Borchard, G., Clark, A.J., Properties of recombinant *Staphylococcus haemolyticus* cystathionine β-lyase (metC) and its potential role in the generation of volatile thiols in axillary malodour. *Chem. Biodiv.*, 5, 2372, 2008.

39. Troccaz, M., Borchard, G., Vuilleumier, C., Raviot-Derrien, S., Niclass, Y., Beccucci, S., Starkenmann, C., Gender-specific differences between the concentrations of nonvolatile (R)/(S)-3-methyl-3-sulfanylhexan-1-ol and (R)/(S)-3-hydroxy-3-methyl-hexanoic acid odor precursors in axillary secretions. *Chem. Senses*, 34, 203, 2009.

40. Emter, R. and Natsch, A., The sequential action of a dipeptidase and a beta-lyase is required for the release of the human body odorant 3-methyl-3-sulfanylhexan-1-ol from a secreted Cys-Gly-(S) conjugate by corynebacteria. *J. Biol. Chem.*, 283, 20645, 2008.

41. Bawdon, D., Cox, D.S., Ashford, D., James, A.G., Thomas, G.H., Identification of axillary *Staphylococcus* sp. involved in the production of the malodorous thioalcohol 3-methyl-3-sufanylhexan-1-ol. *FEMS Microbiol. Lett.*, 362, fnv111, 2015.

42. Kloos, W.E. and Musselwhite, M.S., Distribution and persistence of *Staphylococcus* and *Micrococcus* species and other aerobic bacteria on human skin. *Appl. Microbiol.*, 30, 381, 1975.

43. Troccaz, M., Gaïa, N., Beccucci, S., Schrenzel, J., Cayeux, I., Starkenmann, C., Lazarevic, V., Mapping axillary microbiota responsible for body odors using a culture-independent approach. *Microbiome*, 3, 1, 2015.

44. James, A.G., Cox, D., Cornmell, R., Carvell, A.-M., Majumdar, A., Manipulating the axillary microbiome for odor control, in: *Skin Microbiome Congress*, Kisaco Research, London, 2019, https://www.kisacoresearch.com/presentations/1018.

45. Minhas, G.S., Bawdon, D., Herman, R., Rudden, M., Stone, A.P., James, A.G., Thomas, G.H., Newstead, S., Structural basis of malodour precursor transport in the human axilla. *eLife*, 7, e34995, 2018.

46. Rudden, M., Herman, R., Rose, M., Cox, D.S., Bawdon, D., Dodson, E., Wilkinson, A.J., James, A.G., Thomas, G.H., The molecular basis of thioalcohol production in human body odor. *Scientific Reports*, 2020.

47. Fredrich, E., Barzantny, H., Brune, I., Tauch, A., Daily battle against body odor: towards the activity of the axillary microbiota. *Trends Microbiol.*, 21, 305, 2013.

48. Natsch, A., What makes us smell: the biochemistry of body odor and the design of new deodorant ingredients. *Chimia*, 69, 414, 2015.

49. Lederberg, J. and McCray, A.T., Ome sweet 'omics – a genealogical treasury of words. *Scientist*, 15, 8, 2001.

50. Jackman, P.J.H., Body odor – the role of skin bacteria. *Sem. Dermatol.*, 1, 143, 1982.

51. Fuller, C.W., Middendorf, L.R., Benner, S.A., Church, G.M., Harris, T., Huang, X., Jovanovich, S.B., Nelson, J.R., Schloss, J.A., Schwartz, D.C., Vezenov, D.V., The challenges of sequencing by synthesis. *Nature Biotech.*, 27, 1013, 2009.

52. Margulies, M., Egholm, M., Altman, W.E. *et al.*, Genome sequencing in microfabricated high-density picolitre reactors. *Nature*, 437, 376, 2005.

53. Turnbaugh, P.J., Ley, R.E., Hamady, M., Fraser-Liggett, C.M., Knight, R., Gordon, J.I., The Human Microbiome Project. *Nature*, 449, 804, 2007.

54. Markowitz, V.M., Chen, I.-M.A., Palaniappan, K., Chu, K., Szeto, E., Grechkin, Y., Ratner, A., Jacob, B., Huang, J., Williams, P., Huntemann, M., Anderson, I., Mavromatis, K., Ivanova, N.N., Kyrpides, N.C., IMG: the integrated microbial genomes database and comparative analysis system. *Nucleic Acids Res.*, 40, D115, 2012.

55. Chen, I.-M.A., Chu, K., Palaniappan, K., Pillay, M., Ratner, A., Huang, J., Huntemann, M., Varghese, N., White, J.R., Seshadri, R., Smirnova, T., Kirton, E., Jungbluth, S.P., Woyke, T., Eloe-Fadrosh, E.A., Ivanova, N.N., Kyrpides, N.C., IMG/M v.5.0: an integrated data management and comparative analysis system for microbial genomes and microbiomes. *Nucleic Acids Res.*, 47, D666, 2019.

56. Bennett, S., Solexa Ltd. *Pharmacogenomics*, 5, 433, 2004.

57. Rothberg, J.M., Hinz, W., Rearick, T.M. *et al.*, An integrated semiconductor device enabling non-optical genome sequencing. *Nature*, 475, 348, 2011.

58. Bleidorn, C., Third generation sequencing: Technology and its potential impact on evolutionary biodiversity research. *Syst. Biodivers.*, 14, 1, 2016.

59. Song, Y., Liu, C., Finegold, S.M., Development of a flow chart for identification of Gram-positive anaerobic cocci in the clinical laboratory. *J. Clin. Microbiol.*, 45, 512, 2007.

60. Callewaert, C., Kerckhof, F.-M., Granitsiotis, M.S., Van Gele, M., Van de Wiele, T., Boon, N., Characterization of *Staphylococcus* and *Corynebacterium* clusters in the human axillary region. *PLOS ONE*, 8, e70538, 2013.

61. Okamoto, H., Koizumi, S., Shimizu, H., Cho, O., Sugita, T., Characterization of the axillary microbiota of Japanese male subjects with spicy and milky odor types by pyrosequencing. *Biocontrol Sci.*, 23, 1, 2018.

62. Lam, T.H., Verzotto, D., Brahma, P., Hui Qi Ng, A., Hu, P., Schnell, D., Tiesman, J., Kong, R., My Uyen Ton, T., Li, J., Ong, M., Lu, Y., Swaile, D., Liu, P., Liu, J., Nagarajan, N., Understanding the microbial basis of body odor in pre-pubescent children and teenagers. *Microbiome*, 6, 213, 2018.

63. Li, M., Budding, A.E., van der Lugt-Degen, M., Du-Thumm, L., Vandeven, M., Fan, A., The influence of age, gender and race/ethnicity on the composition of the human axillary microbiome. *Int. J. Cosmet. Sci.*, 41, 371, 2019.

64. Keller, A., Zhuang, H., Chi, Q., Vosshall, L.B., Matsunami, H., Genetic variation in a human odorant receptor alters odor perception. *Nature*, 449, 468, 2007.

65. Rennie, P.J., Gower, D.B., Holland, K.T., Mallet, A.I., Watkins, W.J., The skin microflora and the formation of human axillary odor. *Int. J. Cosmet. Sci.*, 12, 197, 1990.

66. Kanlayavattanakul, M. and Lourith, N., Body malodours and their topical treatment agents. *Int. J. Cosmet. Sci.*, 33, 298, 2011.

67. Starkenmann, C., Mayenzet, F., Brauchli, R., Troccaz, M., 5α-Androst-16-en-3α-ol β-D-glucuronide, precursor of 5α-androst-16-en-3α-ol in human sweat. *Chem. Biodiv.*, 10, 2197, 2013.

68. Zeng, C., Spielman, A.I., Vowels, B.R., Leyden, J.J., Biemann, K., Preti, G., A human axillary odorant is carried by apolipoprotein D. *Proc. Natl. Acad. Sci. U.S.A.*, 93, 6626, 1996.

69. Cavaggioni, A. and Mucignat-Caretta, C., Major urinary proteins, $\alpha_{2\mu}$-globulins and aphrodisin. *Biochim. Biophys. Acta*, 1482, 218, 2000.

70. Akiba, S., Arai, N., Kusuoku, H., Takagi, Y., Hagura, T., Takeuchi, K., Fuji, A., The N-terminal amino acid of apolipoprotein D is putatively covalently bound to 3-hydroxy-3-methyl hexanoic acid, a key odor compound in axillary sweat. *Int. J. Cosmet. Sci.*, 33, 283, 2011.

71. Veloo, A.C.M., de Vries, E.D., Jean-Pierre, H., van Winkelhoff, A.J., *Anaerococcus nagyae* sp. nov., isolated from human clinical specimens. *Anaerobe*, 38, 111, 2016.

72. Tominaga, T., Peyrot des Gachons, C., Dubourdieu, D., A new type of flavour precursors in *Vitis vinifera* L. cv. Sauvignon Blanc: S-cysteine conjugates. *J. Agric. Food Chem.*, 46, 5215, 1998.

73. Zdych, E., Peist, R., Reidl, J., Boos, W., MalY of *Escherichia coli* is an enzyme with the activity of a beta C-S lyase (cystathionase). *J. Bacteriol.*, 177, 5035, 1995.

74. Tauch, A., Kaiser, O., Hain, T., Goesmann, A., Weisshaar, B., Albersmeier, A., Bekel, T., Bischoff, N., Brune, I., Chakraborty, T., Kalinowski, J., Meyer, F., Rupp, O., Schneiker, S., Viehoever, P., Pühler, A., Complete genome sequence and analysis of the multiresistant nosocomial pathogen *Corynebacterium jeikeium* K411, a lipid-requiring bacterium of the human skin flora. *J. Bacteriol.*, 187, 4671, 2005.

75. Brune, I., Barzantny, H., Klotzel, M., Jones, J., James, G., Tauch, A., Identification of McbR as a transcription regulator of aecD and genes involved in methionine biosynthesis in *Corynebacterium jeikeium* K411. *J. Biotechnol.*, 151, 22, 2010.

76. Bawdon, D., *Identification of bacterial transporters for hydroxyalkylcysteinylglycines*, PhD Thesis, University of York, 2014.

77. Christensen, G.J.M. and Brüggemann, H., Bacterial skin commensals and their role as host guardians. *Benef. Microbes*, 5, 201, 2014.

78. Byrd, A.L., Belkaid, Y., Segre, J.A., The human skin microbiome. *Nat. Rev. Microbiol.*, 16, 143, 2018.

79. Nakatsuji, T., Chiang, H.-I., Jiang, S.B., Nagarajan, H., Zengler, K., Gallo, R.L., The microbiome extends to subepidermal compartments of normal skin. *Nat. Commun.*, 4, 1431, 2013.

80. Jahns, A.C. and Alexeyev, O.A., Microbial colonization of normal skin: Direct visualization of 194 skin biopsies. *Anaerobe*, 38, 47, 2016.

81. Hopwood, D., Farrar, M.D., Bojar, R.A., Holland, K.T., Microbial colonization dynamics of the axillae of an individual over an extended period. *Acta Derm. Venereol.*, 85, 363, 2005.

82. Callewaert, C., Hutapea, P., Van de Wiele, T., Boon, N., Deodorants and antiperspirants affect the axillary bacterial community. *Arch. Dermatol. Res.*, 306, 701, 2014.

83. Makin, S.A. and Lowry, M.R., Deodorant Ingredients, in: *Antiperspirants and Deodorants, Second Edition*, K. Laden (Ed.), pp. 169–214, Marcel Dekker, Inc., New York, 1999.

84. Standard Guide for Sensory Evaluation of Axillary Deodorancy, ASTM E1207 – 14, 2014.

85. Standard Test Method for Recovery of Microorganisms From Skin using the Cup Scrub Technique, ASTM E1874 – 14, 2014.

86. Urban, J., Fergus, D.J., Savage, A.M., Ehlers, M., Menninger, H.L., Dunn, R.R., Horvath, J.E., The effect of habitual and experimental antiperspirant and deodorant product use on the armpit microbiome. *PeerJ*, 4, e1605, 2016.

87. Bouslimani, A., da Silva, R., Kosciolek, T. *et al.*, The impact of skin care products on skin chemistry and microbiome dynamics. *BMC Biol.*, 17, 47, 2019.

88. Mathapathi, M.S., Mallemalla, P., Vora, S., Iyer, V., Tiwari, J.K., Chakrabortty, A., Majumdar, A., Niacinamide leave-on formulation provides long-lasting protection against bacteria *in vivo*. *Exp. Dermatol.*, 26, 827, 2017.

89. Callewaert, C., Plaquet, T., Bostoen, J., Van de Wiele, T., Boon, N., Axillary bacterial transplantation and bacteriotherapy as a promising technique to treat bromhidrosis. *J. Invest. Dermatol.*, 133, S207, 2013.

90. Callewaert, C., Lambert, J., Van de Wiele, T., Towards a bacterial treatment for armpit malodor. *Exp. Dermatol.*, 26, 388, 2017.

91. Kuhn, F. and Natsch, A., Body odor of monozygotic human twins: a common pattern of of odorant carboxylic acids released by a bacterial aminoacylase from axilla secretions contributing to an inherited body odour type. *J. R. Soc. Interface*, 6, 377, 2009.

92. Natsch, A., Kuhn, F., Tiercy, J.-M., Lack of evidence for HLA-linked patterns of odorous carboxylic acids released from glutamine conjugates secreted in the human axilla. *J. Chem. Ecol.*, 36, 837, 2010.

93. Martin, A., Saathoff, M., Kuhn, F., Max, H., Terstegen, L., Natsch, A., A functional *ABCC11* allele is essential in the biochemical formation of human axillary odor. *J. Invest. Dermatol.*, 130, 529, 2010.

94. Yoshiura, K., Kinoshita, A., Ishida, T. *et al.*, A SNP in the *ABCC11* gene is the determinant of human earwax type. *Nat. Genet.*, 38, 324, 2006.

95. Fleming, A., On a remarkable bacteriolytic element found in tissues and secretions. *Proc. R. Soc. Lond. [Biol.]*, 93, 306, 1922.

96. Prokop-Prigge, K.A., Greene, K., Varallo, L., Wysocki, C.J., Preti, G., The effect of ethnicity on human axillary odorant production. *J. Chem. Ecol.*, 42, 33, 2016.

97. Egert, M., Höhne, H.M., Weber, T., Simmering, R., Banowski, B., Breves, R., Identification of compounds inhibiting the C-S lyase activity of a cell extract from a *Staphylococcus* sp. isolated from human skin. *Lett. Appl. Microbiol.*, 57, 534, 2013.

6

Infant Skin Microbiome

Georgios N. Stamatas

Johnson & Johnson Santé Beauté France, Issy-les-Moulineaux, France

Abstract

Infancy is probably the most dynamic period of life characterized by a rapid, concordant and well-coordinated development of all tissues and systems in our body. These include the cutaneous tissue and the immune system, both of which undergo a maturation process during the first years of life. The composition of skin microbiome, the ensemble of microflora living on the skin surface and in its appendages are highly dependent on both the skin and immune system maturation processes. It is not surprising then that the skin microbiome undergoes its own maturation process before it becomes relatively stable over time for an individual. In this chapter we will review recent findings from studies advancing our knowledge on the skin and immune system maturation processes, as well as the infant skin microbiome dynamics and the role of microbial bi-directional transmission between the mother and the infant.

Keywords: Infant skin maturation, microbial diversity, microbial richness

6.1 Introduction

Being the largest organ of the body and the principal interface with the environment, skin plays an important role in the overall health of an individual. The skin barrier is the first line of defense of the body [1]. Emerging science demonstrates that the microorganisms that colonize the skin surface play a decisive role in battling skin disease, maintaining skin immunity and supporting a healthy skin barrier. On the other hand, transient

---

Email: gstamata@its.jnj.com

Nava Dayan (ed.) Skin Microbiome Handbook: From Basic Research to Product Development, (131–142) © 2020 Scrivener Publishing LLC

colonization by opportunistic microbial invaders can be the root cause of infections. Moreover, even the long-term "benign" microbial residents of the skin surface may change to a virulent phenotype once provided with the right microenvironment, for example, when given access to the well-hydrated area of the layers of the viable epidermis [2].

At birth the infant is forced to transition and rapidly adapt from the almost sterile aqueous environment of the womb to a dry atmospheric environment where microorganisms are present everywhere. The skin has a double task of forming a competent barrier to dehydration, while at the same time provides the niche for commensal and mutualistic microorganisms to grow and guard against opportunistic parasites. Both of these processes continue through the first years of life and can critically affect the immune development of the child and the risk of developing immune-related diseases such as atopic dermatitis [3]. In the sequence of allergic diseases, skin atopy develops earlier in life and may lead to subsequent food allergies, asthma, hay fever and allergic rhinitis, a sequence that has been termed "the atopic march" [4, 5]. Therefore, research to better understand the skin microbiome and its function early in life is warranted.

6.2   Infant Skin Maturation

Baby skin is often considered as the cosmetic ideal for adult skin care. Its mechanical suppleness and high moisture content [6] contribute to a sensorially pleasant perception. Despite the higher water content compared to adult skin, infant skin's water barrier function is not fully mature, characterized by relatively higher water loss rates per unit area [7]. An immature inside-out barrier (acting against water loss) is also mirrored by an immature outside-in barrier (acting against irritant and allergen penetration). In fact, infant epidermal structure is characterized by smaller cells and thinner layers [8], both of which shorten the effective length that an externally applied substance needs to travel to penetrate through the epidermis. Overall, infant skin differs from that of an adult in structure, function, and composition (Table 6.1).

The realization by the scientific community that infant skin barrier is immature has led to reconsideration of guidelines for infant skin care, such as recommendations for surfactant mildness [9]. Moreover, it helps explain the sensitivity of infant skin to irritant dermatitis (e.g., diaper dermatitis) and is a key parameter to consider in the study of the development of atopic dermatitis early in life [10].

Table 6.1 During the first years of life infant skin undergoes a maturation process characterized by significant differences compared to adult skin with parameters relating to its structure, function, and composition.

Structure	Function	Composition
• Stratum Corneum and Epidermal thickness	• Water content	• Water handling properties
• Corneocyte size	• Natural moisturizing factor	• Barrier function
• Surface roughness	• Melanin	• Skin reactivity
• Collagen in the dermis	• Lipid content and organization	• Cell proliferation
• Elasticity		

6.3   Infant Immune System Maturation

The immune system is understood to be composed of two components that can be considered independent of each other, the innate and the adaptive immunity [11]. In a healthy organism, innate immunity is ready to function at any moment and protect it against external molecular and microbial intruders. On the other hand, adaptive immunity by definition requires time to activate cellular memory for a newly encountered antigen. Therefore, early in life the importance of innate immunity is greater while adaptive immunity is still being trained.

Being the first line of defense against noxious factors of the external environment, skin plays an important role in both innate and adaptive immunity. The structural architecture of the *stratum corneum* that involves the corneocytes, the corneodesmosomes and the intercellular lipid "mortar" could be considered as the first barrier to microbial access to tissues, where they could cause infections. Moreover, antimicrobial peptides and lipids, synthesized in the viable epidermal layers and secreted into the stratum corneum reinforce its innate and constitutive defense mechanisms [12, 13]. Viable keratinocytes can also synthesize cytokines such as interleukins, growth factors and other elements that can signal the recruitment and activation of the cellular compartment of the immune system [14]. Even during the early period of life when the adaptive immunity is still immature and still lacking epitope "education," these components of innate immunity are fully functional. In fact, it has been demonstrated that two groups of antimicrobial peptides, the defensins and the cathelicidins, are constitutively produced in newborn skin [15]. More recently our research group at Johnson & Johnson reported that the surface concentration of human beta defensin-1 on infant skin is high particularly in the perinatal period and gradually deceases by the second and third year of life [16]. In the same study it was demonstrated that infant keratinocytes constitutively produce interleukin-1 alpha and its receptor antagonist, two important modulators of cellular immunity. Thus, enhanced innate immunity early in life may in part compensate for the developmental immaturity of the adaptive immune system.

An important aspect relating to innate immunity at the time of birth is the presence of vernix caseosa. This waxy material covers the surface of the newborn during birth and is known to serve several functions, including lubricating the passage through the birth canal, moisturizing the infant skin, conserving the infant's temperature and in general protecting the infant during the early hours to days after birth [17]. Vernix is a mixture of sebaceous lipids and "ghost" keratinocyte cells, a composition that gives its unique properties [18]. Its composition is loaded with antimicrobial peptides and lipids that are thought to protect the infant skin at the first contact with microbes *ex utero* [19] and is expected to play an important role in shaping the developing skin microbiome.

As the infant grows, its adaptive immune system needs to be trained through exposure to foreign epitopes. Based on epidemiological data on the rising incidence of allergic diseases, the "hygiene hypothesis" as it was first proposed in 1989 [20] states that early childhood exposure to particular microorganisms can have a protective effect against allergic diseases by contributing to the timely training of the adaptive immunity. Inversely, lack of microbial exposure may lead to a defective immune development. The hygiene hypothesis has been challenged by the argument that correlation does not prove causality, but cannot be fully discredited either, as the underlying mechanisms are multiple and complex [21]. In any case, understanding the mechanisms can reveal new therapeutic perspectives in the prevention of allergic diseases.

6.4   Infant Skin Microbiome Dynamics

The presence of a microbial colony on a tissue itself implies that the particular microbial species comprising the colony gains some benefit to be able to grow and thrive in that niche. However, this may not always be the case for the host. For a given symbiosis (for example, between the human host and a microbial species) there can be three possible types of relationships

[22]: a) parasitic, when the presence of the microbes are to the detriment of the host tissue, b) commensal, when the microbial presence is indifferent to the health of the host tissue, and c) mutualistic, when the host receives a benefit from the presence of the particular microbes. In the latter case the benefit may be direct (e.g., the microbes may generate metabolites that stimulate or enhance the function of the host tissue) or indirect (e.g., the microbial presence inhibits colonization by a parasite).

Until almost a decade ago any microbial presence on the skin was associated with a risk of infection. In fact, it has been demonstrated that certain skin diseases are linked to the presence of specific bacterial species such as *Staphylococcus aureus* in atopic eczema [23] and *Propionibacterium acnes* (recently renamed *Cutibacterium acnes*) in acne vulgaris [24]. While such parasitic relationships between microbes and host were well established, any consideration of a potential commensal or even mutualistic relationship was rare or even nonexistent, at least in dermatology.

It is now well known that the human skin is colonized by a diversity of microorganisms, including bacteria, fungi and viruses [25]. The skin microbiome confers a number of benefits to the host, including protection from colonization by opportunistic parasites, training of the adaptive immune system, modulation of the immune response, effect on metabolic processes, etc. [26].

A key concept that has attracted attention in the microbiome research community is that of microbial richness and diversity. While richness refers to the total number of species present in an ecosystem, diversity also accounts for the evenness of the relative abundances of such species. For example, a system of two species where the relative abundance of each is 50% is more diverse than a system where one of the two species is dominating (e.g., 90% of species A and 10% of species B).

The healthy state of a tissue, in which microbiome plays a role, is typically correlated with increased diversity. This concept is also found in ecology and can be easily understood considering that a genetically diverse system would have more mechanisms (e.g., feedback loops, even with some level of redundancy) to resist external perturbations. This idea has been applied to skin microbiome research and indeed disease states, including acne, rosacea and atopic dermatitis, are characterized by decreased microbial diversity compared to healthy cohorts [27].

A second important concept is the effects of skin surface pH on skin microbiome. Many commensal bacterial species show an optimum for growth at the slightly acidic environment of skin (about pH 5), whereas certain opportunistic parasitic species prefer conditions of neutral to alkali pH [28]. Skin surface pH also affects the enzymatic activity in the stratum corneum, the outermost layer of the epidermis composed of keratinized cells called corneocytes. The corneocytes are held together by crosslinked protein complexes known as corneodesmosomes. The latter are broken down by specific pH-dependent enzymes at the surface of the stratum corneum. The rate of this enzymatic activity is critical for maintaining a healthy skin barrier that allows microbes to colonize the skin surface but does not give access to the viable layers of the epidermis, where they would potentially cause infections. Recently, we reported that the caseinolytic specific activity of stratum corneum enzymes is higher in infant skin compared to that of an adult [29]. This observation is consistent with the relatively higher turnover rate of keratinocytes in infant epidermis [8] and could play an indirect role in controlling the microbial colonization and growth on infant skin.

Finally, it is important to note that in adults, although the composition of the skin microbiome is relatively stable in time, with some studies showing stability over 2 years, it is quite variable if we sample different body sites. In fact, the microbiome composition has been shown to uniquely characterize dry, moist or oily skin areas [30–32].

The dynamic processes of structural and functional alterations of infant skin coupled with immune system maturation, as discussed above, are expected to impact the dynamics of microbial colonization and composition on an infant's skin. Our research group at Johnson & Johnson therefore embarked on the study of the skin microbiome of healthy infants during the first year of life [33]. At the phylum level we reported that while adult skin is colonized primarily by Actinobacteria (about 50%), followed by Firmicutes and Proteobacteria (about 20% each), infant skin microbiome is dominated by Firmicutes (about 50%) followed by Actinobacteria and Bacteroidetes (about 20% each). At the genus analysis level more than half of the bacterial sequences obtained from infants were either *Streptococcus*, *Staphylococcus*, *Propionibacterium*, *Prevotella*, or *Corynebacterium*. On adult skin, *Propionibacterium*, *Staphylococcus*, and *Streptococcus* comprised more than 60% of the total skin microbiome. Over time, a continuous gradual shift in the most dominant members of the skin microbiome was observed with *Streptococcus* becoming less dominant in adults as *Propionibacterium* abundance increased. The prevalence of Actinobacteria (notably of *Propionibacterium* genus) in adults and their relative dearth in infants is likely ascribed to the presence of sebum in adult skin, as sebaceous glands remain inactive throughout childhood and get activated by hormones that are released in adolescence.

Interestingly, the species richness and diversity increase with an infant's age during the first year of life, presumably due to increased activity and

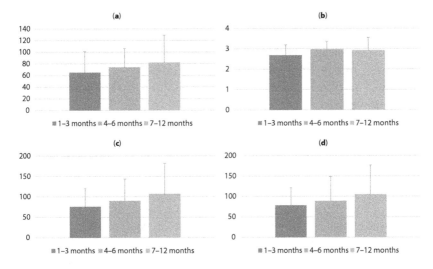

Figure 6.1 Microbial diversity and richness on the forehead site as a function of infant age, presented here at the 3% divergence level corresponding roughly to the species level (a) Rarefaction, (b) Shannon index, (c) Ace index, and (d) Chao1 index maximum observed estimates. The bar graphs show average values and error bars represent one standard deviation. (Data from Capone *et al.*, 2011.)

ample opportunities for contact with new environments. This increased diversity is thought to confer a better protection and parallel the maturation process of the skin barrier (Figure 6.1).

Similar to the findings of studies in adult skin, the composition of infant skin microbiome demonstrates site specificity [33]. However, the microenvironments of various skin sites differ between infants and adults, which affects the microbial population composition. Infants lack "oily" skin sites due to the lack of sebaceous activity. Principal component analysis did not show statistical differences between the face and the arm sites in infants, which has been demonstrated in adults [30]. There were, however, differences in infants between the buttock skin microbiome and the face/arm sites [33]. The presence of several gut-related species on the buttock site is thought to be associated with the use of baby diapers.

6.5   Mother-Infant Microbial Transmission

Since the womb is generally regarded as a sterile environment, the first colonization of skin is thought to occur during birth. The mode of delivery has been shown to determine a child's skin microbiome for as long as several years, with a microbial composition that is defined by bacteria that normally are found on the vaginal epithelium for children born passing through the birth canal and by microbes associated with skin (notably Firmicutes) for babies born by Caesarian section [34, 35].

The first months following birth is a period of intense physical interaction between the infant and the mother. A recent study showed that during this period there is a bi-directional microbial transmission within the mother-infant dyad [36]. The number of bacteria genera isolated per individual varied during the first year of life in a parallel fashion between mothers and infants and peaked around the sixth month of life for both groups. Moreover, the time-dependent changes in isolation rates of the most frequently isolated genera were closely matched between mothers and infants. Indeed, there were no significant differences in the isolation rates between the two groups. The idea of "shared" skin microbial composition in the mother-infant dyad early in life was demonstrated by analyzing the concordance of the isolation of each genus over the first-year postpartum. The concordance rate was highest during the first weeks and tended to decline towards the end of the first year of the infant's life. This decline can be expected to be due to the increased physical activity of the infant (e.g., crawling) and therefore more diverse environmental input contributing to the skin microflora. Therefore, this gradual transition towards exposure to a more diverse environment is thought to contribute to the progressively rising infant skin microbial diversification [33].

6.6   Conclusion

Understanding the dynamic processes of infant skin maturation can help us explain the equally dynamic alterations in the composition of the skin microbiome. Parameters like skin surface pH, stratum corneum water content, levels of enzymatic activity, and concentrations of innate immunity markers, all of which are changing with infant age, have a direct effect on which microbes can attach and form colonies on the skin surface (Figure 6.2).

The question of at what age the skin becomes fully mature is often asked and depends on the parameter of interest. For example, the levels of skin surface hydration and water barrier function (as measured by TEWL) seem to reach adult levels around 4-5 years of age [37]. However, skin function is dynamically changing even later, for example, during puberty with the androgen-activated production of sebum, as well as throughout life due

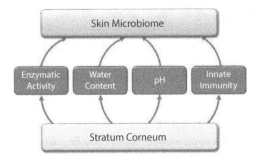

Figure 6.2 Infant skin maturation processes can influence the composition of microbes colonizing the skin surface.

to aging- and photoaging-related processes. Such processes are known to affect the composition of skin microbiome as well.

Future research combining different omics approaches are expected to shed light on the interdependencies between host tissue function and microbiome and provide novel insights for designing appropriate products for supporting skin health during infancy, a time of dynamic physiological changes.

References

1. Madison, K.C., Barrier function of the skin: "la raison d'etre" of the epidermis. *J. Invest. Dermatol.*, 121, 231–241, 2003. https://doi.org/10.1046/j.1523-1747.2003.12359.x.

2. Duckney, P., Wong, H.K., Serrano, J., Yaradou, D., Oddos, T., Stamatas, G.N., The role of the skin barrier in modulating the effects of common skin microbial species on the inflammation, differentiation and proliferation status of epidermal keratinocytes. *BMC Res. Notes*, 6, 474, 2013. https://doi.org/10.1186/1756-0500-6-474.

3. Leung, D.Y.M., New insights into atopic dermatitis: Role of skin barrier and immune dysregulation. *Allergol. Int. Off. J. Jpn. Soc. Allergol.*, 62, 151–161, 2013. https://doi.org/10.2332/allergolint.13-RAI-0564.

4. Spergel, J., Atopic dermatitis and the atopic march. *J. Allergy Clin. Immunol.*, 112, S118–S127, 2003. https://doi.org/10.1016/j.jaci.2003.09.033.

5. Dharmage, S.C., Lowe, A.J., Matheson, M.C., Burgess, J.A., Allen, K.J., Abramson, M.J., Atopic dermatitis and the atopic march revisited. *Allergy*, 69, 17–27, 2014. https://doi.org/10.1111/all.12268.

6. Stamatas, G.N., Nikolovski, J., Mack, M.C., Kollias, N., Infant skin physiology and development during the first years of life: a review of recent findings

based on *in vivo* studies. *Int. J. Cosmet. Sci.*, 33, 17–24, 2011. https://doi.org/10.1111/j.1468-2494.2010.00611.x.

7. Nikolovski, J., Stamatas, G.N., Kollias, N., Wiegand, B.C., Barrier function and water-holding and transport properties of infant stratum corneum are different from adult and continue to develop through the first year of life. *J. Invest. Dermatol.*, 128, 1728–1736, 2008. https://doi.org/10.1038/sj.jid.5701239.

8. Stamatas, G.N., Nikolovski, J., Luedtke, M.A., Kollias, N., Wiegand, B.C., Infant skin microstructure assessed *in vivo* differs from adult skin in organization and at the cellular level. *Pediatr. Dermatol.*, 27, 125–131, 2010. https://doi.org/10.1111/j.1525-1470.2009.00973.x.

9. Blume-Peytavi, U., Lavender, T., Jenerowicz, D., Ryumina, I., Stalder, J.-F., Torrelo, A., Cork, M.J., Recommendations from a European Roundtable Meeting on Best Practice Healthy Infant Skin Care. *Pediatr. Dermatol.*, 33, 311–321, 2016. https://doi.org/10.1111/pde.12819.

10. Kelleher, M., Dunn-Galvin, A., Hourihane, J.O., Murray, D., Campbell, L.E., McLean, W.H.I., Irvine, A.D., Skin barrier dysfunction measured by transepidermal water loss at 2 days and 2 months predates and predicts atopic dermatitis at 1 year. *J. Allergy Clin. Immunol.*, 135, 930–935.e1, 2015. https://doi.org/10.1016/j.jaci.2014.12.013.

11. Basha, S., Surendran, N., Pichichero, M., Immune responses in neonates. *Expert Rev. Clin. Immunol.*, 10, 1171–1184, 2014. https://doi.org/10.1586/1744666X.2014.942288.

12. Aberg, K.M., Man, M.-Q., Gallo, R.L., Ganz, T., Crumrine, D., Brown, B.E., Choi, E.-H., Kim, D.-K., Schröder, J.M., Feingold, K.R. *et al.*, Co-regulation and interdependence of the mammalian epidermal permeability and antimicrobial barriers. *J. Invest. Dermatol*, 128, 917–925, 2008.

13. Bibel, D.J., Miller, S.J., Brown, B.E., Pandey, B.B., Elias, P.M., Shinefield, H.R., Aly, R., Antimicrobial activity of stratum corneum lipids from normal and essential fatty acid-deficient mice. *J. Invest. Dermatol.*, 92, 632–638, 1989.

14. Pasparakis, M., Haase, I., Nestle, F.O., Mechanisms regulating skin immunity and inflammation. *Nat. Rev. Immunol.*, 14, 289–301, 2014. https://doi.org/10.1038/nri3646.

15. Dorschner, R.A., Lin, K.H., Murakami, M., Gallo, R.L., Neonatal skin in mice and humans expresses increased levels of antimicrobial peptides: innate immunity during development of the adaptive response. *Pediatr. Res.*, 53, 566–572, 2003. https://doi.org/10.1203/01.PDR.0000057205.64451.B7.

16. Kirchner, F., Capone, K.A., Mack, M.C., Stamatas, G.N., Expression of cutaneous immunity markers during infant skin maturation. *Pediatr. Dermatol.*, 35, 468–471, 2018. https://doi.org/10.1111/pde.13516.

17. Visscher, M.O., Narendran, V., Pickens, W.L., LaRuffa, A.A., Meinzen-Derr, J., Allen, K., Hoath, S.B., Vernix caseosa in neonatal adaptation. *J. Perinatol.*, 25, 440, 2005.

18. Rissmann, R., Groenink, H.W., Weerheim, A.M., Hoath, S.B., Ponec, M., Bouwstra, J.A., New insights into ultrastructure, lipid composition and organization of vernix caseosa. *J. Invest. Dermatol.*, 126, 1823–1833, 2006.

19. Yoshio, H., Tollin, M., Gudmundsson, G.H., Lagercrantz, H., Jörnvall, H., Marchini, G., Agerberth, B., Antimicrobial polypeptides of human vernix caseosa and amniotic fluid: implications for newborn innate defense. *Pediatr. Res.*, 53, 211, 2003.

20. Strachan, D.P., Hay fever, hygiene, and household size. *Br. Med. J.*, 299, 1259, 1989. https://doi.org/10.1136/bmj.299.6710.1259.

21. Okada, H., Kuhn, C., Feillet, H., Bach, J.-F., The "hygiene hypothesis" for autoimmune and allergic diseases: an update. *Clin. Exp. Immunol.*, 160, 1–9, 2010. https://doi.org/10.1111/j.1365-2249.2010.04139.x.

22. Leung, T.L.F. and Poulin, R., Parasitism, commensalism, and mutualism: Exploring the many shades of symbioses. *Vie Milieu*, 58, 107–115, 2008.

23. Totte, J.E.E., van der Feltz, W.T., Hennekam, M., van Belkum, A., van Zuuren, E.J., Pasmans, S.G.M.A., Prevalence and odds of *Staphylococcus aureus* carriage in atopic dermatitis: A systematic review and meta-analysis. *Br. J. Dermatol.*, 175, 687–695, 2016. https://doi.org/10.1111/bjd.14566.

24. Dreno, B., Pecastaings, S., Corvec, S., Veraldi, S., Khammari, A., Roques, C., Cutibacterium acnes (Propionibacterium acnes) and acne vulgaris: A brief look at the latest updates. *J. Eur. Acad. Dermatol. Venereol. JEADV*, 32 Suppl 2, 5–14, 2018. https://doi.org/10.1111/jdv.15043.

25. Schommer, N.N. and Gallo, R.L., Structure and function of the human skin microbiome. *Trends Microbiol.*, 21, 660–668, 2013. https://doi.org/10.1016/j.tim.2013.10.001.

26. Byrd, A.L., Belkaid, Y., Segre, J.A., The human skin microbiome. *Nat. Rev. Microbiol.*, 16, 143–155, 2018. https://doi.org/10.1038/nrmicro.2017.157.

27. Grice, E.A., Kong, H.H., Renaud, G., Young, A.C., Bouffard, G.G., Blakesley, R.W., Wolfsberg, T.G., Turner, M.L., Segre, J.A., A diversity profile of the human skin microbiota. *Genome Res.*, 18, 1043–1050, 2008. https://doi.org/10.1101/gr.075549.107.

28. Grice, E.A. and Segre, J.A., The skin microbiome. *Nat. Rev. Microbiol.*, 9, 244–253, 2011. https://doi.org/10.1038/nrmicro2537.

29. Liu, Q., Zhang, Y., Danby, S.G., Cork, M.J., Stamatas, G.N., Infant Skin Barrier, Structure, and Enzymatic Activity Differ from Those of Adult in an East Asian Cohort. *BioMed Res. Int.*, 2018, 1–8, 2018. https://doi.org/10.1155/2018/1302465.

30. Costello, E.K., Lauber, C.L., Hamady, M., Fierer, N., Gordon, J.I., Knight, R., Bacterial community variation in human body habitats across space and time. *Science*, 326, 1694–1697, 2009. https://doi.org/10.1126/science.1177486.

31. Grice, E.A., Kong, H.H., Conlan, S., Deming, C.B., Davis, J., Young, A.C., Bouffard, G.G., Blakesley, R.W., Murray, P.R., Green, E.D., Turner, M.L., Segre, J.A., Topographical and temporal diversity of the human skin microbiome. *Science*, 324, 1190–1192, 2009. https://doi.org/10.1126/science.1171700.

32. Oh, J., Byrd, A.L., Deming, C., Conlan, S., Kong, H.H., Segre, J.A., Biogeography and individuality shape function in the human skin metagenome. *Nature*, 514, 59–64, 2014. https://doi.org/10.1038/nature13786.

33. Capone, K.A., Dowd, S.E., Stamatas, G.N., Nikolovski, J., Diversity of the human skin microbiome early in life. *J. Invest. Dermatol.*, 131, 2026–2032, 2011. https://doi.org/10.1038/jid.2011.168.

34. Dominguez-Bello, M.G., Costello, E.K., Contreras, M., Magris, M., Hidalgo, G., Fierer, N., Knight, R., Delivery mode shapes the acquisition and structure of the initial microbiota across multiple body habitats in newborns. *Proc. Natl. Acad. Sci. U. S. A.*, 107, 11971–11975, 2010. https://doi.org/10.1073/pnas.1002601107.

35. Mueller, N.T., Bakacs, E., Combellick, J., Grigoryan, Z., Dominguez-Bello, M.G., The infant microbiome development: mom matters. *Trends Mol. Med.*, 21, 109–117, 2015. https://doi.org/10.1016/j.molmed.2014.12.002.

36. Gaitanis, G., Tsiouri, G., Spyridonos, P., Stefos, T., Stamatas, G.N., Velegraki, A., Bassukas, I.D., Variation of cultured skin microbiota in mothers and their infants during the first year postpartum. *Pediatr. Dermatol.*, 36, 460–465, 2019. https://doi.org/10.1111/pde.13829.

37. Mack, M.C., Chu, M.R., Tierney, N.K., Ruvolo, E., Stamatas, G.N., Kollias, N., Bhagat, K., Ma, L., Martin, K.M., Water-Holding and Transport Properties of Skin Stratum Corneum of Infants and Toddlers Are Different from Those of Adults: Studies in Three Geographical Regions and Four Ethnic Groups. *Pediatr. Dermatol.*, 33, 275–282, 2016. https://doi.org/10.1111/pde.12798.

Part 3

SKIN MICROBIOME IN
DISEQUILIBRIUM AND DISEASE

7

Microbiome of Compromised Skin

Sara Farahmand

The Clorox Company, Pleasanton, California

Abstract

The skin microbiome of normal human skin is characterized by a high diversity and high inter-individual variation. Microbiota of diseased skin with compromised barrier shows distinct differences relative to healthy skin. The dynamic communication between immune cells and microbiota is disturbed when the skin barrier is compromised in patients with inflammatory diseases, such as atopic dermatitis, and such inflammatory reactions are often accompanied by a reduction in the diversity of microbial communities and outgrowth of certain species, such as *Staphylococcus aureus*. The findings of microbiota studies in atopic dermatitis, psoriasis, acne, dandruff, seborrheic dermatitis, irritant and allergic contact dermatitis are reviewed in this chapter. Because understanding skin microbiome of compromised skin is crucial for identification and development of therapeutic targets for skin diseases, future research should address the current data gaps through: using larger cohorts, unified and more advanced sampling protocols and analytical techniques such as metatranscriptomics, characterizing the impact of environmental pollutants and chemicals on skin microbiome, and a focus on understanding dynamics of the skin microbiome and recolonization pattern following skin damage.

Keywords: Acne, atopic dermatitis, compromised skin, dandruff, dysbiosis, exposome, psoriasis, seborrheic dermatitis

Email: sara.farahmandseilab@clorox.com

Nava Dayan (ed.) *Skin Microbiome Handbook: From Basic Research to Product Development,* (145–170) © 2020 Scrivener Publishing LLC

Skin is a complex ecosystem made up of many different habitats and microbial communities. Advances in DNA sequencing analysis such as bacterial 16S ribosomal RNA (rRNA) gene sequencing have provided insights into the skin microbiome composition and function, and its inter-individual and intra-individual variations depending on the specific skin site. Research has demonstrated that skin microbiome contributes to host immunity through maintenance of the epidermal barrier. Evidence from germ-free mice also suggests that communication between commensal microbes and skin-resident cells is important for proper tuning of the local inflammatory environment [1].

As it is becoming clear that the microbiota makes important contributions to skin barrier function, it is logical that disruptions to skin barrier can be correlated with alterations in microbial communities. Several descriptive studies have identified differences in the microbes present in diseased skin with compromised barrier versus those present in healthy skin. The findings of these studies in atopic dermatitis, psoriasis, acne, dandruff and seborrheic dermatitis, irritant and allergic contact dermatitis are reviewed in this chapter. While studies indicate that an imbalance of microorganisms, termed dysbiosis, exists in numerous skin diseases, it is not entirely clear whether alterations in the microbiome lead to disease, or whether underlying conditions result in an imbalance in microbial communities.

Further research is needed to identify the dynamics of the skin microbiome and recolonization pattern following skin damage, using simple models such as tape stripped skin [2]. Such studies will contribute to an in-depth understanding of host and skin microbiome interactions and may lead to identification of new therapeutic targets and strategies for treatment of skin barrier impairment.

7.1   Atopic Dermatitis

Atopic dermatitis (AD) is a multifactorial inflammatory skin disease with a characteristic disturbance of skin barrier function. While pathogenesis of this common disease is not well understood, the complex role of the skin microbiome in the pathogenesis and progression of atopic dermatitis is being elucidated [3]. Several factors have been identified to play a role in AD, including host genetics (e.g. mutations in the gene that encodes for filaggrin) [4–6], immunological abnormalities [5], decreased expression of antimicrobial proteins in the skin [5, 6], and environmental factors including excessive exposure to irritants and allergens or exposure to specific pathogens such as *Staphylococcus aureus* [5, 6].

Various methods of microbiome analysis (e.g. 16S and metagenomic analyses) have shown that dysbiosis (disruption of the structure of the microbial community, often reflected as dominance by one microbe and decrease in richness and diversity of microbes) is the hallmark of atopic dermatitis [4, 5, 7–9]. Alteration of microbial community structure and dysbiosis has been attributed to host demographics and genetics, human behavior, local and regional environmental characteristics, and transmission events may all potentially drive human skin microbiota variability [10, 11].

The human skin regulates colonization by microbial organisms by producing molecules, such as cathelicidin and beta defensin Anti-microbial Peptides (AMPs), fatty acids, and reactive oxygen species that directly inhibit growth of bacteria. Therefore, disruption of these innate defense mechanisms increases the risk of dysbiosis [12]. Using the bacterial 16S rRNA sequenced data, it was shown that in healthy subjects, across the four sampling sites (forehead, antecubital fossa, volar forearm, and extensor forearm), filaggrin deficiency correlates with decreased bacterial diversity and a distinct bacterial colonization pattern [6]. The skin microbiome composition of healthy filaggrin-deficient subjects was more similar to that of patients with AD than healthy filaggrin-competent subjects [6]. But in addition to filaggrin, other epidermal barrier proteins, such as envoplakin, periplakin, and involucrin may as well play a role in pathogenesis of AD by controlling bacterial penetration across the epidermal barrier and providing a pathway for inflammatory activation [12, 13]. Furthermore, a strong association between microbiome and skin lipid composition has been demonstrated [13]. These findings explain the beneficial outcome of skin barrier function restorative therapies using optimized lipid mixture (cholesterol, ceramide, and free fatty acids) and improved clinical symptoms in AD patients [4, 12, 14, 15].

Another characteristic of AD skin microbiome is the relative abundance of *Staphylococcus aureus* in vast majority of patients, despite induction of antimicrobial peptides in AD lesions [5–7, 12, 16].

Whether the *S. aureus* precedes the onset of clinical manifestations of AD remains unclear. In a longitudinal study of 149 infants who were sampled in the axillae and the antecubital fossae seven times during the first 2 years of life, AD developed in 36 of these subjects and *S. aureus* was detected before clinical onset of AD [12, 17]. There is also abundant evidence that *S. aureus* is highly influential in disease pathogenesis, is associated with severe disease flares, and significantly influences the disease phenotype [18]. It is understood that Staphylococci exo-proteins and super-antigens evoke inflammatory reactions in the host [12, 19]. Moreover, by producing various proteases and enhancing production of dermal fibroblasts and keratinocytes' proteases, *S. aureus* disrupts the proteolytic balance in the skin [5]. In another research work, however, Kennedy *et al.* [20], studied 50 infants from birth to 2 years of age who were swabbed at four different skin sites at three time points in their first six months of life. Using 16S ribosomal RNA gene DNA sequencing, the researchers did not detect significant increase in *S. aureus* colonization on the 10 infants who developed AD, which led them to conclude that *S. aureus* colonizes skin after onset of AD. However, a potential causal association of AD was found with other non-identified members of the *Staphylococcus* genus, and their presence correlated with a better outcome of AD [20].

While there is evidence indicating that the relative abundance of some strains of skin coagulase-negative *Staphylococcus* (CoNS) such as *Staphylococcus epidermidis* and *Staphylococcus hominis* was elevated in non-lesional AD skin (with skin site-dependent variability) [6, 7], high-throughput screen of CoNS species found that these antimicrobial strains are deficient on acute and chronic lesional AD skin [6, 12, 21]. Recent studies have demonstrated that antimicrobials from these strains of CoNS in normal microbiome of skin could be beneficial to the host and selectively fight against pathogens, such as *S. aureus* by bactericidal activity or destroying the biofilm through production of antimicrobial peptides or serine proteases [5, 12, 16, 21]. The lack of protective CoNS explains the higher rate of *S. aureus* survival and colonization in AD skin. Furthermore, data from human and mice suggest that exposure to beneficial CoNS at an early age may protect against later development of AD [12, 20, 22]. The limited efficacy of antibiotics in management of AD by inhibiting *S. aureus* is therefore attributed to the negative impact of these chemicals on beneficial strains such as CoNS strains [12].

Reduction of Malassezia spp. and high non-Malassezia fungal diversity were demonstrated by three studies of AD skin microbiome [7]. A decrease in abundance of *Actinobacteria*, *Corynebacterium* and *Propionibacterium* species in AD skin was also reported in several studies [4, 6, 7].

These findings suggest that an impaired skin barrier due to the dysregulation of innate antimicrobial defense system together with low colonization by CoNS, enable survival and dominance of *S. aureus* in AD skin [12, 18].

7.2 Psoriasis

In the first half of 20th century, investigations of the possible link between commensal nasopharyngeal streptococci and psoriasis were started and later work successfully correlated streptococcal pharyngitis with guttate psoriasis as well as exacerbations of stable chronic plaque psoriasis, which suggests a microbial contribution to the disease [23, 24].

In recent years, a number of studies have investigated the association between skin microbiome and psoriasis [23–30]. While the evidence shows that skin microbiota may have a role in the pathogenesis of psoriasis, there is a lack of consensus on the degree of microbiome diversity and composition of the psoriatic skin mircobiome. The conflicting results of psoriasis microbiome studies could be attributed to the variations in the sampling sites, sampling techniques (swab, biopsy, scraping), methods for studying microbiome (whole genome shotgun, 16S rRNA sequencing), and analysis of different regions of bacterial 16S rRNA, subject ethnicity, and inherent heterogeneity of microbial species that promote immune dysfunction in psoriatic patients [24, 29–31]. Moreover, it still remains unclear whether disease-associated changes in the microbiota composition have a causal role in disease development.

7.2.1 Diversity

Several studies evaluated the alpha and beta diversity of skin microbiome in psoriatic lesions, uninvolved skin of psoriasis patients and healthy individuals and reached different conclusions. Alpha diversity[1] describes that variety of microbial community in each sample and is described in terms of evenness (Simpson diversity index), the distribution of species in a sample, and richness or the number of species in a sample [29]. Beta diversity describes how similar microbial communities of psoriatic individuals are to one another [29].

The largest study evaluating alpha and beta diversity was conducted by Alekseyenko *et al.* (2013) in which a total of 199 subjects (75 patients with psoriasis and 124 healthy controls) were enrolled [25]. Using skin swabs and high-throughput 16S rRNA gene sequencing (focused on V3-V5 gene regions), they assayed the cutaneous bacterial communities of 51 matched

---

[1] In ecology, alpha diversity (α-diversity) is the mean species diversity in sites or habitats at a local scale. The term was introduced by R. H. Whittaker together with the terms beta diversity (β-diversity) and gamma diversity (γ-diversity). In microbiome studies, alpha diversity is defined as the variance *within* a particular sample. Usually measured as a single number from 0 (no diversity) to infinity, or sometimes as a percentile. Beta diversity (β-diversity or true beta diversity) is the ratio between regional and local species diversity. In microbiome studies, beta diversity looks at how samples vary against each other to explain differences between sites on the body, or microbiomes across geographic locations, etc. Gamma diversity (γ-diversity) is the total species diversity in a landscape and is determined by alpha and beta diversity [90].

triplets and found decreased taxonomic and species (OTU) level diversity in terms of both evenness and richness of the microbiome. This study also found a progressive increase in intragroup diversity (beta diversity) from control to unaffected skin sites to lesions [25]. In addition, Alekseyenko *et al.* followed the skin microbiome of a subset of 15 healthy controls and 17 psoriasis patients who were on a variety of systemic therapies, including methotrexate and TNF-alpha inhibitors and found that with systemic treatment, the richness initially declined in lesional and unaffected skin at 12 weeks. At 36 weeks, the richness of the unaffected skin rebound to baseline levels, while that the lesional skin did not [25, 29].

Using skin biopsy samples (epidermis and dermis) from lesional skin of 10 patients and 12 healthy controls (unmatched, non-flexural sites) and 16S rRNA gene sequencing (focused on V3-V4 gene regions), Fahlen *et al.* (2012) found a similar alpha diversity between psoriatic and normal skin, but a reduced beta diversity in the psoriatic lesions [26, 29, 32].

Contrary to the findings of these two studies [25, 26], other published work with smaller sample sizes and various sampling and analysis techniques have indicated an increased alpha and beta diversity of skin microbiome in psoriatic skin as compared to the healthy skin. The earliest study by Gao *et al.* (2008) [27], compared skin swabs from lesional and non-lesional skin sites on 6 psoriasis patients with those from unmatched areas of healthy skin from 6 controls, using 16S rRNA (nearly full length) method and demonstrated an increased alpha and beta diversity in lesional skin of psoriatic skin. Analyzing V1-V3 region of 16S rRNA, which is thought to provide more accurate bacterial identities of the skin microbiome at the genus and species levels compared to V4, Chang *et al.* (2018) [24] surveyed the microbiome of 28 psoriasis patients and 26 healthy subjects at 6 different skin sites which included dry, moist and sebaceous regions. This study demonstrated increasing alpha diversity in all measures, which led the investigators to conclude that the skin microbiome of psoriatic skin is more diverse, heterogeneous and unstable than microflora of the healthy skin. Increasing beta diversity for all dry psoriatic skin sites was also observed. This observation was consistent with the findings of Tett *et al.* (2017), who showed that there was increased alpha diversity of skin microbiome on psoriasis skin of elbows but not on ear (sebaceous rich skin site) and hypothesized that sebum provides an antibacterial barrier hence reduced microbiome diversity [28]. This is contrary to the general notion that a higher degree of skin microbiome diversity is associated with healthier skin and highlights that there is a need for further multi-center research with harmonized sequencing methods, using larger sample sizes and more careful control of environmental factors to better characterize the skin microbiome of healthy and damaged skin. It is not known if these alterations in the diversity of microbiome in psoriasis are a consequence of the disease or contributes to its pathogenesis.

Most recent analysis of 34 psoriasis patients and 25 healthy control, using three sampling techniques (swab, biopsy, or scraping) and 16S rRNA (V1V2 and V3V4) gene sequencing revealed insignificant differences between the psoriatic and healthy skin in terms of skin microbiome diversity and confirmed the impact of environmental differences between skin microhabitats on the skin microbiome (dry vs. oily skin) [30]. In line with the data on healthy skin, the evidence from this study indicated that the microbiome profile was comparable in all sampling techniques.

7.2.2   Microbiome Composition

Skin microbiome composition of psoriatic and healthy individuals, is described by several investigators. The weight of evidence indicates that the lesional psoriatic microbiome differs significantly to control and unaffected skin, but the changes in particular microbes differ depending on the study [29]. For example while Fahlen [26] and Stehlikova [30] described lower abundance of *Staphylococcus* in psoriatic skin biopsies, other studies found that psoriasis skin microbiota is enriched for *Staphylococcus aureus* and *Staphylococcus pettenkoferi* [24, 25, 28]. The differences of *Staphylococcus* abundance in different studies could be attributed to the sampled skin sites, since it is more prevalent in moist areas [29]. Overall, there was a trend towards an increased relative abundance of *Streptococcus* and a decreased level of *Propionibacterium* in psoriasis patients compared to controls [24–31].

A few studies suggested a higher fungal diversity in psoriatic skin and showed higher abundance of the fungus *Malassezia* species on different sites of psoriatic skin [24, 29–31]. *Malassezia's* role in psoriasis could be due to its ability to up-regulate the expression of tumor growth factor-beta 1, integrin chain and HSP70, thereby promoting immune cell migration and keratinocyte hyperproliferation in patients with psoriasis [31].

The role of viruses in psoriasis is not well understood. While there are no studies that have profiled the skin microbiome in psoriasis as a whole, multiple studies have identified several HPV subtypes (e.g. HPV5 and HPV38) in psoriasis [29].

The conflicting findings of psoriasis skin microbiome have been attributed to the variations in sampling sites (dry, moist, sebaceous), the microbiome analysis method, sampling method, study design, ethnicity, and alterations of microbe-microbe interactions with disease progression. It should also be noted that none of these studies address the skin microbiome in psoriasis arthritis and how it may differ from skin-limited psoriasis [29]. The implications of gut-skin axis and alterations of gut microbiota in psoriasis should also be taken into account when studying the variations of skin microbiome in psoriasis.

Few studies have demonstrated that clinical improvement of psoriatic plaques after treatments is associated with an alteration of lesional skin microbiota as it becomes more closely resembling that of unaffected skin after therapy [33, 34]. It has yet to be understood whether changes of skin microbiome are a cause or consequence of psoriasis.

7.3   Acne

Existing research suggests that Acne Vulgaris (AV) is associated with inherent abnormalities and changes in epidermal barrier function as well as follicular epithelial barrier [35] and thus acne should be viewed as a skin disease since the follicle is a living structure that changes and proliferates with the entire tissue. Yamamato *et al.* [36] examined sebum secretion, Stratum Corneum (SC) lipids, Transepidermal Water Loss (TEWL), and conductance (directly correlated with epidermal hydration) within the Stratum Corneum of 36 male patients with mild-to-moderate AV and 29 male control subjects. They found that the patients with AV exhibited significantly higher sebum secretion, greater Transepidermal Water Loss (TEWL), decreased SC conductance (hydration) and deficient intercellular lipid membrane as evidenced by reduced free sphingosine and total ceramides. These findings in the patients with AV compared to controls support epidermal permeability barrier impairment associated with AV [35, 36].

A few of the structural changes in untreated facial skin affected by AV include: increased filaggrin expression in follicular keratinocytes [37], increased sebum secretion, increased size of sebaceous glands, increased flow of sebum and consequent dilution of linoleic acid and subclinical inflammation associated with pro-inflammatory sebum lipid fractions (monounsaturated fatty acid and lipoperoxides) [35, 36]. The role of skin microbiome in occurrence of some of these structural changes of skin and pathophysiology of acne has been understood [38].

Androgen hormones lead to an increase in production of sebum and a high colonization of *Propionibacterium acnes* in the sebaceous gland which is an important factor in pathophysiology of AV [35, 39]. Using immunohistochemistry technique both on Normal Human Epiderminal Keratinocytes (NHEK) and on deep-frozen sections of normal human skin explants incubated with three different *P. acnes* extracts, Jarrousse *et al.*

[40] demonstrated that *P. acnes* extracts increased filaggrin expression by suprabasal layer of epidermis of explants. In addition, *P. acnes* interacts with the innate immune system to promote inflammation in two different ways: a) identifying pathogen recognition patterns and activating innate immune response via Toll-like receptors, peroxisome-activated receptors, intracellular NOD-like and AMPs; b) quantitatively and qualitatively modifying the skin microbiome [38]. Sequencing of the bacterial rRNA gene indicates that certain strains of *P. acnes* may be associated with acne and contain unique genetic elements that contribute to their virulence [38, 41, 42]. However, it's noteworthy that acne is a multifactorial disease with contributions from the immune system, genetics, and the environment and acne is not necessarily the result of proliferation of *P. acne* [38, 41].

In addition to *P. acnes*, other skin microbiota such as *S. epidermidis*, *S. aureus* and some *Streptococcal* species were found to be involved in the pathophysiology of acne [41, 43].

The comparison of unaffected skin with non-inflammatory and inflammatory lesions sampled from acne patients revealed similar skin microbiome at phyla level. Quantitatively, the level of actinobacteria was similar across the three sampled sites, however, propionobacteria made up 38% of the phyla in the healthy individuals versus less than 2% in the acne patients. The abundance of proteobacteria was lower for both lesions compared to unaffected skin, and firmicutes were more abundant in lesions due to a significant increase of staphylococci in both lesions compared to unaffected areas [38, 44].

Using 16S rRNA sequencing techniques, it has been shown that follicular microbiota of acne patients is more diverse than follicles from healthy skin. Bek-Thomsen *et al.* [45] showed that the follicles from healthy skin were exclusively colonized by *P. acnes*, whereas the follicular microbiota of acne patients included, in addition, *Staphylococcus epidermidis* and minor proportions of other species. The severity of acne has been attributed to the proportion of staphylococci on the microbiota of the skin surface [38].

7.4   Rosacea

Rosacea may occur in patients with dry skin or skin with important seborrheic levels, not being necessarily linked to a skin type. Studies assessing some parameters of the skin barrier in patients with rosacea are rare. The study of lipids from the sebaceous glands showed an imbalance in the fatty acid concentration in sebum in patients with papulopustular rosacea: which might have implications for skin barrier impairment. Moreover, epidermal inflammation leads to disruption of stratum corneum lipid synthesis affecting skin barrier function and resulting in classic symptoms of rosacea, such as itching, burning and stinging [46].

Research supports the contribution of skin and gut microbiome as trigger factors or potentiators of rosacea pathogenesis or inflammation [47].

Demodex folliculorum, a species of commensal saprophytic mite that colonizes pilosebaceous follicles of human skin has been found to be more abundant on the cheeks of patients with papulopostular rosacea (PPR) [47, 48]. Additional reports demonstrated a 5.7-fold increase in *Demodex* density across erythmetotelangiectatic rosacea (ETR) and PPR and significantly higher *Demodex* infestation rates, typically ranging from 35% to 50% and as high as 90% in 1 PPR study [47, 49–51].

A recent evidence-based meta-analysis of the prevalence and degrees of *Demodex* mite infestation in patients with rosacea revealed that patients with rosacea had significantly higher prevalence and degrees of *Demodex* mite infestation than did control patients and the fact that *Demodex* mites may play a role in both erythematotelangiectatic rosacea and papulopustular rosacea [52]. Ability of dust mite allergens to activate NOD-like receptors *in vitro*, has been proposed as *Dermodex's* mechanism of action in rosacea. Significantly increased levels of NALP3 or cryoporin protein (a component of inflammasome), is directly involved in activation of interlukin-1β inflammasome and may explain activation of the innate immune response in rosacea [47, 49, 53].

Bacillus oleronius are non-motile gram-negative endospore forming bacteria not currently recognized as microbiome of human skin, with unknown pathogenic potential. This bacteria has been cultured from *Demodex* mite isolated from a patient with rosacea and several patients with blepharitis [47]. Lacey *et al.* [54] showed that proteins isolated from *B oleronius* trigger a proliferative response in peripheral blood mononuclear cells of 73% of patients with PPR but only 29% of control subjects. Innate immune mediators induced by this bacteria have not been measured in patients with rosacea [47]; however, neutrophils isolated from healthy volunteers and exposed to *B oleronius* proteins exhibited increased migration and production of matrix metalloproteinase-9, interlukin-8, and tumor necrosis factor which mirrors inflammatory activation in patients with PPR [55–57].

Limited evidence has also linked *Staphylococcus epidermidis,* the most prevalent commensal bacteria of healthy human skin, to rosacea through an altered secretory profile [47, 58–60]. In one study, bacterial swabs were taken and cultured from an incised rosacea pustule, the ipsilateral cheek skin, and the eyelid margin of 15 patients with pustular rosacea. Swabs were also taken from the cheek skin and ipsilateral eyelid margin of 15 matched control subjects. A pure growth of *S. epidermidis* was isolated from a pustule of 9 of 15 patients with pustular rosacea, and no pure growth of *S. epidermidis* was isolated from their ipsilateral cheek skin (P = .0003). A pure growth of *S. epidermidis* was isolated from the eyelid margins of 4 of 15 patients with pustular rosacea, and no pure growth was isolated from the eyelids of age- and sex-matched control subjects (P = .05) [60]. *S. epidermidis* isolates from rosacea pustules were also beta-hemolytic, which may indicate secretion of virulence factors not present in control isolates [61].

In a single uncontrolled study of 10 patients with rosacea, *Chlamidya pneumonia* (obligate intracellular pathogens) antigen was detectable in 40% of malar skin biopsy specimens, and *Chlamidya pneumonia*-reactive antibodies were present in 80% of serum samples [47, 62].

While further research is needed to clarify the role of skin microbiome in rosacea pathophysiology and progression, the weight of evidence suggests skin microbiome if not central in rosacea pathogenesis, may act as a trigger factor of inflammation in these patients.

7.5   Seborrheic Dermatitis and Dandruff

Dandruff has been associated with an impaired skin barrier function. Harding *et al.* [63] analyzed total amounts and relative ratios of stratum corneum lipids in scalp stratum corneum samples collected during studies conducted in the UK and Thailand in order to examine ethnic differences. In both populations, dandruff was associated with a dramatic decrease in free lipid levels, with significant decreases in ceramides, fatty acids, and cholesterol. Detailed sub-analysis of the major ceramide species within the total ceramide fraction revealed a decrease in ceramide 1 and increased proportions of ceramide 6i and 6ii [63]. The skin barrier function in seborrheic dermatitis and dandruff is also impacted by the metabolic activities of the skin fungal community, specifically *Malassezia*.

Malassezia degrade sebum, freeing multiple fatty acids from triglycerides. They consume the very specific saturated fatty acids necessary for their proliferation, leaving behind the unsaturated fatty acids. Experimentally, it can be shown that the changes in sebum composition overtime are a direct result of Malassezia metabolism [64, 65]. By removing the microorganisms, the antimicrobial shampoos bring the sebum composition back to near normal levels of triglycerides and free fatty acids [64]. Penetration of the modified sebaceous secretions into the stratum corneum disrupts the skin barrier function and leads to inflammation, irritation, and the resultant scalp flaking [64]. It has been suggested that dandruff patients display an underlying difference in skin barrier permeability, relative to non-dandruff individuals, that makes them more susceptible to fatty acid-induced barrier disruption [65].

A large scale amplicon and shotgun metagenome-based study of an Indian cohort consisting of 140 women of similar age range has provided insights into the composition and potential role of scalp microbiome of equal number of healthy and dandruff afflicted individuals [66]: It was observed that the alpha-diversity (Shannon diversity index) for the fungal population was significantly lower in the healthy scalp compared to the dandruff scalp. The uncultured *Malassezia* was found to be significantly abundant in dandruff scalp relative to healthy scalp. Unknown species of *Malassezia* and species close to *M. restrica* were also significantly higher in the dandruff scalp. Other investigators also found a high abundance of *Malassezia* in the dandruff scalp samples of different ethnicities [67–69]. The ratio of *M. restrica* to *M. globosa* was significantly higher in the dandruff scalp samples [66, 70]. These findings highlight the key role of this fungal species on pathogenesis of dandruff. While overgrowth of *Malassezia* has been linked to the inflammation in seborrheic dermatitis, some investigators found similar amount of this microorganism in seborrehic dermatitis patients and control groups [71, 72].

Saxena *et al.* [66] found that among the bacterial populations, the alpha diversity did not show a significant difference between the healthy and dandruff scalp. In this study, it was also observed that the abundance of *S. epidermidis* is significantly higher in dandruff than in healthy scalp. This observation is in agreement with findings of other studies utilizing different sampling and analytical techniques [70, 73]. Studies also found a reduced level of *Propionibacterium acne* in dandruff skin and therefore an increased ratio of *S. epidermidis/P. acne* in dandruff scalp skin [66, 70]. Dandruff has also been associated to a difference in the balance between the fungal and bacterial populations on the scalp [70].

Among the *Malassezia* subgroups, *Malassezia sp.* and uncultured *Malassezia* showed significant positive correlation with dandruff scores and itching, whereas, *M. globosa*, which showed a higher abundance in the healthy scalp, was negatively correlated with these parameters. Uncultured *Malassezia* also showed a significant negative correlation with hydration. These findings yet again suggest that the uncharacterized *Malassezia* subgroups share a positive relationship with dandruff. Among the bacterial population, *S. epidermidis and Staphylococcus sp.* displayed a significant positive correlation with dandruff scores, TEWL and itching. These species also correlated negatively with hydration [66]. Furthermore, functional analyses of scalp microbiome revealed that N-glycan biosynthesis, which are implicated in cell-host interaction, were enriched in the dandruff scalp. Also a higher fungal metabolic diversity was found in dandruff scalp relative to the healthy scalp which was consistent with the higher alpha diversity of the fungal population in the dandruff scalp [66].

7.6   Exposome, Skin Barrier, and Skin Microbiome

It's well known that everything that people touch, bathe in, breathe, eat and drink is reflected in in their microbial ecosystems including the skin [74]. The average skin microbial diversity and skin health of healthy Western subjects was found to be much less than that of caveman skin or healthy subjects with little or no exposure to Western practices [75]. A few studies have linked synthetic cosmetic ingredients to skin barrier damage and consequent reduction of skin microbiome diversity [75]. However, these studies have significant limitations and further research is needed to illustrate the impact of chemicals and products on skin microbiome when these materials result in skin barrier damage and conditions such as irritant contact dermatitis and allergic contact dermatitis.

7.6.1   Skin Irritation and Microbiome

Diaper dermatitis and occupational hand dermatitis following hand hygiene practices among healthcare workers are two examples for cases in which the skin microbiome following skin irritation caused by chemicals or personal care products has been characterized.

7.6.2   Diaper Dermatitis

Diaper dermatitis, or diaper rash, describes any of the various inflammatory reactions of the skin within the diaper area, including the buttocks, perianal area, genitals, inner thighs and waistline [76]. The predominant form of diaper dermatitis is irritant contact dermatitis, the most common rash of the diaper area caused by a combination of factors such as: extended periods of wetness and urine in the diaper, friction, and mechanic abrasion; the presence of bile salts and other irritants in feces that breakdown the protective lipids and proteins in the top layer of skin; the increase in the skin pH levels by a mixture of urine and feces; and occasionally the presence of microorganisms [76]. An early colonization within the diaper area with *Clostridium spp.* and other gut-derived bacteria, coupled with a significant increase in Bacteroides, is a direct result of proximity of this area to the gastrointestinal tract and the fact that it is covered with a diaper that may change the oxygen availability, pH, and water-holding capacity of the skin [76, 77]. The study by Capone *et al.* showed that *Staphylococcus spp, Streptococcus spp, Enterococcus spp* as well as other variable or transient microorganisms such as *Prevotella spp, Veillonella spp,* and *Clostridium spp* were present at the buttock site. In one study that included neonates during the first 6 days of life, bifidobacteria and bacteroides were most commonly isolated from the diaper area, followed by enterobacteria, eubacteria, lactobacilli, and others [78]. Normal microbiota favors acidic pH levels, and any rise of skin pH in the diaper area allows the overgrowth of pathogenic microorganisms, including *C. albicans* and *S. aureus,* which play a predominant role in diaper dermatitis [76]. Severe diaper dermatitis is strongly correlated with the presence of *C. albicans,* and the frequency of dermatitis is inversely correlated with the diaper change frequency. On the other hand, in children without diaper rash, *S. epidermidis* was the most abundant organism isolated. Other microorganisms including streptococcal species, *Escherichia coli,* or non–*E. coli* fermenters were seen less often, and *C. albicans* was only rarely isolated from the skin.

Even though pathogenic microorganisms have been isolated from the skin affected by diaper dermatitis, the compromised skin that allows pathogenic microorganisms to gain access to the epidermis seems to be a prerequisite for the development of this condition. Furthermore, microorganisms from the feces of the infant can easily gain access through the damaged stratum corneum, leading to more severe diaper dermatitis together with secondary infection [76].

In one study the possible correlation between the exposure to chemical cleansing compounds in baby wet wipes and changes in infantile periurethral flora was investigated in one study with 173 infants who were cleaned with baby wet wipe (group A, 96 infants) and water and napkin (group B, 77 infants) after diaper soiling. No statistically significant difference was found between the two groups in terms of the type of isolated bacteria and their frequency of occurrence [79].

7.6.3   Occupational Hand Dermatitis

Frequent hand washing and wearing gloves as seen among healthcare workers have been associated with a higher prevalence of irritant contact dermatitis and skin barrier damage [80]. It was found by several investigators that dry, fissured skin as seen in hand dermatitis is associated with increased probability of bacterial growth [80, 81]. Studying small cohorts and using classic culture-based methods, several investigators observed a higher total microbial counts and a higher rate of colonization by *S. aureus* and gram-negative bacteria in the damaged skin of healthcare workers [41, 80]. Larson *et al.* found that nurses with damaged skin on their hands were twice as likely to have enterococci and *Candida* present on the hands [80]. They also observed that damaged skin on hands of nurses were significantly more likely to be colonized with *Staphylococcus hominis* [80]. Rocha *et al.* found same frequencies of yeast on both damaged and healthy hands without recovering any *C. albicans* isolated [82].

Overall, these findings indicated a higher diversity of microorganisms in hands of nurses who frequently wash hands because of consequent skin irritation. However, contradictory results have also been reported by other researchers: Borges *et al.* did not find a statistically significant difference in microbial count and composition between damaged and healthy hands of nurses; however, they observed that washing with soap and water was effective in removing microbial contamination only for healthy hands [83]. Further studies with larger cohorts and DNA sequencing techniques are needed to characterize the differences between the irritated and healthy skin of healthcare workers.

7.6.4   Allergic Contact Dermatitis (ACD) and Skin Microbiome

Eczema, the name for a group of conditions (including atopic dermatitis and contact dermatitis) that cause the skin to become red, itchy and inflamed, is typically the first manifestation of skin allergy and is linked to epithelial barrier dysfunction [74]. As discussed in the atopic dermatitis section, increased colonization with *S. aureus* is observed in filaggrin-deficient and cathelicidin-deficient mice, mimicking the atopic dermatitis skin. Entry of *S. aureus* under the epidermis was shown to increase pro-inflammatory cytokines, thus enhancing the potential for environmental allergen exposure through barrier disruption.

The role of skin microbiome in development of skin sensitization is not completely understood. Skin commensals have been shown to play an important role in T helpers type 1 and 2 (Th1 and Th2) balance along with the regulation of anti-inflammatory responses to chemical allergens [84–86]. Furthermore, oral administration of probiotics, e.g. orally administered *L. casei*, efficiently alleviates T cell-mediated skin inflammation without causing immune suppression, via mechanisms that include control of CD8$^+$ effector T cells and involve regulatory CD4$^+$ T cells [87].

Therefore, despite lack of data on changes in microbiome of allergic contact dermatitis skin, dysbiosis in ACD is possible as also evidenced by studies of skin microbiome in animals. In a study aimed at describing the skin microbiota of cats and determine whether bacterial dysbiosis occurs on the skin of allergic cats, the skin surfaces on various regions of 11 healthy cats and 10 allergic cats were sampled and the V4 region of the bacterial 16S rRNA were analyzed by Older *et al.* [88]. It was demonstrated that the number of bacterial species was not significantly different between the healthy and allergic cats, however, the abundances of these bacterial species were different between healthy and allergic skin, and *Staphylococcus* was more abundant in allergic skin [88]. A similar study with 12 healthy and 6 allergic dogs revealed lower species richness relative to healthy dogs. Also the allergic dogs had lower proportions of the Betaproteobacteria *Ralstonia spp.* when compared to the healthy dogs [89].

Taken together, current evidence suggests skin commensals play a role in regulation of anti-inflammatory responses to chemical allergens. Future microbiome research can potentially shed light on possibility of managing skin sensitization reactions to chemicals through use of probiotics or therapies that target skin commensals and balance their immunomodulatory functions.

7.7   Conclusion

The skin microbiome of normal human skin is characterized by a high diversity and high inter-individual variation. While some studies in psoriasis and acne have found higher microbial diversity in skin lesions, several lines of evidence suggest that maintaining microbial diversity is beneficial to support the homeostasis of skin immunity. For instance, certain key microbes can elicit specific types of immune cells to the skin [18]. One of the key factors of skin barrier impairment, filaggrin deficiency, correlates with decreased bacterial diversity and a distinct bacterial colonization pattern. The dynamic communication between immune cells and microbiota is disturbed when the skin barrier is compromised in patients with inflammatory diseases, such as atopic dermatitis, and such inflammatory reactions are often accompanied by a reduction in the diversity of microbial communities and outgrowth of certain species, such as *Staphylococcus aureus*. Some examples of distinct differences in microbiota composition of diseased skin relative to the normal skin include but are not limited to: enhanced colonization by *S. aureus* in atopic and irritant contact dermatitis, and abundance of *P. acne* and *S. epidermidis* in acne, *Demodex* and *S. epidermidis* in rosacea, and *Malassezia* in dandruff scalp skin. A summary of various skin barrier impairments and associated changes in skin microbiome is shown in Table 7.1.

Table 7.1 Overview of skin barrier impairments and associated changes in microbiota.

Skin barrier impairment/disease	Changes in skin microbiome	References
Atopic Dermatitis	*S. aureus* ↑ Coagulase-negative *Staphylococcus* (CoNS) (e.g. *S. epidermidis*) ↓ *Malassezia* spp. ↓ *Actinobacteria* spp. ↓ *Corynebacterium* spp. ↓ *Propionibacterium* spp. ↓ Low diversity	[3–22]
Psoriasis	*Streptococcus* ↑ *Propionibacterium* ↓ *Malassezia* spp. ↑ *Staphylococcus* (↑ or ↓) *Firmicutes* (↑ or ↓) Lower, higher and unchanged diversity relative to normal skin reported in different studies	[23–34]
Acne	*Propionibacterium acnes* ↑ *S. epidermidis* ↑ *S. aureus* ↑ Firmicutes ↑ Proteobacteria ↓ High diversity	[35–45]
Rosacea	*Demodex folliculorum* ↑ (*bacillus oleronius* is cultured from this mite) *S. epidermidis* (with an altered secretory profile) ↑ *Chlamidya pneumonia* ↑ Low diversity	[46–62]
Seborrheic dermatitis and dandruff	*Malassezia* sp. and uncultured ↑ *Malassezia restrica* ↑ *Malassezia globosa* ↓ *S. epidermidis* ↑ *Staphylococcus* sp. *Propionibacterium acne* ↓ High diversity of fungal population	[62–73]

(Continued)

Table 7.1 Overview of skin barrier impairments and associated changes in microbiota. (*Continued*)

Skin barrier impairment/disease	Changes in skin microbiome	References
Diaper dermatitis	*Clostridium* spp. ↑ *Staphylococcus* spp. ↑ *Streptococcus* spp. ↑ *Enterococcus* spp. ↑ *C. albicans* ↑ *S. aureus* ↑	[76–79]
Occupational hand dermatitis	*S. aureus* ↑ Gram negative bacteria ↑ *Enterococci* ↑ *Candida* ↑ *S. hominis* ↑ Yeast ↑ Lower and higher diversity relative to normal skin reported in different studies	[80–83]

Understanding the skin microbiome of damaged and compromised skin is crucial for identification and development of therapeutic strategies for skin diseases. It is well known that microbiome findings are strongly influenced by study design and this should be a key consideration in evaluating skin microbiome studies aimed at comparing intact and compromised skin barrier. For instance, microbiome is not uniformly distributed in the stratum corneum. In diseased or injured skin, the transient microbiome of top layers is replaced by the microbiome that inhabits the deeper layers in a few weeks. Therefore utilizing sampling techniques that enable identification of the microbiome of deeper skin layers rather than that of superficial skin layer, may provide more accurate information [2]. Future research could address the current data gaps by using larger sample sizes, unified and more advanced sampling protocols and analytical techniques such as metatranscriptomics, which is utilized in understanding gut microbiome and provides an analysis of total RNA (both mRNA and rRNA) isolated from a microbial ecosystem [31], characterizing the impact of environmental pollutants and chemicals on skin microbiome, and a focus on understanding dynamics of the skin microbiome and recolonization pattern following skin damage.

References

1. Sanford, J.A. and Gallo, R.L., Functions of the skin microbiota in health and disease. *Semin. Immunol.*, 25, 370–377, 2013.
2. Zeeuwen, P.L., Boekhorst, J., van den Bogaard, E.H., de Koning, H.D., van de Kerkhof, P.M., Saulnier, D.M., van Swam, I.I., van Hijum, S.A., Kleerebezem, M., Schalkwijk, J., Timmerman, H.M., Microbiome dynamics of human epidermis following skin barrier disruption. *Genome Biol.*, 13, R101, 2012.
3. Powers, C.E., McShane, D.B., Gilligan, P.H., Burkhart, C.N., Morrell, D.S., Microbiome and pediatric atopic dermatitis, *J. Dermatol.*, 42, 1137–1142, 2015.
4. Lynde, C.W., Andriessen, A., Bertucci, V., McCuaig, C., Skotnicki, S., Weinstein, M., Wiseman, M., Zip, C., The skin microbiome in atopic dermatitis and its relationship to emollients, *J. Cutan. Med. Surg.*, 20, 21–28, 2016.
5. Nakatsuji, T. and Gallo, R.L., The role of the skin microbiome in atopic dermatitis. *Ann. Allergy, Asthma Immunol.*, 122, 263–269, 2019.
6. Baurecht, H., Rühlemann, M.C., Rodríguez, E., Thielking, F., Harder, I., Erkens, A.S., Stölzl, D., Ellinghaus, E., Hotze, M., Lieb, W., Wang, S., Heinsen-Groth, F.A., Franke, A., Weidinger, S., Epidermal lipid composition, barrier integrity, and eczematous inflammation are associated with skin microbiome configuration. *J. Allergy Clin. Immunol.*, 141, 1668–1676.e16, 2018.
7. Bjerre, R.D., Bandier, J., Skov, L., Engstrand, L., Johansen, J.D., The role of the skin microbiome in atopic dermatitis: A systematic review. *Br. J. Dermatol.*, 177, 1272–1278, 2017.
8. Williams, M.R. and Gallo, R.L., Evidence that Human Skin Microbiome Dysbiosis Promotes Atopic Dermatitis. *J. Invest. Dermatol.*, 137, 2460–2461, 2017.
9. Kong, H.H., Oh, J., Deming, C., Conlan, S., Grice, E.A., Beatson, M.A., Nomicos, E., Polley, E.C., Komarow, H.D., Murray, P.R., Turner, M.L., Segre, J.A., Segre, J.A., Temporal shifts in the skin microbiome associated with disease flares and treatment in children with atopic dermatitis. *Genome Res.*, 22, 850–859, 2012.
10. Clausen, M.L., Agner, T., Lilje, B., Edslev, S.M., Johannesen, T.B., Andersen, P.S., Association of disease severity with skin microbiome and filaggrin gene mutations in adult atopic dermatitis. *JAMA Dermatology.*, 154, 293–300, 2018.
11. Rosenthal, M., Goldberg, D., Aiello, A., Larson, E., Foxman, B., Skin microbiota: Microbial community structure and its potential association with health and disease. *Infect. Genet. Evol.*, 11, 839–848, 2011.
12. Williams, M. and Gallo, R., Role of the skin microbiome in atopic dermatitis. *Clin. Transl. Allergy*, 65, 15, 2015.
13. Natsuga, K., Cipolat, S., Watt, F.M., Increased bacterial load and expression of antimicrobial peptides in skin of barrier-deficient mice with reduced cancer susceptibility. *J. Invest. Dermatol.*, 136, 99–106, 2016.

14. Seité, S., Zelenkova, H., Martin, R., Clinical efficacy of emollients in atopic dermatitis patients - relationship with the skin microbiota modification. *Clin. Cosmet. Investig. Dermatol.*, 10, 25–33, 2017.

15. Chamlin, S., Frieden J., Fowler A., Ceramide-dominant, barrier-repair lipids improve childhood atopic dermatitis. *Arch. Dermatol.*,137, e1112, 2001.

16. Salava, A. and Lauerma, A., Role of the skin microbiome in atopic dermatitis, *Clin. Transl. Allergy*, 4, 33–38, 2014.

17. Meylan, P., Lang, C., Mermoud, S., Johannsen, A., Norrenberg, S., Hohl, D., Vial, Y., Prod'hom, G., Greub, G., Kypriotou, M., Christen-Zaech, S., Skin Colonization by *Staphylococcus aureus* Precedes the Clinical Diagnosis of Atopic Dermatitis in Infancy. *J. Invest. Dermatol.*, 137, 2497–2504, 2017.

18. Paller, A.S., Kong, H.H., Seed, P., Naik, S., Scharschmidt, T.C., Gallo, R.L., Luger, T., Irvine, A.D., The microbiome in patients with atopic dermatitis. *J. Allergy Clin. Immunol.*, 143, 26–35, 2019.

19. Wollina, U., Microbiome in atopic dermatitis, *Clin. Cosmet. Investig. Dermatol.*, 10, 51–56, 2017.

20. Kennedy, E.A., Connolly, J., Hourihane, J.O., Fallon, P.G., McLean, W.H.I., Murray, D., Jo, J.-H., Segre, J.A., Kong, H.H., Irvine, A.D., Skin microbiome before development of atopic dermatitis: Early colonization with commensal staphylococci at 2 months is associated with a lower risk of atopic dermatitis at 1 year. *J. Allergy Clin. Immunol.*, 139, 166–172, 2017.

21. Paller, A.S., Kong, H.H., Seed, P., Naik, S., Scharschmidt, T.C., Gallo, R.L., Luger, T., Irvine, A.D., The microbiome in patients with atopic dermatitisfile:///Users/Sara/Desktop/skin microbiome-2018/Bjerre_et_al-2017-British_Journal_of_Dermatology.pdf. *J. Allergy Clin. Immunol.*, 143, 26–35, 2019.

22. Scharschmidt, T.C., Vasquez, K.S., Truong, H.A., Gearty, S.V., Pauli, M.L., Nosbaum, A., Gratz, I.K., Otto, M., Moon, J.J., Liese, J., Abbas, A.K., Fischbach, M.A., Rosenblum, M.D., A Wave of Regulatory T Cells into Neonatal Skin Mediates Tolerance to Commensal Microbes. *Immunity.*, 43, 1011–1021, 2015.

23. Benhadou, F., Mintoff, D., Schnebert, B., Thio, H., Psoriasis and Microbiota: A Systematic Review. *Diseases.*, 6, 47, 2018.

24. Chang, H.W., Yan, D., Singh, R., Liu, J., Lu, X., Ucmak, D., Lee, K., Afifi, L., Fadrosh, D., Leech, J., Vasquez, K.S., Lowe, M.M., Rosenblum, M.D., Scharschmidt, T.C., Lynch, S.V., Liao, W., Alteration of the cutaneous microbiome in psoriasis and potential role in Th17 polarization. *Microbiome.*, 6, 1–27, 2018.

25. Alekseyenko, A.V., Perez-Perez, G.I., De Souza, A., Strober, B., Gao, Z., Bihan, M., Li, K., Methé, B.A., Blaser, M.J., Community differentiation of the cutaneous microbiota in psoriasis. *Microbiome.*, 1, 31, 2013.

26. Fahlén, A., Engstrand, L., Baker, B.S., Powles, A., Fry, L., Comparison of bacterial microbiota in skin biopsies from normal and psoriatic skin. *Arch. Dermatol. Res.*, 304, 15–22, 2012.

27. Gao, Z., Tseng, C., Strober, B.E., Pei, Z., Blaser, M.J., Substantial alterations of the cutaneous bacterial biota in psoriatic lesions. *PLoS One.*, 3, e2719, 2008.

28. Tett, A., Pasolli, E., Farina, S., Truong, D.T., Asnicar, F., Zolfo, M., Beghini, F., Armanini, F., Jousson, O., De Sanctis, V., Bertorelli, R., Girolomoni, G., Cristofolini, M., Segata, N., Unexplored diversity and strain-level structure of the skin microbiome associated with psoriasis. *NPJ Biofilms Microbiomes*, 3, 14, 2017.

29. Yan, D., Issa, N., Afifi, L., Jeon, C., Chang, H.W., Liao, W., The Role of the Skin and Gut Microbiome in Psoriatic Disease. *Curr. Dermatol. Rep.*, 6, 94–103, 2017.

30. Stehlikova, Z., Kostovcik, M., Kostovcikova, K., Kverka, M., Juzlova, K., Rob, F., Hercogova, J., Bohac, P., Pinto, Y., Uzan, A., Koren, O., Tlaskalova-Hogenova, H., Jiraskova Zakostelska, Z., Dysbiosis of Skin Microbiota in Psoriatic Patients: Co-occurrence of Fungal and Bacterial Communities. *Front. Microbiol.*, 10, 438, 2019.

31. Zeeuwen, P.L.J.M., Kleerebezem, M., Timmerman, H.M., Schalkwijk, J., Microbiome and skin diseases. *Curr. Opin. Allergy Clin. Immunol.*, 13, 514–520, 2013.

32. Zeeuwen, P.L.J.M., Ederveen, T.H.A., van der Krieken, D.A., Niehues, H., Boekhorst, J., Kezic, S., Hanssen, D.A.T., Otero, M.E., van Vlijmen-Willems, I.M.J.J., Rodijk-Olthuis, D., Falcone, D., van den Bogaard, E.H.J., Kamsteeg, M., de Koning, H.D., Zeeuwen-Franssen, M.E.J., van Steensel, M.A.M., Kleerebezem, M., Timmerman, H.M., van Hijum, S.A.F.T., Schalkwijk, J., Gram-positive anaerobe cocci are underrepresented in the microbiome of filaggrin-deficient human skin. *J. Allergy Clin. Immunol.*, 139, 1368–1371, 2017.

33. Martin R, Henley JB, Sarrazin P, Seité S., Skin microbiome in patients with psoriasis before and after balneotherapy at the thermal care center of La Roche-Posay. *J. Am. Acad. Dermatol.*, 14, 1400–1405, 2016.

34. Assarsson, M., Duvetorp, A., Dienus, O., Söderman, J., Seifert, O., Significant changes in the skin microbiome in patients with chronic plaque psoriasis after treatment with narrowband ultraviolet B. *Acta Derm. Venereol.*, 2018.

35. Thiboutot, D. and Del Rosso, J.Q., Acne Vulgaris and the Epidermal Barrier: Is Acne Vulgaris Associated with Inherent Epidermal Abnormalities that Cause Impairment of Barrier Functions? Do Any Topical Acne Therapies Alter the Structural and/or Functional Integrity of the Epidermal Barrier? *J. Clin. Aesthet. Dermatol.*, 6, 18–24, 2013.

36. Yamamoto, A., Takenouchi, K., Ito, M., Impaired water barrier function in acne vulgaris. *Arch. Dermatol. Res.*, 287, 214–8, 1995.

37. Kurokawa, I., Mayer-da-Silva, A., Gollnick, H., Orfanos, C.E., Monoclonal antibody labeling for cytokeratins and filaggrin in the human pilosebaceous unit of normal, seborrhoeic and acne skin. *J. Invest. Dermatol.*, 91, 566–71, 1988.

38. Dreno, B., Martin, R., Moyal, D., Henley, J.B., Khammari, A., Seité, S., Skin microbiome and acne vulgaris: *Staphylococcus*, a new actor in acne. *Exp. Dermatol.*, 26, 798–803, 2017.

39. Findley, K. and Grice, E.A., The Skin Microbiome: A Focus on Pathogens and Their Association with Skin Disease. *PLoS Pathog.*, 10, e1004436, 2014.

40. Jarrousse, V., Castex-Rizzi, N., Khammari, A., Charveron, M., Dréno, B., Modulation of integrins and filaggrin expression by Propionibacterium acnes extracts on keratinocytes. *Arch. Dermatol. Res.*, 299, 441–447, 2007.

41. Rocha, M.A. and Bagatin, E., Skin barrier and microbiome in acne. *Arch. Dermatol. Res.*, 310, 181–185, 2018.

42. Fitz-Gibbon, S., Tomida, S., Chiu, B.H., Nguyen, L., Du, C., Liu, M., Elashoff, D., Erfe, M.C., Loncaric, A., Kim, J., Modlin, R.L., Miller, J.F., Sodergren, E., Craft, N., Weinstock, G.M., Li, H., Propionibacterium acnes strain populations in the human skin microbiome associated with acne. *J. Invest. Dermatol.*, 133, 2152–2160, 2013.

43. Wang, Y., Kuo, S., Shu, M., Yu, J., Huang, S., Dai, A., Two, A., Gallo, R.L., Huang, C.-M., *Staphylococcus epidermidis* in the human skin microbiome mediates fermentation to inhibit the growth of Propionibacterium acnes: Implications of probiotics in acne vulgaris. *Appl. Microbiol. Biotechnol.*, 98, 411–24, 2014.

44. Numata, S., Akamatsu, H., Akaza, N., Yagami, A., Nakata, S., Matsunaga, K., Analysis of Facial Skin-Resident Microbiota in Japanese Acne Patients. *Dermatology.*, 228, 86–92, 2013.

45. Bek-Thomsen, M., Lomholt, H.B., Kilian, M., Acne is not associated with yet-uncultured bacteria. *J. Clin. Microbiol.*, 46, 3355–60, 2008.

46. Falay Gur, T., Erdemir, A.V., Gurel, M.S., Kocyigit, A., Guler, E.M., Erdil, D., The investigation of the relationships of demodex density with inflammatory response and oxidative stress in rosacea. *Arch. Dermatol. Res.*, 310, 759–767, 2018.

47. Holmes, A.D., Potential role of microorganisms in the pathogenesis of rosacea. *J. Am. Acad. Dermatol.*, 69, 1025–1032, 2013.

48. Forton, F., Germaux, M.A., Brasseur, T., De Liever, A., Laporte, M., Mathys, C., Sass, U., Stene, J.J., Thibaut, S., Tytgat, M., Seys, B., Demodicosis and rosacea: Epidemiology and significance in daily dermatologic practice. *J. Am. Acad. Dermatol.*, 2005.

49. Casas, C., Paul, C., Lahfa, M., Livideanu, B., Lejeune, O., Alvarez-Georges, S., Saint-Martory, C., Degouy, A., Mengeaud, V., Ginisty, H., Durbise, E., Schmitt, A.M., Redoulès, D., Quantification of Demodex folliculorum by PCR in rosacea and its relationship to skin innate immune activation. *Exp. Dermatol.*, 21, 906–907, 2012.

50. Roihu, T. and Kariniemi, A.L., Demodex mites in acne rosacea. *J. Cutan. Pathol.*, 25, 550–552, 1998.

51. Bonamigo, R.R., Bakos, L., Edelweiss, M., Cartellt, A., Could matrix melalloproteinase-9 be a link between Demodex folliculorum and rosacea?, *J. Eur. Acad. Dermatol. Venereol.,* 19, 646–647, 2005.

52. Chang, Y.-S. and Huang, Y.-C., Role of Demodex mite infestation in rosacea: A systematic review and meta-analysis. *J. Am. Acad. Dermatol.,* 77, 441–447. e6, 2017.

53. Dai, X., Sayama, K., Tohyama, M., Shirakata, Y., Hanakawa, Y., Tokumaru, S., Yang, L., Hirakawa, S., Hashimoto, K., Mite allergen is a danger signal for the skin via activation of inflammasome in keratinocytes. *J. Allergy Clin. Immunol.,* 127, 806–814, 2011.

54. Lacey, N., Delaney, S., Kavanagh, K., Powell, F.C., Mite-related bacterial antigens stimulate inflammatory cells in rosacea. *Br. J. Dermatol.,* 157, 474–481, 2007.

55. O'Reilly, N., Bergin, D., Reeves, E.P., McElvaney, N.G., Kavanagh, K., Demodex-associated bacterial proteins induce neutrophil activation. *Br. J. Dermatol.,* 166, 753–760, 2012.

56. Yamasaki, K., Di Nardo, A., Bardan, A., Murakami, M., Ohtake, T., Coda, A., Dorschner, R.A., Bonnart, C., Descargues, P., Hovnanian, A., Morhenn, V.B., Gallo, R.L., Increased serine protease activity and cathelicidin promotes skin inflammation in rosacea. *Nat. Med.,* 13, 975–980, 2007.

57. Yamasaki, K., Kanada, K., MacLeod, D.T., Borkowski, A.W., Morizane, S., Nakatsuji, T., Cogen, A.L., Gallo, R.L., TLR2 expression is increased in rosacea and stimulates enhanced serine protease production by keratinocytes. *J. Invest. Dermatol.,* 131, 688–697, 2011.

58. Dahl, M.V., Ross, A.J., Schlievert, P.M., Temperature regulates bacterial protein production: Possible role in rosacea. *J. Am. Acad. Dermatol.,* 50, 266–272, 2004.

59. Holmes, A.D. and Steinhoff, M., Integrative concepts of rosacea pathophysiology, clinical presentation and new therapeutics. *Exp. Dermatol.,* 26, 659–667, 2017.

60. Whitfeld, M., Gunasingam, N., Leow, L.J., Shirato, K., Preda, V., *Staphylococcus epidermidis:* A possible role in the pustules of rosacea. *J. Am. Acad. Dermatol.,* 64, 49–52, 2011.

61. Cheung, G.Y.C., Duong, A.C., Otto, M., Direct and synergistic hemolysis caused by *Staphylococcus* phenol-soluble modulins: Implications for diagnosis and pathogenesis. *Microbes Infect.,* 14, 380–386, 2012.

62. Fernandez-Obregon, A. and Patton, D.L., The role of Chlamydia pneumoniae in the etiology of acne rosacea: Response to the use of oral azithromycin. *Cutis.,* 79, 163–167, 2007.

63. Harding, C.R., Moore, A.E., Rogers, S.J., Meldrum, H., Scott, A.E., McGlone, F.P., Dandruff: A condition characterized by decreased levels of intercellular lipids in scalp stratum corneum and impaired barrier function. *Arch. Dermatol. Res.,* 294, 221–230, 2002.

64. Ro, B.I. and Dawson, T.L., The Role of Sebaceous Gland Activity and Scalp Microfloral Metabolism in the Etiology of Seborrheic Dermatitis and Dandruff. *J. Investig. Dermatology Symp. Proc.*, 10, 194–197, 2005.

65. DeAngelis, Y.M., Gemmer, C.M., Kaczvinsky, J.R., Kenneally, D.C., Schwartz, J.R., Dawson, T.L., Three Etiologic Facets of Dandruff and Seborrheic Dermatitis: Malassezia Fungi, Sebaceous Lipids, and Individual Sensitivity. *J. Investig. Dermatology Symp. Proc.*, 10, 295–297, 2005.

66. Saxena, R., Mittal, P., Clavaud, C., Dhakan, D.B., Hegde, P., Veeranagaiah, M.M., Saha, S., Souverain, L., Roy, N., Breton, L., Misra, N., Sharma, V.K., Comparison of Healthy and Dandruff Scalp Microbiome Reveals the Role of Commensals in Scalp Health. *Front. Cell. Infect. Microbiol.*, 8, 346, 2018.

67. Soares, R.C., Camargo-Penna, P.H., de Moraes, V.C.S., De Vecchi, R., Clavaud, C., Breton, L., Braz, A.S.K., Paulino, L.C., Dysbiotic Bacterial and Fungal Communities Not Restricted to Clinically Affected Skin Sites in Dandruff. *Front. Cell. Infect. Microbiol.*, 6, 157–166, 2016.

68. Xu, Z., Wang, Z., Yuan, C., Liu, X., Yang, F., Wang, T., Wang, J., Manabe, K., Qin, O., Wang, X., Zhang, Y., Zhang, M., Dandruff is associated with the conjoined interactions between host and microorganisms. *Sci. Rep.*, 6: 24877, 2016.

69. Tajima, M., Sugita, T., Nishikawa, A., Tsuboi, R., Molecular analysis of Malassezia microflora in seborrheic dermatitis patients: Comparison with other diseases and healthy subjects. *J. Invest. Dermatol.*, 128, 345–51, 2008.

70. Clavaud, C., Jourdain, R., Bar-Hen, A., Tichit, M., Bouchier, C., Pouradier, F., El Rawadi, C., Guillot, J., Ménard-Szczebara, F., Breton, L., Latgé, J.-P., Mouyna, I., Dandruff Is Associated with Disequilibrium in the Proportion of the Major Bacterial and Fungal Populations Colonizing the Scalp. *PLoS One.*, 8, e58203, 2013.

71. Gupta, A. and Bluhm, R., Seborrheic dermatitis. *J. Eur. Acad. Dermatology Venereol.*, 18, 13–26, 2004.

72. Dessinioti, C. and Katsambas, A., Seborrheic dermatitis: Etiology, risk factors, and treatments: Facts and controversies. *Clin. Dermatol.*, 4, 343–351, 2013.

73. Tamer, F., Yuksel, M.E., Sarifakioglu, E., Karabag, Y., *Staphylococcus aureus* is the most common bacterial agent of the skin flora of patients with seborrheic dermatitis. *Dermatol. Pract. Concept.*, 8, 80–84, 2018.

74. Prescott, S.L., Larcombe, D.L., Logan, A.C., West, C., Burks, W., Caraballo, L., Levin, M., Etten, E.V., Horwitz, P., Kozyrskyj, A., Campbell, D.E., The skin microbiome: Impact of modern environments on skin ecology, barrier integrity, and systemic immune programming. *World Allergy Organ. J.*, 10, 1–16, 2017.

75. Wallen-Russell, C., The Role of Every-Day Cosmetics in Altering the Skin Microbiome: A Study Using Biodiversity. *Cosmetics.*, 6, 2, 2018. Wallen-Russell, Christopher.

76. Šikić Pogačar, M., Maver, U., Marčun Varda, N., Mičetić-Turk, D., Diagnosis and management of diaper dermatitis in infants with emphasis on skin microbiota in the diaper area, 2018.

77. Capone, K.A., Dowd, S.E., Stamatas, G.N., Nikolovski, J., Diversity of the Human Skin Microbiome Early in Life. *J. Invest. Dermatol.*, 131, 2026–2032, 2011.

78. Grice, E.A. and Segre, J.A., The skin microbiome, *Nat. Rev. Microbiol.*, 9, 244–253, 2011.

79. Şenses, D.A., Öztürk, C.E., Yar, N.E., Acar, S., Bahçebaşi, T., Kocabay, K., Kaya, D., Do baby wet wipes change periurethral aerobic flora? *Jpn. J. Infect. Dis*, 12, 59–67, 2007.

80. Larson, E.L., Hughes, C.A.N., Pyrek, J.D., Sparks, S.M., Cagatay, E.U., Bartkus, J.M., Changes in bacterial flora associated with skin damage on hands of health care personnel. *Am. J. Infect. Control.*, 26, 513–521, 1998.

81. Larson, E., Effects of handwashing agent, handwashing frequency, and clinical area on hand flora. *AJIC Am. J. Infect. Control.*, 12, 76–82, 1984.

82. Rocha, L.A., Ferreira de Almeida e Borges, L., Gontijo Filho, P.P., Changes in hands microbiota associated with skin damage because of hand hygiene procedures on the health care workers. *Am. J. Infect. Control.*, 37, 155–159, 2009.

83. Borges, L.F. d A. e, Silva, B.L., Gontijo Filho, P.P., Hand washing: Changes in the skin flora. *Am. J. Infect. Control.*, 35, 417–420, 2007.

84. Knaysi, G., Smith, A.R., Wilson, J.M., Wisniewski, J.A., The Skin as a Route of Allergen Exposure: Part II. Allergens and Role of the Microbiome and Environmental Exposures, *Curr. Allergy. Asthma. Rep.*, 17, 7–19, 2017.

85. Schommer, N.N. and Gallo, R.L., Structure and function of the human skin microbiome. *Trends Microbiol.*, 21, 660–668, 2013.

86. Shane, H.L., Long, C.M., Anderson, S.E., Novel cutaneous mediators of chemical allergy, *J. Immunotoxicol.*, 16,13–27, 2019.

87. Hacini-Rachinel, F., Gheit, H., Le Luduec, J.B., Dif, F., Nancey, S., Kaiserlian, D., Oral probiotic control skin inflammation by acting on both effector and regulatory T cells. *PLoS One.*, 4, e4903, 2009.

88. Older, C.E., Diesel, A., Patterson, A.P., Meason-Smith, C., Johnson, T.J., Mansell, J., Suchodolski, J.S., Hoffmann, A.R., The feline skin microbiota: The bacteria inhabiting the skin of healthy and allergic cats. *PLoS One.*, 12, e0178555, 2017.

89. Hoffmann, A.R., Patterson, A.P., Diesel, A., Lawhon, S.D., Ly, H.J., Stephenson, C.E., Mansell, J., Steiner, J.M., Dowd, S.E., Olivry, T., Suchodolski, J.S., The skin microbiome in healthy and allergic dogs. *PLoS One.*, 9, e83197, 2014.

90. Alpha diversity, https://en.wikipedia.org/wiki/Alpha_diversity.

8

Human Cutaneous Ectoparasites: A Brief Overview and Potential Therapeutic Role for Demodex

Stephen L. Strobel

Mercy Health - St. Vincent Medical Center, Toledo, OH

Abstract

Ectoparasites of human skin, which include chiggers, bed bugs, lice, scabies and Demodex (folliculorum and brevis) are discussed. A more detailed focus is directed to Demodex, particularly Demodex folliculorum (DF), with regard to its purported role in rosacea and blepharitis, it's potential beneficial role in the maintenance of skin (hair follicle) health and its possible application as a drug delivery agent for early skin cancers. Limitations to this hypothetical application are addressed, as well as potential future directions for this concept.

Keywords: Demodex, ectoparasite, pilosebaceous unit, antibody drug complex

8.1 Introduction

Cutaneous ectoparasites are tiny animals (mites, related to spiders, ticks and fleas), that comprise a relatively minor component of the human microbiome. These include: chiggers, bed bugs, lice, scabies and Demodex (folliculorum and brevis). Most exist as transient pathogens that require blood or tissue meals for reproduction and sustenance. Our immune system naturally reacts against these foreign invaders, attempting to expel them from our skin into the surrounding environment. Our affiliation with the majority of these organisms is neither symbiotic nor entirely benign [1],

Email: Skullman57@AOL.com

Nava Dayan (ed.) *Skin Microbiome Handbook: From Basic Research to Product Development*, (171–184) © 2020 Scrivener Publishing LLC

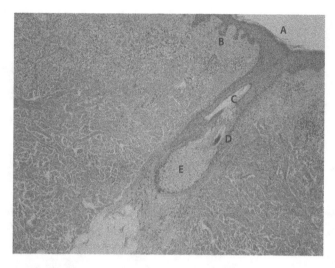

Figure 8.1 Histologic section of a Demodex mite in a pilosebaceous unit of human skin. A) skin surface, B) dermal-epidermal junction, C) hair shaft, D) Demodex mite, E) sebaceous gland. (Hematoxylin and eosin stain, 40x).

as they can transmit several potentially serious blood borne diseases. Therefore, although our association is ancient, it also contentious.

Demodex [2, 3] represents the exception, having evolved with us in an essentially harmonious and symbiotic relationship. As differences in our skin features evolved with our migrations around the world thousands of years ago to acclimate to different climates and sun exposure, our Demodex partners evolved to successfully coexist with us [4]. The vast majority of us complete our lives totally unaware that these specific mites even exist, a testimony to their adaptation.

In this chapter, the life cycle and clinical significance of each of these ectoparasites is briefly discussed. Greater focus is directed to Demodex (see Figure 8.1), addressing features of our intimate relationship and their potential use as a cutaneous drug delivery agent. Limitations and benefits are considered, with the hope of stimulating future research, interest and applications.

8.2   Chiggers (Trombiculidae)

Chiggers [5, 6] also known as berry bugs, red bugs and harvest mites, are common inhabitants of low level of vegetation. Their prevalence is greatest in the late spring to early summer, when grasses, weeds and other low-level vegetation flourish. Their life cycle (egg to larva to nymph to adult) occurs predominately on vegetation, with only the larval stage requiring animal contact. The larval stage attaches to the skin of animals, including humans, that come into contact with infested vegetation. The nymphs feed on host skin via a stylostome, a channel which they create in the skin and inject digestive enzymes to feed on nutrients in the skin cells. These digestive enzymes induce a localized pruritic reaction.

In the United States and Mexico, T. Alfreddugesi (berry mite) predominates, in Western Europe and Eastern Asia, T. autumnalis (harvest mite), and in Australia T. hirsti (scrub-itch mite). Chiggers do not transmit other diseases in North America or Western Eurasia, but are a vector for scrub typhus (Orientia tsutsugamushi) in Eastern Asia and the South Pacific.

8.3   Bedbugs (Cimex lectularius and Hemipterus)

Bedbugs [7-9] prey on a wide variety of warm blooded animals. These two species preferentially seek human hosts. Adults are approximately 0.25 inches in length, flat, oval and range from whitish to tan to brown. After a blood meal, they can double in size and become reddish (blood colored). As their name implies, these mites have evolved to reside close to humans in beds, couches and similar structures that permit close proximity for feeding, mainly at night. Their bites can cause irritation (pruritus), but the effect is usually self-limited. Secondary infections are uncommon. They are cold blooded and prefer to reside away from the natural warmth of our bodies, except when feeding. Adult females, when fertile, usually lay a single egg per day. Eggs require 10 days to hatch. Nymphs cycle through five stages toward maturity and require a blood meal to successfully molt through each stage.

After World War 2, bedbugs appeared to be essentially eradicated through improved hygiene and the widespread use of pesticides. However, with increased human population densities, more prevalent travel patterns, and evolving mite pesticide residence, the number and distribution of bedbugs has rapidly expanded in recent decades. Eradication is difficult since bedbugs can reside on almost any surface in a room when not feeding. They are not known to transmit blood borne diseases.

8.4   Lice

Human lice infestations occur in three forms: body lice (Pediculus humanus corporus), head lice (Pediculus capitis) and pubic lice (Pthirus pubis)

[10, 11]. These subtypes have evolved slight variations in body and leg morphology that allow them to inhabit and exploit certain body regions while coexisting without direct competition: hair on the head (Pediculus capitis), body clothing (Pediculus corporus) and pubic hair (Pthirus pubis). They occur worldwide and are readily transmitted through close physical bodily contact and association with infected clothing.

Lice lay their eggs (nits) on hairs or on clothing and visit the skin periodically for blood meals. By colonizing hair shafts and clothing slightly removed from the skin surface, they benefit from the thermal energy of their host while minimizing host immune response. Eradication can be achieved through clean hygiene (cleansing of clothing at temperatures exceeding 130 degrees Fahrenheit) and avoiding contact with other infected individuals.

Symptoms of infestation are generally mild. Localized pruritus and cutaneous rash may occur as allergic reactions to their bites and waste products. However, body lice can also serve as vectors for potentially serious diseases, which include: epidemic typhus, relapsing fever and trench fever, caused by Rickettsia prowazekii, Borrelia recurrentis and Bartonella quintana, respectively. Depending on severity, these diseases may be self-limited or require systemic medical therapy.

8.5   Scabies (Sarcoptes scabiei) [12, 13]

Scabies are a highly contagious infestation spread through skin-to-skin contact [14]. Adults are 0.2-0.4 mm in length, straw colored and eyeless. Fifteen to twenty female mites may occupy a single host, and are viable for only several hours if removed from the host. Their life cycle is 14-17 days. Infections may be present in the initial phase for 4-6 weeks before symptoms occur. During this time, the host is infectious and can unknowingly transmit the disease to other hosts. Subsequent infections elicit a more rapid (anamnestic) response within 3-4 days.

Female scabies mites burrow into the epidermis and lay 2-3 eggs per day within cutaneous tunnels. Larvae hatch in 48 hours. Developing mites progress through a six legged larval phase and two eight legged nymphal phases within the skin. Adult females and immature forms feed on nutrients in the skin and hair follicles.

Immune reaction to the mites, eggs, larvae and waste products elicit intense pruritus, leading to the nickname "itch mite," with a pimple-like rash occurring at the affected site. Extreme excoriation can cause secondary bacterial infections. Severe consequences are uncommon, but may occur in immunocompromised hosts. Hyperinfestation can result in numerous adjacent tunnels with crusted skin, referred to as crusted or Norwegian scabies. Hyperinfested individuals are highly contagious and may serve as a reservoir for infecting numerous hosts in hospitals and nursing homes. No systemic pathogens have been associated with this mite.

8.6   Demodex

Demodex mites are ubiquitous throughout the animal populations of the world and have been shown to exist in nearly all mammals, with the exception of monotremes (platypus and echidna) [15]. The type of mite is generally specific to their animal host. Demodex are obligate ectoparasites which exist in or near pilosebaceous units in the skin.

Two species occur in humans: Demodex folliculorum (DF) and Demodex brevis (DB), with DF numerically representing the dominant species. DF tend to concentrate in the facial region (cheeks, nose, chin, forehead, eyelashes and eyebrows), but may also populate other hair bearing regions. DB typically occupy the pilosebaceous units (PSU) of the trunk and extremities. The prevalence of both species varies in different studies, but recent analyses that examine Demodex DNA suggest that essentially all humans acquire these mites via contact with close relatives and carry them from adolescence (when the PSU matures) through the remainder of life, with increasing density observed with advancing age and sun exposure. Their coevolution with humans has been highly successful and they generally exist unnoticed (asymptomatic).

Demodex belong to the family Demodicidae, class Arachnida, order Acarina. Adult DF measure 0.3-0.4 mm in length. DB are slightly shorter, 0.15-0.2 mm in length. Because of their small size, the mites are invisible to the naked eye and require microscopic examination for identification. Each mite is composed of two fused body segments, with eight short segmented legs attached to the first body segment. External scales are present over the body, which appear to assist in anchoring the mites in hair follicles for feeding and resting. DF appears to feed predominately on follicular lining cells, while DB consumes sebum and fatty acids that accumulate in the follicles.

Male Demodex mites are slightly longer than their female counterparts. Both sexes have genital openings. Mating occurs on the skin surface near the openings of the hair follicles at night and fertilization is internal. The fertilized eggs are laid inside of the follicles or in sebaceous glands. Larvae hatch after approximately 3-4 days and develop into mature adults in 7 days. Mites typically live for 14 days, although some may live slightly longer if local competition and stress are low. Demodex have no anus, so digestive waste products and bacteria accumulate throughout each mite's life. These are released into the follicle and surrounding tissue when the mites die and decompose.

DF occupy the upper region of the PSU canal. DB burrows more deeply in to the canal where the sebaceous glands exist. Several DF typically occupy a single PSU, with a density of up to 5 mites/square centimeter in healthy skin. Higher density suggests pathogenic potential. Single DB generally occupy involved PSU and are therefore less often implicated with disease symptoms.

8.7 The Association Between Demodex, Rosacea and Blepharitis

Demodex mites necessarily coexist with a plethora of other cutaneous microfauna, including bacteria, fungi and viruses. Under normal conditions, this balanced coexistence goes unnoticed by the host and acts as natural biological barrier against potentially pathogenic agents. Under conditions of altered host immunity (immunosuppression), the normally innocuous microfauna can increase in density to a level that elicits a symptomatic cutaneous infection. The inciting cause of the immunosuppression can be localized (topical steroids) or systemic (HIV/AIDS, antineoplastic chemotherapy, congenital immune deficiency).

On the face, the cutaneous reaction manifests as rosacea [16]. Rosacea is characterized by localized erythema (redness), swelling and pimples (hair follicles plugged with sebum, bacteria and cellular debris). The clogged follicles may become secondarily infected and contain purulent material.

When the localized reaction occurs around the eyelids, it is known as blepharitis [17]. Although similar to rosacea, the inflammation and infection occur in and around meibomian glands, specialized oil glands in the eyelids. In the setting of Demodex hyper infestation, both rosacea and blepharitis appear to have allergic and inflammatory/infectious components.

Augmented Demodex mite density has been implicated in these conditions. However, recent studies have suggested that coexistent bacterial overgrowth and infection may represent the dominate culprit [18]. Bacillus oleronius, a symbiotic gram negative bacteria that resides in Demodex hindgut, and *Staphylococcus epidermidis*, a gram positive coccus indigenous in the skin and skin appendages, are the primary infectious bacterial agents. Therapeutic response (resolution) of these conditions with antibacterial medications supports this supposition, although Demodex may also be sensitive to these agents. Therefore, the potential contributory role of these mites cannot be entirely excluded.

Demodex mites demonstrate different genetic signatures [19], corresponding to our ancestral migration out of Africa about 100,000 years ago to inhabit multiple regions throughout the earth. Several different clades of mites have been identified that are slightly different among individuals from various geographic regions, corresponding to adaptive changes in our skin related to environmental differences (temperature, sun exposure, humidity) in these regions. This has anthropological significance (permitting the study of human migration patterns via Demodex DNA analysis). It also strongly suggests adaptive coevolution by Demodex to maximize efficiency and survival in these slightly varied PSU, which may differ in hair structure, sebum production, and pH, in humans of these different regions. Within given areas, mites are typically more genetically similar among related individuals when compared those who are not closely related. While the geographic variations in mite DNA offer selective advantage to the Demodex, it should also be considered that these variations could also benefit the human hosts by establishing more robust hair follicles.

8.8   Hypothesis

Demodex folliculorum could be used in tandem to deliver topical medications directly to the dermal-epidermal junction, via PSU, to maximize efficiency, minimize systemic toxicity and limit the need for surgical intervention in certain early skin cancers, and possibly certain forms of dermatosis/dermatitis. Diseases to consider for investigation include early melanoma and nonmelanoma skin cancers, alopecia, acne (rosacea), and blepharitis.

8.9   Demodex Folliculorum as a Drug Delivery Agent for Early Skin Cancer

DF provides a potentially unique mechanism for drug delivery to the dermal-epidermal junction for the treatment of early skin cancer [20]. Tumor cells targeted with drug linked antibodies directed to specific cellular antigens (antibody drug complex methodology, referred to as ADC) [21] would permit focused cytolysis in a restricted therapeutic zone in the skin (see Figure 8.2). Drug-antibody complexes can function through a variety of mechanisms, including induced tumor cell apoptosis, immune mediated cytotoxicity and phagocytosis, and tumor cell growth arrest. Monoclonal antibody therapies directed against basal cell carcinoma, squamous cell carcinoma and melanoma currently exist as systemic therapies [22, 23]. This proposed drug delivery system would employ these agents via local application, allowing high drug concentration at the tumor site with presumably limited systemic toxicity.

The ADC could be passively attached to DF at night (when the mites visit the skin surface), with the ADC embedded in a topical cream or ointment. Linkage of the ADC directly to the mites via antibodies directed to specific Demodex antigens could also be investigated, to enhance sufficient mite labeling with the drug complexes before the return of the mites into the PSU. Activating agents for the ADC, such as photo or thermal activation, could also be investigated to augment tumor cell destruction (see Figure 8.3).

Paradoxically, if DF can be successfully labeled with ADC, its potential use in the treatment of rosacea and blepharitis at the level of the PSU might be investigated. Although DF does not appear to represent a significant

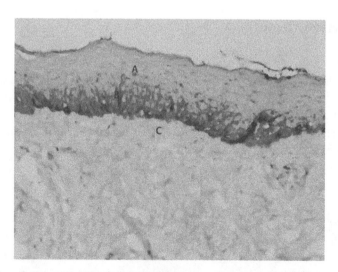

Figure 8.2 Immunohistochemical stain of human skin highlighting melanoma cells at the dermal-epidermal junction. A) normal epithelial cells (gray), B) melanoma cells (red), C) dermal epidermal junction. Melanoma triple cocktail (HMB45/A103/T311), mouse monoclonal antibodies, Roche Diagnostics. 40x.

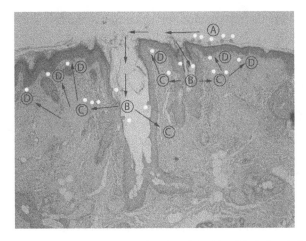

Figure 8.3 A) Demodex mites (represented with red dots) are labeled with drug complexes (represented with white dots) on skin surface, B) mites return into hair follicles below the dermal-epidermal junction (DEJ) with attached medication, C) activated drug diffuses into the upper dermis to the DEJ in the region of the hair follicles, D) activated drug selectively reacts with and destroys tumor cells at the DEJ. 20x Figure 8.3 depicts the utilization of the natural nocturnal migration of DF mites to the skin surface for the initial drug complex labeling of the mites. By day they return to the mid portion of the PSU (with drug complex attached) for feeding and egg laying. Here the drug complex can be released into the PSU and surrounding dermis at a concentration corresponding to the local mite density. Contact of the drug complex with the predetermined epidermal epitope(s) leads to selective cytolysis at the DF. With sufficient mite density, an intense but localized antineoplastic response could theoretically be achieved.

causative factor of alopecia, it could serve as a delivery agent for medications that stimulate hair growth, such as minoxidil, directly in to the PSU.

8.10   Limitations

Under current conditions, consideration of DF as a drug delivery agent has significant limitations. Research that successfully addresses these limitations would be necessary before drug development and clinical trials could be implemented. Several of these potential limitations are outlined below.

- Sufficient mite density necessary to provide adequate drug concentration for a desired cytotoxic effect at a give site must be defined and achievable.
- DF cannot currently be grown outside of the human host (*in vitro*), so artificial enhancement of mite density would

need to occur in patient host's skin. This may be difficult and potentially locally irritating to the skin. Labeling of naturally occurring commensal bacteria in the DF hind-gut (Bacillus oleronius), which can be cultivated in the laboratory and applied to the skin, might serve as an alternative.

- Drugs utilized for the treatment of early skin cancers could potentially be toxic to DF. Mites would need to retain sufficient viability to migrate from the skin surface into PSU for the drug delivery and activation to function appropriately.
- The extent of diffusion of drugs between PSU (diffusion coefficient) would be dependent on the density of and distance between PSU at a given site. Insufficient medication concentration and therapeutic response could result if PSU are present in low density and/or widely spaced.
- The potential for the therapy related release of neoplastic cells in to dermal lymphatics, and ultimately into systemic circulation, would need to be ruled out.
- Treatment applications are currently limited to cutaneous sites naturally inhabited by Demodex mites.
- The treatment must be aesthetically acceptable to patients and cost effective when compared to current therapeutic modalities.

8.11   Conclusion

DF and DB are the only permanent cutaneous ectoparasites in humans. Through millions of years of adaptive coevolution with our hominid ancestors, these mites are virtually ideal symbiotic copartners that typically exist with us without negative consequence to the host or parasite. Their consistent presence in and on regions of our hair bearing skin suggests the opportunity to explore their use as a drug delivery system for selected cutaneous conditions; in particular, early skin cancer. A variety of delivery mechanisms could be considered, including microparticles, nanoparticles and ADC, which are already established as delivery mechanisms in other settings.

The ubiquitous existence of Demodex organisms throughout the majority of mammalian species provides a plethora of options for animal experimenting prior to human trials. Animal studies would help to define focused enhancement of the Demodex population at a chosen site, viability of drug delivery systems, achievable and desirable intradermal drug concentrations, diffusion coefficients for selected drugs in the dermis, and the efficiency of the selective destruction of specific types of cells at the dermal-epidermal junction. Rigorous histologic assessment of these cutaneous sites, focused on the selected cell types pre and post therapy would define the efficacies of the drugs evaluated.

Ultimately, human trials would be refined, based upon the results of these animal studies, before implementation. In its current construct, this proposed drug delivery system is conjectural and hypothetical. Definite limitations exist, as outlined previously. However, the potential significant benefits of a non-surgical treatment for early skin cancer, which might include reduced local morbidity and scarring, should be considered. If successful, this application could benefit many patients worldwide.

8.12   Future Considerations

If the proposed utilization of DF is proven to be a valid mechanism for cutaneous drug delivery, the establishment of sufficient local mite density would remain as a major limitation. Investigation of laboratory (*in vitro*) methods of growing and harvesting mites would be warranted. To achieve this, several factors would need to be successfully addressed. Demodex mites thrive in their natural host skin micro environment. Cultivation of the host's own skin cells would permit the greatest potential for extracorporeal mite growth.

An artificial nutrient media that allows the extra corporeal growth and reproduction of the Demodex mites could be identified. While this is not currently available, commercial production of specialized human tissues, including skin, is on the horizon. A substrate that effectively matches human skin is necessary to support the complex life cycle of these ectoparasites. The lack of a host immune response in the artificial setting would enhance mite viability.

Transfer of mites from host skin to growth substrate for cultivation and drug labeling and return to host skin is required. Temporary direct contact between host skin and substrate may represent the most efficient means. Transport via cutaneous patch might be less efficient but more esthetically acceptable. Ultimately, if high DF concentration can be created in an artificial setting, antibodies directed to specific mite antigens could ensure linkage to carrier mites.

Even if these developments are successful, the issue of patient acceptance must be addressed. The concept of mites living on and in our skin for the majority of our lives is uncomfortable to accept, even though it is natural and potentially beneficial. But awareness of our complex microbiome and its role in health maintenance is increasing rapidly, particularly via internet media. Widespread use of bacteria as probiotics and the utility of bacteria and viruses for drug delivery is already accepted by many individuals. Education about use of our own cutaneous microfauna for beneficial purposes should enhance its endorsement.

The author would like to thank Amy L. Steele for typeset and copyedit of this chapter.

References

1. Mathison, B. and Pritt, B., Laboratory Identification of Arthropod Ectoparasites. *Clin. Microbiol. Rev*, 27, 1, 48–67, 2014 Jan.
2. Rather, P.A. and Hassan, I., Human *Demodex* Mite: The Versatile Mite of Dermatological Importance. *Indian J Dermatol.*, 59, 60–6, 2014.
3. Thoemmes, M.S., Fergus, D.J., Urban, J., Trautwein, M., Dunn, R.R., Ubiquity and Diversity of Human-Associated Demodex Mites. *PLoS ONE*, 9, 8, e106265, 2014. https://doi.org/10.1371/journal.pone.0106265.
4. Palopoli, M.F., Fergus, D.J., Minot, S., Pei, D.T., Simison, W.B., Fernandez-Silva, I., Thoemmes, M.S., Dunn, R.R., Trautwein, M., Global divergence of the human follicle mite Demodex folliculorum: Persistent associations between host ancestry and mite lineages. *PNAS*, 112, 52, 15958–15963, December 29, 2015.
5. Stöppler, MD, Medical Author: M C and Shiel, Medical Editor: W C., MD, FACP, FACR. Jr., Chiggers (Bites) Symptoms, Pictures, Home Remedies, Medicine, and Cure. https://www.medicinenet.com/chiggers_bites/article.htm#chiggers_definition_and_facts, May 16, 2017.
6. Hohenberger, M., M.D. and Elston, D., M.D., Environmental Dermatology What's Eating You? Chiggers. *Cutis.*, 99, 6, 386–388, 2017 June.
7. Woloski, J.R., Burman, D., Adebona, O., Mite and bed bug infections. *Prim Care*, 45, 3, 409–421, 2018.
8. Doggett, S., Dwyer, D., Pablo, P., Russell, R., Bed Bugs: Clinical Relevance and Control Options. *Clin Microbiol Rev*, 25, 1, 164–192, 2012 Jan.
9. Wang, C., Singh, N., Zha, C., Cooper, R., Bed Bugs: Prevalence in Low-Income Communities, Resident's Reactions, and Implementation of a Low-Cost Inspection Protocol. *J. Med. Entomol.*, 53, 3, 639–646, 1 May 2016. https://doi.org/10.1093/jme/tjw018.
10. Bonilla, D.L., Durden, L.A., Eremeeva, M.E., Dasch, G.A., The Biology and Taxonomy of Head and Body Lice—Implications for Louse-Borne Disease Prevention. *PLOS Pathogens*, 9, 11, e1003724, 2013. https://doi.org/10.1371/journal.ppat.1003724.

11. Sangaré, A.K., Doumbo, O.K., Raoult, D., Management and Treatment of Human Lice. *BioMed Res Int*, 2016, 12, 2016. Article ID 8962685 https://doi.org/10.1155/2016/8962685.
12. Thomas, J., Peterson, G.M., Walton, S.F., Carson, C.F., Naunton, M., Baby, K.E., Scabies: An ancient global disease with a need for new therapies. *BMC Infectious Diseases*, 15, 250, 2015.
13. Seidelman MD, J., Garza MD, R.M., Smith MD, C.M., Fowler, V.G., MD, MHS Jr., More than a Mite Contagious: Crusted Scabies. *Am J Med*, 130, 9, 1042–1044, 2017-09-01.
14. Chandler, D.J. and Fuller, L.C., A Review of Scabies: An Infestation More Than Skin Deep. *Dermatology* (Review Article), 235, 79–90, 2019.
15. Litwin, D., Chen, W.C., Dzika, E., Korycinska, J., Human Permanent Ectoparasites; Recent Advances on Biology and Clinical Significance of Demodex Mites: Narrative Review Article. *Iran J Parasitol*, 12, 1, 12–21, 2017 Jan-Mar.
16. Gonzalez-Hinojosa, D., Jaime-Villalonga, A., Aguilar-Montes, G., Lammoglia-Ordiales., L., Demodex and rosacea: Is there a relationship? *Indian J Ophthalmol*, 66, 1, 36–38, 2018.
17. Liu, J., Sheha, H., Tseng, S.C.G., Pathogenic role of Demodex mites in blepharitis. *Curr Opin Allergy Clin Immunol*, 10, 5, 505–510, 2010 Oct.
18. Jarmuda, S., McMahon, F., Żaba, R., O'Reilly, N., Jakubowicz, O., Holland, A., Szkaradkiewicz, A., Kavanagh, K., Correlation between serum reactivity to Demodex associated Bacillus oleronius proteins, and altered sebum levels and Demodex populations in erythematotelangiectatic rosacea patients. *J Med Microbiol*, 63, 258–262, 2014.
19. Palopoli, M.F., Fergus, D.J., Minot, S., Pei, D.T., Simison, W.B., Fernandez-Silva, I., Thoemmes, M.S., Dunn, R.R., Trautwein, M., Global divergence of the human follicle mite *Demodex folliculorum*: Persistent associations between host ancestry and mite lineages. *PNAS*, 112, 52, 15958–15963, December 29, 2015. Published online ahead of print December 14, 2015. https://doi.org/10.1073/pnas.1512609112.
20. Strobel, S.L., Demodex as a Delivery Vector for Topical Targeted Medications in the Skin for Early Melanoma and Non-Melanoma Skin Cancer. *Ann Clin Lab Sci.*, 47, 5, 604–605, 2017.
21. Diamantis, N. and Banerji, U., Antibody-drug conjugates – an emerging class of cancer treatment. *Br J Cancer*, 114, 4, 362–367, 2016.
22. Falchook, G.S., Leidner, R., Stankevich, E., Piening, B., Bifulco, C., Lowy, I., Fury, M., Responses of metastatic basal cell and cutaneous squamous cell carcinomas to anti-PD1 monoclonal antibody REGN2810. Published online 2016 Nov 15. *J Immunother Cancer.*, 4, 7–0, 2016.
23. Malas, S., Harrasser, M., Lacy, K.E., Karagiannis, S.N., Antibody therapies for melanoma: New and emerging opportunities to activate immunity (Review). *Oncol Rep*, 32, 3, 875–886, 2014.

9

Dysbiosis of the Skin Microbiome in Atopic Dermatitis

Joyce Cheng and Tissa Hata*

Department of Dermatology, University of California, San Diego, CA, USA

Abstract

The human skin microbiome is a complex ecosystem of microorganisms that serves both as a protective barrier against foreign assault and as a fundamental pillar of skin innate defense. Dysbiosis of the skin microbiome is increasingly recognized to play a key role in the pathogenesis of atopic dermatitis (AD). This chapter seeks to summarize what is known about a healthy skin microbiome, to describe what is known about alterations of the skin microbiome in AD, and to explore the role of commensal skin microorganisms and their potential therapeutic implications in AD.

Keywords: Atopic dermatitis, commensal, dysbiosis, microbiome, *staphylococcus aureus*

9.1 Introduction

The human skin microbiome is a complex ecosystem of microorganisms that serves both as a protective barrier against foreign assault and as a fundamental pillar of skin innate defense. The composition of the microbial community varies across skin sites. Dysbiosis of the skin microbiome is increasingly recognized to play a key role in the pathogenesis of atopic dermatitis (AD). This chapter seeks to summarize what is known about a healthy skin microbiome, to describe what is known about alterations

Corresponding author: thata@mail.ucsd.edu

Nava Dayan (ed.) Skin Microbiome Handbook: From Basic Research to Product Development, (185–202) © 2020 Scrivener Publishing LLC

of the skin microbiome in AD, and to explore the role of commensal skin microorganisms and their potential therapeutic implications in AD.

9.2   The Healthy Skin Microbiome

Understanding what makes up a healthy skin microbiome is crucial to unraveling how alterations in the microbiome may lead to clinical disease. Technological advances in molecular methods of microorganism identification have revolutionized our understanding of the healthy skin microbiome. Numerous studies examining 16S ribosomal RNA gene sequences from distinct skin sites of healthy humans enable characterization of the microbial composition on the skin at the species and strain levels. These studies show that a healthy skin microbiome is not only diverse and complex within and between individuals—but also relatively stable across physiologically similar sites within an individual, despite constant exposure to the external environment [1–4]. Single-nucleotide variant level analysis reveals that individuals maintain their own stable microbial population, rather than reacquiring microbes from the environment [3].

Host-intrinsic factors, such as immunity or hygiene, and environmental factors, such as cosmetics, have as of yet unclear effects on the composition of a healthy microbial community. Two et al. found that short-term use of commercial soaps has relatively little effect on the skin microbiome [5]. However, addition of antimicrobial compounds such as benzalkonium chloride or triclocarban to soap before washing reduced Group A Streptococcus growth applied after a rinse [5].

Different skin bacteria prefer different microenvironments created by natural variations in skin pH, temperature, topography, density of hair follicles and glands, and other features [3, 6]. Sebaceous sites, such as those on the face or upper trunk, host the most stable and least diverse microbial populations at the species level. These relatively anoxic microenvironments are predominantly colonized by lipophilic Propionibacterium and some Staphylococcal species [1]. Meanwhile, moist sites such as the axilla and antecubital fossa harbor a more diverse microbial community in comparison but primarily host Gram-positive Corynebacterium species and some Staphylococcal species [1]. In contrast, dry sites are occupied by very diverse populations of mostly Gram-negative bacteria from the Proteobacteria, Firmicutes, Bacteroidetes, and Actinobacteria phyla [1]. The microbiome of dry sites like the palm was surprisingly stable over time despite frequent environmental interaction, while foot sites were found to be the least stable [3].

9.3   The Skin Microbiome in Atopic Dermatitis

Atopic dermatitis (AD) is a common chronic inflammatory skin disease. Presentation can be heterogeneous, but patients typically present with relapsing inflamed and pruritic skin lesions; they also often have concomitant atopic diseases such as asthma or hay fever [7, 8]. In infancy, lesions often involve the cheeks, forehead, neck, and scalp, progressing in childhood and adolescence to the antecubital and popliteal fossae, face, neck and hands (Figures 9.1 and 9.2). In adulthood, locations tend to be less characteristic and more diverse [9]. Diverse presentations and the subjective nature of the diagnosis make the epidemiology of AD challenging to pinpoint. However, AD is now estimated to affect approximately 15-30% of children and up to 10.2% of adults in the world [10–13]. Prevalence varies widely by region. For example, the prevalence of severe eczema in the U.S. state of Michigan was found to be 12.6% in the 2007-2008 National Survey of Children's Health (NSCH), while prevalence of severe eczema in the U.S. state of California was 5.9%. The International Study of Asthma and Allergies in Childhood (ISAAC) found that the prevalence of AD at ages 6 to 7 years of age was 0.9% in India, while it was 22.5% in Ecuador for the same age cohort [10, 12, 14–16]. Data on the epidemiology of adult AD is limited; however, the 1-year prevalence of eczema as determined by the 2010 National Interview Health Survey was much higher than expected at 10.2%, suggesting that AD may persist into adulthood more than previously thought [10, 17]. While

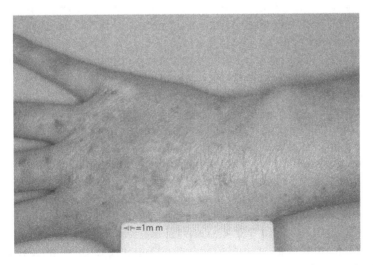

Figure 9.1 Atomic dermatitis lesions involving the hands. Note the erythema and scaling present.

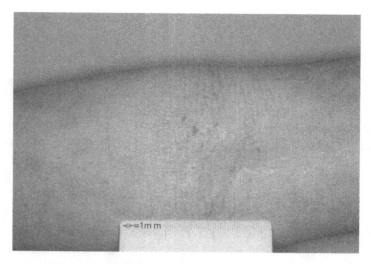

Figure 9.2 Atomic dermatitis lesions involving the antecubital fossae. Note the erythema and scaling with mild lichenification.

incidence appears to be plateauing in countries with the highest prevalence (20-30%), such as the UK and New Zealand, prevalence continues to increase globally, especially in young children and in developing countries [18].

Multiple prior studies have revealed the environment of the skin of atopics to have defective barrier function, increased colonization with *Staphylococcus aureus* (*S. aureus*), a Th2-predominant environment with increased expression of IL-4 and IL-13, increased expression of thymic stromal lymphopoietin (TSLP), and a suppressed innate response with decreased expression of antimicrobial peptides (AMPs) such as LL-37 and human β-defensins 2 and 3 [19–24]. This complex milieu of findings together contributes to the unique microbiome seen in atopic dermatitis patients (Figure 9.3).

Barrier dysfunction in AD has been well characterized, with increase in transepidermal water loss (TEWL) noted even in the non-lesional skin of atopic patients [25, 26]. Although loss-of-function mutations in the filaggrin gene have been associated with AD, only 27% of humans with the filaggrin-null mutation develop AD, suggesting that other barrier proteins and factors must play a role in AD pathogenesis [23, 27]. Studies in mice with loss-of-function filaggrin mutations have shown that these mice were more easily infected with *S. aureus*, and this correlated with increased expression of IL-4, IL-13, and TSLP, as well as decreased expression of AMPs [28]. Application of a ceramide-triple lipid mixture to these mice restored barrier function as measured by TEWL, improved antimicrobial peptide expression, and decreased penetration of *S. aureus* [28]. The importance

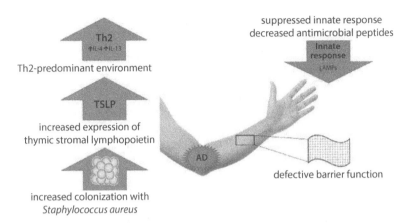

Figure 9.3 Pathophysiology of AD. The skin of an AD patient is a Th2-predominant immune environment with increased expression of interleukin-4 and interleukin-13, increased expression of thymic stromal lymphopoietin (TSLP), and a suppressed innate response with decreased expression of antimicrobial peptides. Defective barrier function is observed in both lesional and non-lesional skin. The microbiome of atopic patients is characterized by increased colonization with *S. aureus*.

of barrier repair was also highlighted in humans with AD; just as in mice with loss-of-function filaggrin mutations, application of lipid mixtures improved skin barrier function and clinical symptoms in patients with AD [29–31]. Further, it has been shown that filaggrin-deficient patients have a deficiency in breakdown products of filaggrin—urocanic acid and pyrrolidone carboxylic acid, components of the natural moisturizing factor (NMF) in the stratum corneum [32]; this decrease in NMF has been associated with increased bacterial adhesion of *S. aureus* to skin corneocytes, contributing to the altered microbiome of atopics [33].

The microbiome in atopic patients typically shows a predominance of *S. aureus*, along with a decrease in bacterial diversity, primarily during flares of AD [15]. *S. aureus* was first noted to be present on the skin of AD patients in 1974 when Leyden and Kligman obtained quantitative aerobic cultures from fifty patients with atopic dermatitis and found that 90% of these patients were colonized with *S. aureus* [34]. Since this time, the central role of *S. aureus* in AD has repeatedly been affirmed [21, 35].

Multiple lines of evidence suggest that *S. aureus* can create an AD-like clinical presentation. *S. aureus* possesses multiple virulence factors (Table 9.1), including lysins, proteases, and toxins. Clumping factors A and B, fibronectin-binding protein, and iron-regulated surface determinant help the bacteria adhere to and colonize its host [36]. *S. aureus* α-toxin is a member of the β-pore forming toxins, which insert a hydrophilic channel

Table 9.1 Summary of the virulence factors of *S. aureus*.

S.aureus virulence factors	
Adherence and colonization	Barrier destruction
• Clumping factors A and B (ClfA and ClfB) • Fibronectin-binding protein (fnBP) • Iron-regulated surface determinants A Isda)	• Alpha toxin • Direct stimulation and endogenous keratinocyte proteases, including KLK6, KLK13, and KLK14 • Lysins • Proteases
Biofilm formation	Pro-Inflammatory
• Alpha toxin	• Delta toxin • Lipoproteins • Phenol-soluble modulins • Protein A • Superantigens (SEA, SEB, SEC, toxic shock syndrome toxin-1)

Clumping factors A and B (ClfA and ClfB), fibronectin-binding protein (fnBP), iron-regulated surface determinant A (IsdA) have all been shown to facilitate adherence and colonization of atopic skin by *S. aureus*. *S. aureus* has numerous mechanisms to effect barrier destruction, including alpha toxin, the direct stimulation of endogenous keratinocyte proteases such as KLK6, KLK13, and KLK14, lysins, and proteases. Alpha toxin has also been implicated in *S. aureus*'s ability to form biofilms. *S. aureus* is capable of effecting pro-inflammatory responses through a variety of effectors such as delta toxin, lipoproteins, phenol-soluble modulins, protein A, and superantigens (SEA, SEB, SEC, toxic shock syndrome toxin-1).

in the lipid bilayer of a cell, thus forming a pore in host cell membranes [37]. Alpha-toxin is also important for *S. aureus* biofilm formation, which makes *S. aureus* much harder to eliminate. Absence of filaggrin and Th2 cytokine skewing further seem to enhance the activity of this toxin [28]. *S. aureus* isolates recovered from AD patients also produce large amounts of δ-toxin, which appears to be a potent inducer of mast cell degranulation [38]. *S. aureus* also produce Protein A and various superantigens, including toxic shock syndrome toxin 1, which can trigger cytokine release and inflammatory responses [39]. In mice, *S. aureus* colonization also appears to disrupt the epidermal barrier by inducing keratinocyte proteases including kallikrein (KLK) 6, KLK13, and KLK14 [40]. In addition, Staphylococcal lipoproteins induce a Th2 imbalance in AD by induction of TSLP though a TLR2/TLR6-dependent manner [41].

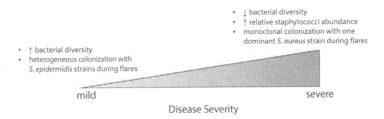

- ↓ bacterial diversity
- ↑ relative staphylococci abundance
- monoclonal colonization with one dominant *S. aureus* strain during flares

- ↑ bacterial diversity
- heterogeneous colonization with *S. epidermidis* strains during flares

mild   severe

Disease Severity

Figure 9.4 Factors influencing AD disease severity: Severe AD is characterized by decreased bacterial diversity, with an increased relative abundance of staphylococci. In particular, monoclonal colonization with a dominant *S. aureus* strain has been noted in severe AD patients during flares. In contrast, comparably more bacterial diversity is noted in mild AD, and mild AD patients are heterogeneously colonized with *S. epidermidis* strains during flares.

Novel shotgun metagenomic sequencing techniques now allow appreciation of strain-level effects in the skin microbiome on clinical presentation of AD. Byrd *et al.* examined the strain diversity of *S. aureus* and *S. epidermidis* in 11 children with moderate to severe AD compared with 7 healthy children [15]. They sampled the microbiome at baseline (off topical medications for at least 7 days), during a flare, and post-flare 14 days after initiation of treatment. They found that bacterial communities shift with progression of AD disease—reduced skin bacterial diversity correlates with worse disease severity (Figure 9.4). The relative abundance of staphylococci increased most during AD disease flares [15]. *S. aureus* predominated in those with more severe disease, and *S. epidermidis* in patients with less severe disease. *S. aureus*-predominant individuals tended to be colonized with a single *S. aureus* strain; however, this dominant strain was largely unique to each individual and was hypothesized to account for differences in disease course and therapeutic responses of AD patients. Presence of a monoclonal *S. aureus* strain was observed in more severe patients, and application of representative strains was sufficient to induce inflammatory response in the skin of germ-free mice [15]. *S. epidermidis* strains observed in less severe AD presentations were heterogeneous but notably possessed more antibiotic resistance genes than those isolated from more severe AD hosts, potentially providing them with a survival advantage [15]. These findings suggest that targeted modulation of an AD patient's particular staphylococci strains could potentially ameliorate development of atopic disorders.

In an effort to determine whether *S. aureus* precedes or is a result of the milieu of atopic dermatitis, Meylan *et al.* conducted a larger prospective longitudinal clinical trial to examine the timing of the relationship between *S. aureus* colonization and clinical diagnosis of AD [42]. They followed 149 Caucasian infants with or without a family history of atopy from birth and sampled their microbiome using culture-based techniques seven times over their first two years of life; 36 of these infants went on to develop AD by two years of age (mean age 9.4 months) [42]. Differences in birth mode-related differences in the microbiome were generally not apparent after age 1 week. At age 3 months, they found that *S. aureus* was more prevalent on the skin of infants who later developed AD compared with on the skin of age-matched, unaffected infants; this increased *S. aureus* prevalence was noted at the time of clinical AD onset and also 2 months before AD onset, suggesting that early-life microbiome alterations with *S. aureus* may actively drive onset of clinical AD in infancy. Interestingly, the commensal *Staphylococcus hominis* appeared to be less abundant in AD and thus potentially protective against AD [42].

In a similar study utilizing 16S ribosomal RNA sequencing instead of culture-based techniques, Kennedy *et al.* swabbed fifty infants at ages 2 days, 2 months, and 6 months and examined the bacterial 16S ribosomal RNA sequences from a randomly selected cohort of patients [43]. Ten patients in this cohort went on to develop AD by one year of age, and these subjects, along with ten age-matched controls, were then analyzed. Mean Shannon Diversity index, an index commonly used to characterize species diversity in a community, was examined, and no differences by birth method or by feeding method (breast-fed, formula-fed, or a combination of the two) were detected. Kennedy *et al.* found that bacterial community structures and the diversity of the skin microbiome change with age. Neither the characteristic dysbiotic changes found in established AD nor *S. aureus* colonization was seen in infantile AD, in contradiction to the study described above. Interestingly, however, infants who developed AD at one year had a statistically significant decrease in their commensal staphylococcus at month two, suggesting that early colonization with commensal staphylococci may be protective against later development of atopic dermatitis [43].

The skin microbiome in adult AD is not as well-characterized as the pediatric skin microbiome. Shi *et al.* found that the diversity of the skin microbiome is much higher in young children than in adults and teenagers with AD, and that this diversity is significantly decreased in lesional skin compared with non-lesional skin in both age cohorts [13]. As in children, *Staphylococcus* is significantly more abundant on both the lesional and non-lesional skin of adult AD patients [13]. Another genome sequencing study comparing the non-lesional skin of adult atopic patients to healthy controls found a relative increase in the abundance of *Gemella* and *Streptococcus* species, while a depletion of *Dermacoccus* was noted. This study also noted that AD samples were enriched in nitrogen, arginine, and proline metabolism pathways that are responsible for metabolizing arginine and citrulline into ammonia. Alkalization by the microbiome would establish a higher pH, which has been seen during atopic flares, and a setting more favorable for growth of *S. aureus* [44]. Further characterization of the presence or absence of age-specific skin commensals with varying potential for pathogen defense and skin health maintenance may account for some of the differences observed between the skin microbiome of pediatric and adult AD patients, but specifics of these differences have yet to be characterized.

Both studies by Kennedy *et al.* and Meylan *et al.*, as well as others, suggest that commensal skin bacteria play an active role in skin homeostasis and may be protective against AD (Table 9.2) [42, 43, 45–47]. As mentioned prior, the commensal *Staphylococcus hominis* appeared to be less abundant in AD and thus potentially protective against AD [42]. *S. epidermidis* plays an important role in immune modulation, as its presence has been shown to be required for effector T cells to produce cytokines such as IL-17A and IFN-γ [48]. Selective strains of *S. epidermidis* have been shown to produce phenol-soluble modulins, which through their alpha helical structure, function like antimicrobial peptides by fatally disrupting microbial membranes through a barrel-stave mechanism. Interestingly, these phenol-soluble modulins effectively inhibit skin pathogens such as *Group A Streptococcus*, *Escherichia coli*, and *S. aureus*, but not the survival of *S. epidermidis*, suggesting that these commensal bacteria are important in maintaining a healthy microbiome [49]. Some strains of *S. epidermidis* have been shown to produce a lipopeptide, which can trigger keratinocyte antimicrobial peptide expression to help the host defend against pathogens [50, 51], while other strains have been shown to express the serine protease glutamyl endopeptidase (Esp), which is able to inhibit *S. aureus* biofilm formation by degrading proteins critical for biofilm formation [52, 53]. *S. epidermidis* can also produce lipotechoic acid, a ligand of TLR2, which can dampen skin inflammation [54]. In addition to *S. epidermidis*, another commensal Staphyloccocus has been shown to produce an autoinducing peptide, which can inhibit *S. aureus* colonization and infection by blocking its quorum sensing ability [55]. *Staphylococcus lugdunensis* has been shown to produce a novel thiazolidine-containing cyclic peptide (lugdunin), which is also able to inhibit growth of *S. aureus* [56]. Interestingly, not all commensal organisms promote a healthy microbiome environment. Certain *Propionibacterium* species can induce *S. aureus* aggregation and biofilm formation [57], suggesting that the balance between commensal organisms in the microbiome is essential for human health.

Table 9.2 Examples of commensal modulation of the skin microbiome.

Examples of commensal modulation of the skin microbiome		
S. epidermidis	Phenol-soluble modulins: α-helical AMP-like peptides that can discrupt bacterial membranes	Inhibit skin pathogens like *Group A Streptococcus, E. coli,* and *S. aureus*
	Lipopeptide (some strains)	Trigger keratinocyte AMP expression to boost host defenses
	Serine protease glutamyl endopeptidase (some strains)	Inhibit *S. aureus* biofilm formation through protein degradation
	Lipoteichoic acid	Suppress skin inflammation
S. caprae	Autoinducing peptide	Inhibit *S. aureus* colonization by blocking *S. aureus* accessory gene regulator Quorum Sensing
S. lugdunensis	Lugdunin: thiazolidine-containing cyclic peptide	Inhibits *S. aureus* growth
S. hominis	Hogocidin: lanthionine-containing antibiotics	Selective activity against *S. aureus*; synergizes with host AMPs
Corynebacterium species	Mycolic acid	Induce IL-17A dermal γδ T cells
Propionibacterium species	Induce *S. aureus* aggregation and biofilm formation	

Commensal species can have both positive and negative effects on the skin microbiome through a variety of mechanisms. *S. epidermidis* influences the skin microbiome through a diverse host of effectors. For example, they have been shown to produce phenol-soluble modulins, which are alpha-helical AMP-like peptides that can disrupt bacterial membranes and inhibit the growth of skin pathogens such as group A *Streptococcus* (group A strep), *E. coli*, and *S. aureus*. Some strains can also produce lipopeptide, which triggers expression of antimicrobial peptides by keratinocytes to boost host defenses. *S. epidermidis* has also been reported to produce serine protease glutamyl endopeptidases, which degrade proteins and thus are able to inhibit *S. aureus* biofilm formation. Finally, *S. epidermidis* has also been shown to produce lipoteichoic acid, which can suppress skin inflammation overall. Another commensal staphylococcal species, *S. caprae*, has been shown to produce autoinducing peptide, which inhibits *S. aureus* colonization by blocking *S. aureus* accessory gene regulator quorum sensing. Similarly, *S. lugdunensis* produces lugdunin, a thiazolidine-containing cyclic peptide that inhibits *S. aureus* growth, and *S. hominis* produces hogocidin, a lanthionine-containing antibiotic that synergizes with host AMPs and exerts selective activity against *S. aureus*. In contrast, Propionibacterium species have been noted to induce *S. aureus* aggregation and subsequent biofilm formation.

9.4   Microbiome-Targeted Treatment Strategies

Topical microbiome transplantation has emerged as a promising rational therapeutic avenue for AD, in light of the growing body of evidence that dysbiosis contributes to disease pathogenesis. Application of *Roseomonas mucosa* (*R. mucosa*), a Gram-negative skin bacteria, isolated from healthy volunteers improved outcomes in animal and cell culture AD models [58], while application of *R. mucosa* isolated from AD patients resulted in worsened outcomes [59]. An open-label phase I/II trial in ten adult AD patients and five pediatric AD patients showed that *R. mucosa* safely and effectively decreases measures of disease severity, steroid requirement, and *S. aureus* burden [59].

In order to examine the balance of commensal organisms in patients with AD, Nakatsuji *et al.* isolated coagulase-negative Staphylococcus species (CoNS) from the skin of healthy and AD patients and functionally screened them for activity against *S. aureus* [60]. Amazingly, antimicrobial activity against *S. aureus* was noted in only 3.6% of randomly selected CoNS isolates from lesional AD skin compared with 23.8% from nonlesional AD skin and 72.6% from healthy skin, suggesting that the defective microbiome in patients with AD was a significant contributor to colonization with *S. aureus* [60]. Subsequently, the source of the antimicrobial activity was identified as two previously unknown antimicrobial peptides (AMPs) known as lantibiotics (lanthionine-containing antibiotics) produced by *S. hominis*. These AMPs are highly potent, synergize with the human AMP LL-37, and exhibit selective activity against *S. aureus* [60]. These findings highlight the defective microbiome of atopic patients, and also the therapeutic potential of CoNS strains with strong anti-*S. aureus* activity.

In order to further test this hypothesis, a randomized, double blind, placebo-controlled trial was conducted to assess the capacity of commensal bacteria to inhibit *S. aureus* on human skin [60]. Clones of CoNS with anti-*S. aureus* activity isolated from the autologous skin of AD patients were expanded in Cetaphil moisturizing lotion. Lotion containing CoNS bacteria from the patient or vehicle was applied to lesional skin on the patient twice a day for one week, targeting a surface density of 10^5 CFU/cm^2 in order to mimic the normal concentration of bacteria on the skin. A single application of CoNS with anti-*S. aureus* activity was noted to decrease *S. aureus* abundance significantly compared to vehicle alone (p = 0.04), suggesting that the microbiome transplant decreases *S. aureus* colonization and is a promising strategy for correction of the dysbiosis seen in AD [60]. A larger multi-center, Phase 1 trial with 54 AD subjects examining the effect of a non-autologous commensal staphylococcus with anti-*S. aureus* properties delivered by cream on AD dysbiosis is currently underway. A 3-month trial is also planned to examine clinical improvement in AD as a result of this treatment strategy.

9.5 Conclusion

Barrier dysfunction, a skewed Th2 phenotype, decreased AMP production, an increase in *S. aureus*, and a relative reduction of commensal organisms all contribute to a dysbiosis of the skin microbiome in AD. The delicate balance of the skin microbiome is essential for human health; however, current treatments with traditional antibiotics create increased bacterial resistance and further skew the microbiome. Topical treatments that alter dysbiosis of the microbiome by transplanting beneficial bacteria, or other agents that promote the growth of the healthy microbiome, will not only improve our understanding of the microbiome that characterize AD but also provide novel options to treat and prevent the ongoing dysbiosis in AD.

References

1. Grice, E.A., Kong, H.H., Conlan, S., Deming, C.B., Davis, J., Young, A.C., Bouffard, G.G., Blakesley, R.W., Murray, P.R., Green, E.D., Turner, M.L., Segre, J.A., Topographical and temporal diversity of the human skin microbiome. *Science.*, 324, 5931, 1190–2, 2009.
2. Grice, E.A. and Segre, J.A., The skin microbiome. *Nat. Rev. Microbiol.*, 9, 4, 244–53, 2011.
3. Oh, J., Byrd, A.L., Park, M., Kong, H.H., Segre, J.A., Temporal Stability of the Human Skin Microbiome. *Cell*, 165, 4, 854–66, 2016.
4. Oh, J., Byrd, A.L., Deming, C., Conlan, S., Program, N.C.S., Kong, H.H., Segre, J.A., Biogeography and individuality shape function in the human skin metagenome. *Nature*, 514, 7520, 59–64, 2014.
5. Two, A.M., Nakatsuji, T., Kotol, P.F., Arvanitidou, E., Du-Thumm, L., Hata, T.R., Gallo, R.L., The Cutaneous Microbiome and Aspects of Skin Antimicrobial Defense System Resist Acute Treatment with Topical Skin Cleansers. *J. Invest. Dermatol.*, 136, 10, 1950–4, 2016.
6. Tagami, H., Location-related differences in structure and function of the stratum corneum with special emphasis on those of the facial skin. *Int. J. Cosmet. Sci.*, 30, 6, 413–34, 2008.

7. Bantz, S.K., Zhu, Z., Zheng, T., The Atopic March: Progression from Atopic Dermatitis to Allergic Rhinitis and Asthma. *J. Clin. Cell. Immunol.*, 5, 2, 2014.

8. Czarnowicki, T., Krueger, J.G., Guttman-Yassky, E., Novel concepts of prevention and treatment of atopic dermatitis through barrier and immune manipulations with implications for the atopic march. *J. Allergy Clin. Immunol.*, 139, 6, 1723–34, 2017.

9. James, W.D., Elston, D.M., Berger, T.G., Andrews, G.C., *Andrews' Diseases of the Skin: Clinical Dermatology*. London, Saunders/Elsevier, 2011.

10. Silverberg, J.I., Public Health Burden and Epidemiology of Atopic Dermatitis. *Dermatologic Clinics*, 35, 3, 283–9, 2017.

11. Nutten, S., Atopic dermatitis: Global epidemiology and risk factors. *Annals Nutr. Metab.*, 66 Suppl 1, 8–16, 2015.

12. Barbarot, S., Auziere, S., Gadkari, A., Girolomoni, G., Puig, L., Simpson, E.L., Margolis, D.J., de Bruin-Weller, M., Eckert, L., Epidemiology of atopic dermatitis in adults: Results from an international survey. *Allergy*, 73, 6, 1284–93, 2018.

13. Shi, B., Bangayan, N.J., Curd, E., Taylor, P.A., Gallo, R.L., Leung, D.Y.M., Li, H., The skin microbiome is different in pediatric versus adult atopic dermatitis. *J. Allergy Clin. Immunol.*, 138, 4, 1233–6, 2016.

14. Drucker, A.M., Wang, A.R., Li, W.-Q., Sevetson, E., Block, J.K., Qureshi, A.A., The Burden of Atopic Dermatitis: Summary of a Report for the National Eczema Association. *J. Invest. Dermatol.*, 137, 1, 26–30, 2017.

15. Byrd, A.L., Deming, C., Cassidy, S.K.B., Harrison, O.J., Ng, W.I., Conlan, S., Program, N.C.S., Belkaid, Y., Segre, J.A., Kong, H.H., *Staphylococcus aureus* and *Staphylococcus epidermidis* strain diversity underlying pediatric atopic dermatitis. *Sci. Transl. Med.*, 9, 397, 2017.

16. Bieber, T., Atopic dermatitis. *Ann Dermatol.*, 22, 2, 125–37, 2010.

17. Garg, N. and Silverberg, J.I., Epidemiology of childhood atopic dermatitis. *Clin. Dermatol.*, 33, 3, 281–8, 2015.

18. Deckers, I.A., McLean, S., Linssen, S., Mommers, M., van Schayck, C.P., Sheikh, A., Investigating international time trends in the incidence and prevalence of atopic eczema 1990-2010: A systematic review of epidemiological studies. *PLoS One*, 7, 7, e39803, 2012.

19. Chieosilapatham, P., Ogawa, H., Niyonsaba, F., Current insights into the role of human beta-defensins in atopic dermatitis. *Clin. Exp. Immunol.*, 190, 2, 155–66, 2017.

20. Brunner, P.M., Leung, D.Y.M., Guttman-Yassky, E., Immunologic, microbial, and epithelial interactions in atopic dermatitis. *Annals Allergy, Asthma Immunol.*, 120, 1, 34–41, 2018.

21. Geoghegan, J.A., Irvine, A.D., Foster, T.J., *Staphylococcus aureus* and Atopic Dermatitis: A Complex and Evolving Relationship. *Trends Microbiol.*, 26, 6, 484–97, 2018.

22. Furue, M., Chiba, T., Tsuji, G., Ulzii, D., Kido-Nakahara, M., Nakahara, T., Kadono, T., Atopic dermatitis: immune deviation, barrier dysfunction, IgE autoreactivity and new therapies. *Allergol. Int.*, 66, 3, 398–403, 2017.

23. Zaniboni, M.C., Samorano, L.P., Orfali, R.L., Aoki, V., Skin barrier in atopic dermatitis: Beyond filaggrin. *An Bras Dermatol.*, 91, 4, 472–8, 2016.

24. Malik, K., Heitmiller, K.D., Czarnowicki, T., An Update on the Pathophysiology of Atopic Dermatitis. *Dermatologic Clinics.*, 35, 3, 317–26, 2017.

25. Gupta, J., Grube, E., Ericksen, M.B., Stevenson, M.D., Lucky, A.W., Sheth, A.P., Assa'ad, A.H., Khurana Hershey, G.K., Intrinsically defective skin barrier function in children with atopic dermatitis correlates with disease severity. *J. Allergy Clin. Immunol.*, 121, 3, 725–30 e2, 2008.

26. Di Nardo, A., Wertz, P., Giannetti, A., Seidenari, S., Ceramide and cholesterol composition of the skin of patients with atopic dermatitis. *Acta Derm. Venereol.*, 78, 1, 27–30, 1998.

27. Morar, N., Cookson, W.O., Harper, J.I., Moffatt, M.F., Filaggrin mutations in children with severe atopic dermatitis. *J. Invest. Dermatol.*, 127, 7, 1667–72, 2007.

28. Nakatsuji, T., Chen, T.H., Two, A.M., Chun, K.A., Narala, S., Geha, R.S., Hata, T.R., Gallo, R.L., *Staphylococcus aureus* Exploits Epidermal Barrier Defects in Atopic Dermatitis to Trigger Cytokine Expression. *J. Invest. Dermatol.*, 136, 11, 2192–200, 2016.

29. Chamlin, S.L., Kao, J., Frieden, I.J., Sheu, M.Y., Fowler, A.J., Fluhr, J.W., Williams, M.L., Elias, P.M., Ceramide-dominant barrier repair lipids alleviate childhood atopic dermatitis: Changes in barrier function provide a sensitive indicator of disease activity. *J. Am. Acad. Dermatol.*, 47, 2, 198–208, 2002.

30. Weidinger, S. and Novak, N., Atopic dermatitis. *Lancet.*, 387, 10023, 1109–22, 2016.

31. Simpson, E.L., Chalmers, J.R., Hanifin, J.M., Thomas, K.S., Cork, M.J., McLean, W.H., Brown, S.J., Chen, Z., Chen, Y., Williams, H.C., Emollient enhancement of the skin barrier from birth offers effective atopic dermatitis prevention. *J. Allergy Clin. Immunol.*, 134, 4, 818–23, 2014.

32. Miajlovic, H., Fallon, P.G., Irvine, A.D., Foster, T.J., Effect of filaggrin breakdown products on growth of and protein expression by *Staphylococcus aureus*. *J. Allergy Clin. Immunol.*, 126, 6, 1184–90.e3, 2010.

33. Feuillie, C., Vitry, P., McAleer, M.A., Kezic, S., Irvine, A.D., Geoghegan, J.A., Dufrene, Y.F., Adhesion of *Staphylococcus aureus* to Corneocytes from Atopic Dermatitis Patients Is Controlled by Natural Moisturizing Factor Levels. *mBio.*, 9, 4, 2018.

34. Leyden, J.J., Marples, R.R., Kligman, A.M., *Staphylococcus aureus* in the lesions of atopic dermatitis. *Br. J. Dermatol.*, 90, 5, 525–30, 1974.

35. Clausen, M.L., Edslev, S.M., Andersen, P.S., Clemmensen, K., Krogfelt, K.A., Agner, T., *Staphylococcus aureus* colonization in atopic eczema and its association with filaggrin gene mutations. *Br. J .Dermatol.*, 177, 5, 1394–400, 2017.

36. Paller, A.S., Kong, H.H., Seed, P., Naik, S., Scharschmidt, T.C., Gallo, R.L., Luger, T., Irvine, A.D., The microbiome in patients with atopic dermatitis. *J. Allergy Clin. Immunol.*, 143, 1, 26–35, 2019.

37. Berube, B.J. and Bubeck Wardenburg, J., *Staphylococcus aureus* alpha-toxin: Nearly a century of intrigue. *Toxins*, 5, 6, 1140–66, 2013.

38. Nakamura, Y., Oscherwitz, J., Cease, K.B., Chan, S.M., Munoz-Planillo, R., Hasegawa, M., Villaruz, A.E., Cheung, G.Y., McGavin, M.J., Travers, J.B., Otto, M., Inohara, N., Nunez, G., Staphylococcus delta-toxin induces allergic skin disease by activating mast cells. *Nature*, 503, 7476, 397–401, 2013.

39. Spaulding, A.R., Salgado-Pabon, W., Kohler, P.L., Horswill, A.R., Leung, D.Y., Schlievert, P.M., Staphylococcal and streptococcal superantigen exotoxins. *Clin. Microbiol. Rev.*, 26, 3, 422–47, 2013.

40. Williams, M.R., Nakatsuji, T., Sanford, J.A., Vrbanac, A.F., Gallo, R.L., *Staphylococcus aureus* Induces Increased Serine Protease Activity in Keratinocytes. *J. Invest. Dermatol.*, 137, 2, 377–84, 2017.

41. Vu, A.T., Baba, T., Chen, X., Le, T.A., Kinoshita, H., Xie, Y., Kamijo, S., Hiramatsu, K., Ikeda, S., Ogawa, H., Okumura, K., Takai, T., *Staphylococcus aureus* membrane and diacylated lipopeptide induce thymic stromal lymphopoietin in keratinocytes through the Toll-like receptor 2-Toll-like receptor 6 pathway. *J. Allergy Clin. Immunol.*, 126, 5, 985–93, 93.e1-3, 2010.

42. Meylan, P., Lang, C., Mermoud, S., Johannsen, A., Norrenberg, S., Hohl, D., Vial, Y., Prod'hom, G., Greub, G., Kypriotou, M., Christen-Zaech, S., Skin Colonization by *Staphylococcus aureus* Precedes the Clinical Diagnosis of Atopic Dermatitis in Infancy. *J. Invest. Dermatol.*, 137, 12, 2497–504, 2017.

43. Kennedy, E.A., Connolly, J., Hourihane, J.O.B., Fallon, P.G., McLean, W.H.I., Murray, D., Jo, J.-H., Segre, J.A., Kong, H.H., Irvine, A.D., Skin microbiome before development of atopic dermatitis: Early colonization with commensal staphylococci at 2 months is associated with a lower risk of atopic dermatitis at 1 year. *J. Allergy Clin. Immunol.*, 139, 1, 166–72, 2017.

44. Chng, K.R., Tay, A.S., Li, C., Ng, A.H., Wang, J., Suri, B.K., Matta, S.A., McGovern, N., Janela, B., Wong, X.F., Sio, Y.Y., Au, B.V., Wilm, A., De Sessions, P.F., Lim, T.C., Tang, M.B., Ginhoux, F., Connolly, J.E., Lane, E.B., Chew, F.T., Common, J.E., Nagarajan, N., Whole metagenome profiling reveals skin microbiome-dependent susceptibility to atopic dermatitis flare. *Nat. Microbiol.*, 1, 9, 16106, 2016.

45. Gallo, R.L. and Nakatsuji, T., Microbial Symbiosis with the Innate Immune Defense System of the Skin. *J. Invest. Dermatol.*, 131, 10, 1974–80, 2011.

46. Scharschmidt, T.C., Vasquez, K.S., Pauli, M.L., Leitner, E.G., Chu, K., Truong, H.A., Lowe, M.M., Sanchez Rodriguez, R., Ali, N., Laszik, Z.G., Sonnenburg, J.L., Millar, S.E., Rosenblum, M.D., Commensal Microbes and Hair Follicle Morphogenesis Coordinately Drive Treg Migration into Neonatal Skin. *Cell Host Microbe.*, 21, 4, 467–77.e5, 2017.

47. Scharschmidt, T.C., Establishing Tolerance to Commensal Skin Bacteria: Timing Is Everything. *Dermatologic Clinics*, 35, 1, 1–9, 2017.

48. Belkaid, Y. and Naik, S., Compartmentalized and systemic control of tissue immunity by commensals. *Nat. Immunol.*, 14, 646, 2013.
49. Cogen, A.L., Yamasaki, K., Sanchez, K.M., Dorschner, R.A., Lai, Y., MacLeod, D.T., Torpey, J.W., Otto, M., Nizet, V., Kim, J.E., Gallo, R.L., Selective antimicrobial action is provided by phenol-soluble modulins derived from *Staphylococcus epidermidis*, a normal resident of the skin. *J. Invest. Dermatol.*, 130, 1, 192–200, 2010.
50. Lai, Y., Cogen, A.L., Radek, K.A., Park, H.J., Macleod, D.T., Leichtle, A., Ryan, A.F., Di Nardo, A., Gallo, R.L., Activation of TLR2 by a small molecule produced by *Staphylococcus epidermidis* increases antimicrobial defense against bacterial skin infections. *J. Invest. Dermatol.*, 130, 9, 2211–21, 2010.
51. Lai, Y., Di Nardo, A., Nakatsuji, T., Leichtle, A., Yang, Y., Cogen, A.L., Wu, Z.-R., Hooper, L.V., Schmidt, R.R., von Aulock, S., Radek, K.A., Huang, C.-M., Ryan, A.F., Gallo, R.L., Commensal bacteria regulate Toll-like receptor 3-dependent inflammation after skin injury. *Nat. Med.*, 15, 12, 1377–82, 2009.
52. Sugimoto, S., Iwamoto, T., Takada, K., Okuda, K., Tajima, A., Iwase, T., Mizunoe, Y., *Staphylococcus epidermidis* Esp degrades specific proteins associated with *Staphylococcus aureus* biofilm formation and host-pathogen interaction. *J. Bacteriol.*, 195, 8, 1645–55, 2013.
53. Iwase, T., Uehara, Y., Shinji, H., Tajima, A., Seo, H., Takada, K., Agata, T., Mizunoe, Y., *Staphylococcus epidermidis* Esp inhibits *Staphylococcus aureus* biofilm formation and nasal colonization. *Nature*, 465, 7296, 346–9, 2010.
54. Lai, Y., Di Nardo, A., Nakatsuji, T., Leichtle, A., Yang, Y., Cogen, A.L., Wu, Z.-R., Hooper, L.V., Schmidt, R.R., von Aulock, S., Radek, K.A., Huang, C.-M., Ryan, A.F., Gallo, R.L., Commensal bacteria regulate Toll-like receptor 3–dependent inflammation after skin injury. *Nat. Med.*, 15, 1377, 2009.
55. Paharik, A.E., Parlet, C.P., Chung, N., Todd, D.A., Rodriguez, E.I., Van Dyke, M.J., Cech, N.B., Horswill, A.R., Coagulase-Negative Staphylococcal Strain Prevents *Staphylococcus aureus* Colonization and Skin Infection by Blocking Quorum Sensing. *Cell Host Microbe.*, 22, 6, 746–56.e5, 2017.
56. Zipperer, A., Konnerth, M.C., Laux, C., Berscheid, A., Janek, D., Weidenmaier, C., Burian, M., Schilling, N.A., Slavetinsky, C., Marschal, M., Willmann, M., Kalbacher, H., Schittek, B., Brotz-Oesterhelt, H., Grond, S., Peschel, A., Krismer, B., Human commensals producing a novel antibiotic impair pathogen colonization. *Nature*, 535, 7613, 511–6, 2016.
57. Wollenberg, M.S., Claesen, J., Escapa, I.F., Aldridge, K.L., Fischbach, M.A., Lemon, K.P., Propionibacterium-produced coproporphyrin III induces *Staphylococcus aureus* aggregation and biofilm formation. *mBio.*, 5, 4, e01286–14, 2014.
58. Myles, I.A., Williams, K.W., Reckhow, J.D., Jammeh, M.L., Pincus, N.B., Sastalla, I., Saleem, D., Stone, K.D., Datta, S.K., Transplantation of human skin microbiota in models of atopic dermatitis. *JCI Insight.*, 1, 10, 2016.

59. Myles, I.A., Earland, N.J., Anderson, E.D., Moore, I.N., Kieh, M.D., Williams, K.W., Saleem, A., Fontecilla, N.M., Welch, P.A., Darnell, D.A., Barnhart, L.A., Sun, A.A., Uzel, G., Datta, S.K., First-in-human topical microbiome transplantation with Roseomonas mucosa for atopic dermatitis. *JCI Insight.*, 3, 9, 2018.

60. Nakatsuji, T., Chen, T.H., Narala, S., Chun, K.A., Two, A.M., Yun, T., Shafiq, F., Kotol, P.F., Bouslimani, A., Melnik, A.V., Latif, H., Kim, J.N., Lockhart, A., Artis, K., David, G., Taylor, P., Streib, J., Dorrestein, P.C., Grier, A., Gill, S.R., Zengler, K., Hata, T.R., Leung, D.Y., Gallo, R.L., Antimicrobials from human skin commensal bacteria protect against *Staphylococcus aureus* and are deficient in atopic dermatitis. *Sci. Transl. Med.*, 9, 378, 2017.

10

The Skin Microbiome of Inverse Psoriasis

Jennifer Chung[1,2*], Bruce E. Strober[3,4] and George M. Weinstock[1,2]

[1]*University of Connecticut School of Medicine, Farmington, CT USA*
[2]*The Jackson Laboratory For Genomic Medicine, Farmington, CT USA*
[3]*Central Connecticut Dermatology, Cromwell, CT USA*
[4]*Yale University, New Haven, CT USA*

Abstract

Inverse psoriasis is a painful and disfiguring immunodysregulatory skin disease with a unknown etiology. This subtype of psoriasis only demonstrates lesions at intertriginous or skin fold sites, where moisture is high. Past experiments have identified microbial differences in healthy intertriginous sites when compared to other healthy skin sites. We hypothesize that a distinct skin microbiome at these moist inverse sites has a role in the pathogenesis of inverse psoriasis. Currently there are not any studies looking into the skin microbiome and its relation to inverse psoriasis. Therefore, we are the first to characterize the skin microbiome at nine inverse sites in three cohorts: plaque psoriatics 1) with inverse psoriasis (n = 13), 2) without inverse psoriasis (n = 11), and 3) healthy non-psoriatics (n = 4). In this pilot study, we determined that the overall bacterial community structure is significantly different at lesional vs. non-lesional sites in subjects with inverse psoriasis at their inframammary, infra-abdominal and inguinal skin sites. We also identified nine bacteria that are significantly different at least two of these sites: four bacteria that are enriched at lesions and five that are enriched at non-lesion sites. Presence or absence of these microbes may be responsible for lesional flares in patients with inverse psoriasis. In addition, the bacterial community structure between the three cohorts in non-lesion sites significantly differ at the axillary, inframammary, and infra-abdominal areas, suggesting that there may be a signature skin microbiome that may help us determine if plaque psoriasis patients will develop inverse psoriasis. Further studies with more subjects and a longitudinal study design will help to elucidate this.

Keywords: Psoriasis, intertriginous, *Corynebacterium*

*Corresponding author: jchung@uchc.edu

Nava Dayan (ed.) Skin Microbiome Handbook: From Basic Research to Product Development, (203–216) © 2020 Scrivener Publishing LLC

10.1   Introduction

Psoriasis is a painful and disfiguring disease that can strongly diminish a person's quality of life. It is estimated as high as one in twenty Americans are affected by psoriasis [1]. This common chronic immuno-dysregulatory skin disease is classified into a few subtypes. Inverse (intertriginous) psoriasis is a subtype that affects only the skin folds, where moisture is high. According to the Nurses' Health Study and Health Professionals Follow-up Study, the frequency of inverse psoriasis among physician-diagnosed psoriasis is 24% [2]. Lesions of inverse psoriasis are clinically diagnosed as shiny, red plaques, and scales are usually absent. These itchy, painful lesions affect very sensitive areas on the body, including the groin, inframammary, and underarm areas. A better understanding of this disease could provide substantial improvement to quality of life in this patient population.

Plaque psoriasis (vulgaris) is another subtype of psoriasis that affects random sites of the body *except* the skin folds. Majority of inverse psoriasis patients also have plaque psoriasis. Interestingly, the reverse is not true; many plaque psoriasis patients do not develop inverse psoriasis [2], suggesting a possible common trigger for inverse lesion development among plaque psoriasis patients. Plaque psoriasis lesions appear as raised, dull-red patches that are covered with a silvery white buildup as opposed to inverse psoriasis lesions that appear to be bright red, smooth, and shiny.

While the complete etiology of psoriasis still remains to be determined, a genetic susceptibility to the disease have been established. Majority of genetic susceptibility have been identified in the psoriasis susceptibility 1 locus (PSORS1), which encompasses variation in the major histocompatibility complex (MHC) genes. Overall, more than 70 genes have been identified to be associated with psoriasis through linkage and genetic association studies, but these genes only account for 30% overall psoriatic heritability [3]. With a lack of clear heritability patterns, environmental stimuli are strongly believed to play a role in disease development [4]. We believe that there is a connection between inverse psoriasis and the skin microbiota. The skin acts as an interface between the body and the environment. It is colonized by microorganisms that outnumber human cells by an order of magnitude [5]. Collectively these microorganisms are called the skin microbiota and may play a role in educating our immune system [6, 7]. Moreover, the cutaneous innate and adaptive immune responses can also modulate the skin microbiota [6, 8]. Disruptions in this balance between the immune system and the skin microbiota can result in skin disorders or infections [6, 8].

We hypothesize that a distinct skin microbiome at moist skin fold sites has a role in the pathogenesis of inverse psoriasis. Inverse psoriasis only occurs at moisture-rich sites. We know that the microbiome within these moisture-rich areas has been characterized to be different from other skin sites on the healthy human body [7]. In particular, metagenomic analysis has revealed an increased amount of *Staphylococcus* and *Corynebacterium* spp. colonizing moist areas when compared to sebaceous and dry sites of the skin [9]. These two types of bacteria result in the characteristic malodor associated with sweat in humans [10]. We believe that inverse psoriasis patients have a different inverse microbiome than plaque psoriatic patients, and that this unique microbial community may predispose them to having inverse lesions.

Currently, there are a few publications on studies of plaque psoriasis and the skin microbiome [11–13], but there have not been any studies on inverse psoriasis and the skin microbiome. Although there are various plaque psoriasis studies, they fail to identify a common microbial community that is particular to plaque lesions. Differences between psoriasis lesions and healthy skin have been seen but there is no consensus of lesional communities among these studies [14]. We believe that this might be due to the fact that plaque psoriasis has a preference for drier skin sites and majority of these studies are focused on dry sites at many different locations on the body. At dry skin sites, there are greater amounts of bacterial diversity and lesser bacterial load than moist sites [7], which may pose as a challenge when trying to identify commonality. We believe that focusing on skin folds, which are moist sites, and studying inverse psoriasis will allows us to have a more definitive dataset into identifying concrete differences between disease state microbiomes.

To investigate this, we have characterized the skin microbiome at intertriginous sites of three cohorts: plaque psoriatics 1) with inverse psoriasis, 2) without inverse psoriasis, and 3) healthy non-psoriatics. Our analyses would bring us one step closer to understanding the skin microbiome roles in the etiology of inverse psoriasis.

10.2   Methods

10.2.1   Subject Population

Between September 2018 and May 2019, we obtained consent and enrolled a total of 28 patients with ethical approval from University of Connecticut Institutional Review Board (IRB# 18-184J-1). These patients were recruited from the same geographic region (central Connecticut) and from two UConn dermatology clinics in Farmington, CT and Canton, CT. All patients were asked if they took antibiotics two weeks prior to sampling, and patients were not enrolled if antibiotics were taken two weeks before sampling.

10.2.2   Patient Diagnosis and Characteristics of Populations

Patients were diagnosed with chronic plaque psoriasis in a dermatology clinic, and psoriasis was clinically classified based on characteristic morphologic features of the individual skin lesions and their distribution on their body. For each patient, age, BMI, sex, ethnicity, family history of psoriasis, disease duration, percentage cutaneous involvement (% BSA), Psoriasis Area and Severity (PASI), and physician global assessment (PGA) scores were recorded. Patients with inverse psoriasis with at least one sampling site lesion would be recruited to be part of Cohort 1 (plaque + inverse psoriasis). Patients with at least 1% BSA of plaque psoriasis without any or past involvement of inverse psoriasis would be recruited to Cohort 2 (plaque psoriasis only). Generally healthy patients without any diagnosis of psoriasis or any inflammatory disease were recruited to be part of Cohort 3 (healthy non-psoriatics). Patients with confounding inflammatory disease, recent or known infection, and/or malignancy were excluded from the study.

10.2.3   Specimen Collection

We obtained nine intertriginous skin swabs: right and left axilla, right and left inframammary sites, right and left infra-abdominal sites, right and left inguinal sites, and the superior intergluteal cleft. These sites were chosen because of their commonality for inverse psoriasis lesions. A 2 x 2 cm area of the skin surface at each of these locations were sampled by swabbing the skin with a sterile polyester flock swab that had been moistened in sterile Specimen Collection Fluid (SCF-1) buffer (50nM Tris-HCl, pH 7.5; 1 mM EDTA, pH 8.0; 0.5% Tween-20) [15]. The subject's skin was stretched with one hand while holding the swab with the other hand so that the shaft is parallel to the skin surface. The swab was rubbed back and forth 50 times applying firm pressure for approximately 30 seconds. The swab heads were placed in to an empty screw-top 2mL tube and immediately placed in dry ice. Within 4 hours, the sample was transferred to and stored in a -80C freezer until further processing.

10.2.4   Sample DNA Extraction and Sequencing

DNA were extracted from the swabs in a biosafety cabinet in a PCR-free clean room using the DNeasy Powersoil Kit (Qiagen) with individual tubes. Extracted DNA was quantified using Quant-iT and Qubit HS. Dual indexed paired-end amplicon libraries of 16S rRNA gene V1-V3 hypervariable regions were generated using inhouse-designed oligonucleotides including universal primers, 27F 5'-AGAGTTTGATCCTGGCTCAG-3' and 534R 5'-ATTACCGCGGCTGCTGG-3'. PCR was performed using standard protocols. PCR mixtures contained 4 ng of purified DNA, 0.75U AccuPrime HiFi Taq polymerase (ThermoFisher Scientific), AccuPrime II PCR buffer (1X), 10 nM each forward and reverse primer, and molecular-grade water to a final volume of 20 uL. Thermal cycler conditions were initial denaturation at 95°C for 2 min; 30 cycles of denaturation at 95°C for 20s, annealing at 56°C for 30s, and extension at 72°C for 1min. The amplified fragments were analyzed on 0.8% agarose gel. The amplified fragments were then purified using AmPure XP beads (Beckman Coulter) in the ratio of 1:1 with PCR reaction volume and quantitated using Qubit HS reagents (Thermofisher Scientific). The purified libraries were then normalized to same molarity and combined to make an equimolar pool. The 16S (V1-V3) pool was purified again using AmPure XP beads and quantitated by Qubit HS reagents for final sequencing on the MiSeq platform using v3-600 cycle reagents (Illumina). Positive/negative controls were included for DNA extraction and amplification.

10.2.5   Downstream Sequence Processing and Analysis

Standard sequence processing was followed from Mahdavinia *et al.* [16] Briefly, Illumina's software handled initial processing of all raw sequences. Adapters and primers from sequences were removed by trimmomatic and then assembled by flash. Chimeric sequences and low quality reads were then filtered out by uchime. Subsequently sequences were then clustered by the operational taxonomic unit (OTU)-based approach with 3% dissimilarity cutoff using usearch. Taxonomic species classification was identified via NCBI refseq database using BLAST. All samples were rarified at 9169 sequences and relative abundance at species level was used for all analysis. Samples were removed from analysis if the sample had less than 9169 sequences. All graphs and statistics from sequencing data were generated with R.

10.3   Results

10.3.1   Cohort Metadata

We recruited 13 patients in cohort 1 (chronic plaque psoriatic patients with inverse psoriasis), 11 patients in cohort 2 (chronic plaque psoriatic patients without inverse psoriasis) and 4 patients in cohort 3 (healthy non-psoriatics). Many patients fulfilled the psoriatic involvement criteria but were not recruited due to their comorbidities. Nine intertriginous sites were swabbed for skin microbiome analysis: right and left axilla, right and left inframammary, right and left infra-abdominal, right and left inguinal and superior intergluteal cleft. Most patients who participated in the study had no problem volunteering to be swabbed at all nine sites, with a couple subjects in cohort 2 not comfortable swabbing the inguinal and superior intergluteal cleft. Table 10.1 tabulates the metadata of the three cohorts.

10.3.2   Sequencing Information

246 samples were extracted and sequenced. The mean number of reads was 21787 +/- 10513, with a range of 3 to 50626 (Figure 10.1). Samples were then rarified at 9169 to include 228 samples for final analysis, excluding 18 samples due to low read count (<4390 reads). We identified 1517 OTUs, which represented 1227 species.

10.3.3   The Skin Microbiome of Intertriginous Lesion and Non-Lesional Sites on Inverse Psoriasis Subjects

10.3.3.1   *Psoriasis Lesional Status is Associated with Relative Abundance and Presence of Specific Species*

We separated out each site to perform our analysis because prior studies have determined that different sites on the body contain a different microbial community [7]. Indeed, in our samples, the microbiome of each site showed different relative abundances of bacteria as shown in Figure 10.2a. However, since all of our sites tend to be high in moisture, all samples shared a large fraction of the same species. The top most abundant species across all samples were *Corynebacterium tuberculostearicum*, *Staphylococcus epidermidis*, *Cutibacterium acnes*, and *Staphylococcus hominis*. *C. tuberculostearicum* is of interest in that it has been reported to often be mis-identified with methods other than used here, and is a clinically relevant, often multidrug resistant bacterium [17]. We also observed that the

Table 10.1 Metadata of all subjects recruited and samples collected.

Cohort	Number of Subjects	Age (Years)	Height (Inches)	Weight (Pounds)	BMI	Sex	Ethnicity	Family history of psoriasis	Duration of psoriasis (Years)	BSA (%)	Number of Samples Collected	Number of Lesion Samples
1: Inverse + Plaque Psoriasis	13	51 +/- 9.6	69 +/- 4.3	220 +/- 65.4	33 +/- 7.1	3 (F) 10 (M)	8 (Caucasian) 3 (Black) 2 (Hispanic)	6 (Yes) 7 (No)	21 +/- 12	10 +/- 11	117	34 (Lesion) 83 (Non-Lesion)
2: Plaque Psoriasis Only	11	54 +/- 18.2	67 +/- 3.7	178 +/- 31.2	29 +/- 3	5 (F) 6 (M)	9 (Caucasian) 0 (Black) 1 (Hispanic) 1 (Other)	6 (Yes) 5 (No)	12 +/- 13	8 +/- 9	93	93 (Non-Lesion)
3: No Psoriasis	4	74 +/- 16.9	70 +/- 4.6	178 +/- 12	26 +/- 4.8	2 (F) 2 (M)	4 (Caucasian) 0 (Black) 0 (Hispanic)	4 (No)	0 +/- 0	0 +/- 0	36	36 (Non-Lesion)

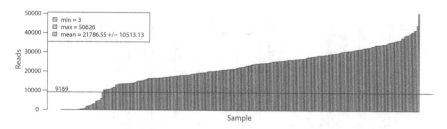

Figure 10.1 Read Distribution. 16S V1-V3 rRNA sequencing. Mean: 21787 ± 10513. Range: 3 – 50626. All samples were rarefied at 9169 for analysis, which excluded 18 out of 248 samples.

left and right sites were very similar to one another in species composition as also shown in Figure 10.2a.

Differences in species composition between lesional and non-lesional sites were evident in our taxa plots (Figure 10.2a). To further determine which species were significantly different between lesional and non-lesional sites, Kruskal Wallis testing was done on each species at each anatomical site. Nine bacteria were determined to be significantly different between lesional and non-lesional samples in cohort 1 in at least two sampling sites (Figure 10.2b), one of which was the eighth most abundant bacteria across all samples (Figure 10.2a, b, highlighted in cyan (*Corynebacterium massiliense*)). *Bartonella coopersplainsensis*, *Acinetobacter baumannii*, *Capnocytophaga ochracea*, *Corynebacterium massiliense*, and *Haematobacter missouriensis* were found to be significantly enriched in lesion sites. Of these, interestingly, *Acinetobacter baumannii* is rarely found as part of the normal skin microbiota [18], and is known to target moist tissues to cause hemorrhagic bullae. *Cutibacterium granulosum*, *Dermacoccus nishinomiyaensis*, *Lawsonella clevelandensis*, and *Sphingomonas olei* were found to be enriched in non-lesional sites. *Cutibacterium granulosum* was also found to be more enriched in healthy skin when compared to a psoriasis-associated skin in another study [19].

10.3.3.2   Psoriatic Lesions Trend to Decrease Taxonomic Diversity

To assess the within sample diversity in each sample, we measured the richness and Shannon diversity at the species taxonomical level (Figure 10.2c). Richness measures the number of species in each sample. Shannon diversity incorporates both richness and evenness of each sample. In both measures, at every site except the superior intergluteal cleft, the non-lesional sites of cohort 1 tend to have higher species diversity than lesion sites, though most sites were not significant (p < 0.05 by Mann-Whitney testing).

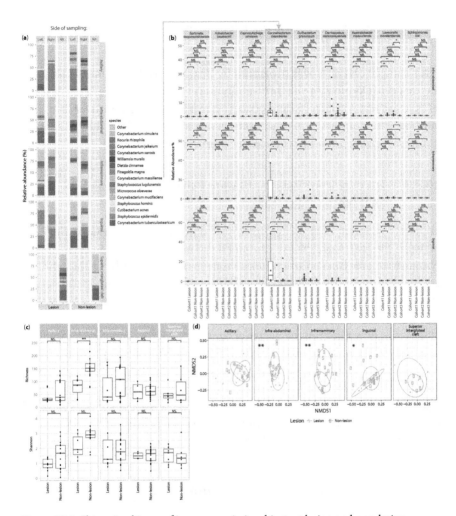

Figure 10.2 Skin microbiome of inverse psoriasis subjects at lesion and non-lesion intertriginous sites. (a) Bar plots of the average relative abundance of the top 15 most abundant species at each sampling site. (b) Nine species that were identified to be significantly different (p < 0.05, Mann-Whitney testing) at more than one site between lesion and non-lesion sites. Cyan highlights one species that was also identified to be one of the top 15 most abundant species as shown in (a). (c) Boxplots of intra-sample diversity between lesion and non-lesion sites as measured by richness and Shannon diversity in cohort 1. Significance testing done by Mann-Whitney testing. (d) NMDS plots of inter-sample diversity between lesion and non-lesion sites in cohort 1 at different sites, measured by Bray Curtis dissimilarity. Ellipses represent the one standard deviation from the center. Adonis testing between lesion status was done for significance. ***p < 0.001, **p < 0.01, *p < 0.05.

10.3.3.3 Psoriatic Lesions are Characterized by Greater Intragroup Variability

Inter-sample diversity was measured by Bray Curtis dissimilarity and plotted in a NMDS plot. At the infra-abdominal, inframammary, and inguinal sites, inverse psoriasis lesions possess a more variable and overall different bacterial composition than non-lesions as demonstrated by the larger diameter ellipses and different center points in Figure 10.2d.

10.3.4 Inverse Psoriasis vs. Plaque Psoriasis vs. Healthy (All Non-Lesion Sites)

To assess whether there is an "intrinsic" skin microbiome that is different between the three cohorts, we examined the non-lesion sites in each cohort. A signature predisposed microbiome may explain why subjects in cohort 1 are more prone to inverse psoriasis involvement. We determined the overall community composition structures of each sample using Bray Curtis dissimilarity. Figure 10.3 shows the PCoA plots of each sample, colored by cohort, to visualize how different the bacterial community structure of each sample is to one another. The ellipses represent the center of the samples in each cohort with the radius representing one standard deviation from the center. From adonis testing, the axillary, inframammary, and infra-abdominal sites showed significant difference between cohorts ($p < 0.05$), suggesting that the overall baseline skin microbiome of healthy non-psoriatics, psoriasis patients with, and without inverse involvement are all different.

10.4 Conclusions & Future Plans

We only began to scratch the surface in understanding the role of the skin microbiome in inverse psoriasis. From this study, we know that the skin microbiota at lesional and non-lesional intertriginous sites are different in patients with inverse psoriasis. Specifically, there are particular bacteria that were found to be significantly different that may influence lesion development. Corynebacterium is known to dominate moist sites on the skin, particular strains may be associated with inverse lesion development in plaque psoriasis patients. Namely, a particular strain of *Corynebacterium massiliense* could be part of inverse psoriasis pathogenesis as we have found this species to be significantly enriched in lesions sites compared to non-lesion sites. More research should be done to investigate the roles non-diphteriae Corynebacterium species play in the skin microbial community as these commensal species have not much been investigated.

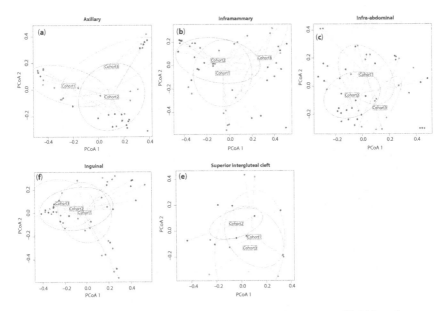

Figure 10.3 Skin microbiome of inverse psoriasis, plaque psoriasis, and healthy subjects at non-lesion intertriginous sites. PCoA plots of inter-sample diversity between different cohorts at (a) Axillary, (b) Inframammary, (c) Infra-abdominal, (d) Inguinal, (e) Superior intergluteal cleft. Measured by Bray Curtis dissimilarity calculated at species level. Ellipses represent one standard deviation from the center. Blue = Cohort1, Red = Cohort2, Green = Cohort3. Adonis testing between cohorts was done for significance. ***p < 0.001, **p < 0.01, *p < 0.05.

Another important finding from this study showed that the intrinsic skin microbiome in psoriatic patients with and without inverse involvement, and healthy non-psoriatics all have distinct microbiomes, which may explain why certain psoriasis patients are more prone to having inverse lesions. One limitation from this study was the low number of subjects recruited and lack of longitudinal information. However, future studies with more subjects and follow up of plaque psoriasis only subjects that later developed inverse psoriasis would provide more power and stronger evidence that particular bacteria or a group of bacteria are responsible for inverse lesions.

Acknowledgements

Jennifer Chung was a recipient of a National Psoriasis Foundation Psoriatic Disease Research Fellowship. We would also like to thank Miguel Rodriguez Reyes for his help in sample DNA extractions and library preparation.

References

1. Michalek I.M., Loring, B., John, S.M., A systematic review of worldwide epidemiology of psoriasis. *J. Eur. Acad. Dermatol. Venereol.*, 31, 2, 205–212, 2017.
2. Merola, J.F., Li, T., Li, W.Q., Cho, E., Qureshi, A.A., Prevalence of psoriasis phenotypes among men and women in the USA. *Clin. Exp. Dermatol.*, 41, 5, 486–9, 2016.
3. Greb, J.E., Goldminz, A.M., Elder, J.T., Lebwohl, M.G., Gladman, D.D., Wu, J.J., Mehta, N.N., Finlay, A.Y., Gottlieb, A.B., Psoriasis. *Nat. Rev. Dis. Primers*, 2, 16082, 2016.
4. Watson, W., Cann, H.M., Farber, E.M., Nall, M.L., The genetics of psoriasis. *Arch. Dermatol.*, 105, 2, 197–207, 1972.
5. Human Microbiome Project C., Structure, function and diversity of the healthy human microbiome. *Nature*, 486, 7402, 207–14, 2012.
6. Belkaid, Y. and Hand, T.W., Role of the microbiota in immunity and inflammation. *Cell.*, 157, 1, 121–41, 2014.
7. Grice, E.A. and Segre, J.A., The skin microbiome. *Nat. Rev. Microbiol.*, 9, 4, 244–53, 2011.
8. Hogenova, H.T., Zakostelska, Z.J., Petanova, J., Kverka, M., Microbiota, immunity and immunologically-mediated diseases. *Vnitr Lek.*, 65, 2, 98–107, 2019.
9. Grice, E.A., Kong, H.H., Conlan, S., Deming, C.B., Davis, J., Young, A.C., Program, N.C.S., Bouffard, G.G., Blakesley, R.W., Murray, P.R., Green, E.D., Turner, M.L., Segre, J.A., Topographical and temporal diversity of the human skin microbiome. *Science*, 324, 5931, 1190–2, 2009.
10. Leyden, J.J., McGinley, K.J., Holzle, E., Labows, J.N., Kligman, A.M., The microbiology of the human axilla and its relationship to axillary odor. *J. Invest. Dermatol.*, 77, 5, 413–6, 1981.
11. Alekseyenko, A.V., Perez-Perez, G.I., De Souza, A., Strober, B., Gao, Z., Bihan, M., Li, K., Methe, B.A., Blaser, M.J., Community differentiation of the cutaneous microbiota in psoriasis. *Microbiome.*, 1, 1, 31, 2013.
12. Fahlen, A., Engstrand, L., Baker, B.S., Powles, A., Fry, L., Comparison of bacterial microbiota in skin biopsies from normal and psoriatic skin. *Arch. Dermatol. Res.*, 304, 1, 15–22, 2012.
13. Tett, A., Pasolli, E., Farina, S., Truong, D.T., Asnicar, F., Zolfo, M., Beghini, F., Armanini, F., Jousson, O., De Sanctis, V., Bertorelli, R., Girolomoni, G., Cristofolini, M., Segata, N., Unexplored diversity and strain-level structure of the skin microbiome associated with psoriasis. *NPJ Biofilms Microbiomes.*, 3, 14, 2017.
14. Yan, D., Issa, N., Afifi, L., Jeon, C., Chang, H.W., Liao, W., The Role of the Skin and Gut Microbiome in Psoriatic Disease. *Curr. Dermatol. Rep.*, 6, 2, 94–103, 2017.

15. Human Microbiome Project C., A framework for human microbiome research. *Nature*, 486, 7402, 215–21, 2012.
16. Mahdavinia, M., Rasmussen, H.E., Botha, M., Binh Tran, T.D., Van den Berg, J.P., Sodergren, E., Davis, E., Engen, K., Gray, C., Lunjani, N., Hlela, C., Preite, N.Z., Basera, W., Hobane, L., Watkins, A., Engen, P., Mankahla, A., Gaunt, B., Thomas, F., Tobin, M.C., Landay, A., Weinstock, G.M., Keshavarzian, A., Levin, M.E., Effects of diet on the childhood gut microbiome and its implications for atopic dermatitis. *J. Allergy. Clin. Immunol.*, 143, 4, 1636–7 e5, 2019.
17. Hinic, V., Lang, C., Weisser, M., Straub, C., Frei, R., Goldenberger, D., Corynebacterium tuberculostearicum: A potentially misidentified and multiresistant Corynebacterium species isolated from clinical specimens. *J. Clin. Microbiol.*, 50, 8, 2561–7, 2012.
18. Howard, A., O'Donoghue, M., Feeney, A., Sleator, R.D., Acinetobacter baumannii: An emerging opportunistic pathogen. *Virulence*, 3, 3, 243–50, 2012.
19. Chang, H.W., Yan, D., Singh, R., Liu, J., Lu, X., Ucmak, D., Lee, K., Afifi, L., Fadrosh, D., Leech, J., Vasquez, K.S., Lowe, M.M., Rosenblum, M.D., Scharschmidt, T.C., Lynch, S.V., Liao, W., Alteration of the cutaneous microbiome in psoriasis and potential role in Th17 polarization. *Microbiome.*, 6, 1, 154, 2018.

Part 4
SKIN'S INNATE IMMUNITY

11

Effects of Endogenous Lipids on the Skin Microbiome

Carol L. Fischer[1] and Philip W. Wertz[2]*

[1] *Waldorf University, Forest City, Iowa, USA*
[2] *University of Iowa, Iowa City, Iowa, USA*

Abstract

The human skin surface serves as the interface between the environment and the rest of the body. As such, the skin provides a barrier against the penetration of environmental chemicals and provides an environment that is not amenable to the colonization and growth of most microorganisms. Yet, it does support the growth of some commensal microorganisms, which help in defending against pathogens. Other factors that influence which microorganisms can live at the skin surface include availability of nutrients and water, the presence of antimicrobial peptides and a relatively low pH. Sebaceous fatty acids can serve as a nutrient source for some microorganisms while being toxic to others. Some of the sebaceous fatty acids and free long-chain bases derived from stratum corneum ceramides have differential antimicrobial activity. Factors influencing microbial growth vary regionally. The head, neck, chest and upper back regions have abundant sebaceous glands, so these areas are oily. The antecubital fossa are moist, while most of the remaining skin surface is relatively dry and contains little sebum. The purpose of this chapter is to examine the roles of certain lipids found at the skin surface in determining the growth of bacteria and fungi.

Keywords: Ceramide, *Cutibacterium acnes*, lauric acid, long-chain base, *Marassezia spp*, sapienic acid, sebum, *Staphylococcus aureus*

11.1   Introduction

It has long been recognized that the human skin surface is colonized by a limited number of bacterial and fungal species that, under most circumstances,

---

Corresponding author: philipwwertz@gmail.com

Nava Dayan (ed.) Skin Microbiome Handbook: From Basic Research to Product Development, (219–236) © 2020 Scrivener Publishing LLC

do no harm [1]. Although the same species are present at most skin sites, numbers vary with characteristics of the skin site. Sebaceous lipid-rich sites favor *Cutibacterium acnes* (formerly *Proprionibacterium acnes*) and *Malassezia spp.* (formerly *Pityrosporum spp.*), whereas dry but less oily sites are more favorable to *Staphylococcus epidermidis* and other *Staphylococcus spp.*. Moist sites tend to include some Gram-negative species [1, 2]. Other microorganisms, such as *Staphylococcus aureus*, that come into contact with the skin are normally transients; however, *S. aureus* does successfully colonize the nares, and subsequently, the skin of approximately one-third of the population [3–6], sometimes causing infection [7–9]. In this population, the colonization of *S. aureus* is generally stable [4]. Certain free fatty acids and long-chain bases present at the skin surface are one major factor in determining the resident microbial populations and preventing

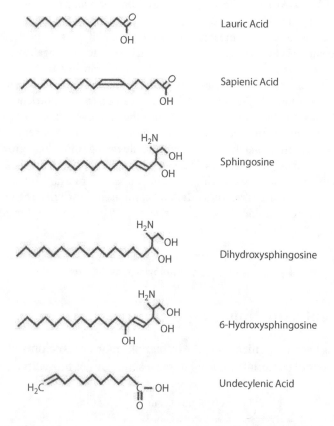

Figure 11.1 Chemical structures of the major antimicrobial lipids from the human skin surface.

colonization by potential pathogens. The major antimicrobial lipids present at the skin surface are shown in Figure 11.1. Perturbations of endogenous lipids can create opportunities for colonization and pathogenesis.

11.2 Sebaceous Lipids -- Source of Fatty Acids

Sebaceous glands are found in all regions of human skin except for the palmar and plantar areas. They are most abundant in the regions of the head, neck, chest and upper back. *In utero*, fetal sebaceous gland activity is high due to stimulation by the mother's ovarian and adrenal androgens [10]. At birth, the sebum secretion rate is still high and remains so for approximately the first week of life, after which it rapidly drops to a very low level where it remains until the onset of puberty [11–13]. The sebum secretion rate reaches a maximum level in both men and women in the late teens or early 20s and declines thereafter until about age 70 [13]. In the elderly population, the sebum secretion rate is again very low as in prepubertal children. Figure 11.2 demonstrates the decline in the availability of free fatty acids at the skin surface with increasing age.

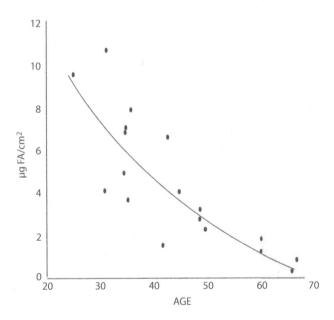

Figure 11.2 Decrease in free fatty acids at the human skin surface with age. Skin surface lipid was extracted into ethanol from the legs of 20 female subjects and analyzed by thin-layer chromatography. Ages ranged from 25 through 68 years.

It was known for some time that skin surface lipids included tri-glycerides and fatty acids, but the complete composition of human sebum was not known until the 1950s. Sebum collected from human hair consists of squalene, wax monoesters, cholesterol esters, triglycerides, fatty acids and small proportions of cholesterol [14, 15]. Sebum from the lumen of sebaceous glands does not contain free fatty acids; however, generation of free fatty acids occurs via hydrolysis of the triglycerides by microbial lipases as sebum flows through the follicle and over the surfaces of skin and hair [16]. The average composition of sebum collected from the fore-head of seventeen subjects determined by quantitative thin-layer chroma-tography is: diglycerides, 2.2 % (by weight); cholesterol, 1.4 %; fatty acids, 16.4 %; triglycerides, 41.0 %; wax esters, 25.0 %; cholesterol esters, 2.1 %; squalene, 12.0 % [17].

Early speculation that the free fatty acids at the skin surface may be anti-microbial brought attention to this lipid fraction. The first determination of human sebaceous fatty acid composition was published in 1947 [18]. For this pioneering study, 45 kg of hair clippings were collected from bar-bershops in Chicago. Boiling ether was used to extract lipids from this hair in a single batch. The free fatty acids were extracted from ether solution into aqueous potassium hydroxide as potassium soaps. The recovered fatty acid soaps were converted to methyl esters by heating in methanol satu-rated with dry hydrochloric acid and extracted into petroleum ether. The petroleum ether was removed by careful distillation through a fractionat-ing column so as not to lose short-chain fatty acid methyl esters. The final fatty acid methyl ester fraction weighed 240 g. The methyl esters were dis-tilled under reduced pressure within an apparatus that measured tempera-ture as a function of volume distilled. This enabled plotting of a distillation curve from which the carbon chain-length distribution of the fatty acid methyl esters could be determined. The fatty acids ranged from 7- through 22-carbons in length, with the 16- and 18-carbon entities being the most abundant. The 7- through 10-carbon and the 22-carbon fractions were saturated. The other fractions contained a mixture of a saturated and one monounsaturated fatty acid, except for the 18-carbon fraction, which con-tained a saturated species, two monounsaturated species and two dienoic species. The saturated species were separated from the unsaturated species by crystallization. Double bonds were located in most of the monoenes, and the most abundant fatty acid proved to be C16:1Δ6, subsequently called sapienic acid [19]. The late Donald T. Downing coined the term sapi-enic acid, which reflects the fact that C16:1Δ6 is uniquely abundant in the sebum of *Homo sapiens*. It also led to the in-house joke that the two-carbon extension product from sapienic acid, C18:1Δ8, is di**homosapien**ic acid.

Several early investigations of human sebaceous fatty acids employing gas-liquid chromatography essentially confirmed the findings of Weitkamp, Smiljanic and Rothman [18, 20, 21]. The short-chain fatty acids, C7 - C13, were also found in sebaceous triglycerides supporting the assertion that they were of sebaceous and not sweat origin. Unfortunately, most subsequent investigators who studied sebaceous fatty acids by gas-liquid chromatography used either boron trichloride or boron trifluoride in methanol to prepare fatty acid methyl esters. With this method, the fatty acids are heated with the reagent in a sealed tube followed by evaporation of the reagent under a stream of nitrogen. This results in loss by evaporation of all of the fatty acids shorter than 14-carbons.

Among the most abundant microorganisms in sebum rich areas of skin are *C. acnes* and *Malassezia spp.*. Both of these lipophilic organisms use sebaceous lipids as nutrients and secrete lipases that hydrolyze sebaceous triglycerides to liberate free fatty acids, some of which limit or prevent the growth of other microorganisms [22, 23]. *C. acnes* also secretes propionic acid, which suppresses the growth of *S. aureus* [24]. The commensal yeast *Malassezia globosa* secretes an aspartyl protease that interferes with biofilm formation by *S. aureus*, thereby providing protection to the host [25].

C. acnes is a commensal traditionally implicated as an opportunistic pathogen in acne vulgaris [26]. Recent genetic analyses have identified three phylogenetic lineages of *C. acnes* [27]. One of these three strains of *C. acnes* becomes dominant in acne vulgaris, and there is also an increase in follicular *Staphylococcus epidermidis*.

Malassezia spp., most abundant on the scalp, have been implicated in the etiology of dandruff [28]. A correlation exists between the severity of dandruff and the number of *Malassezia spp.* organisms present on the scalp; however, other factors are probably also involved including bacteria and host-related physiological factors.

11.3 Stratum Corneum Lipids - Source of Long-Chain Bases

Epidermal keratinocytes differentiate as they move out of the basal layer and toward the skin surface [29]. Part of the differentiation process involves the accumulation of glucosylceramides, phospholipids including sphingomyelin and phosphoglycerides and cholesterol in small organelles called lamellar granules [30]. Lamellar granules are round to ovoid in shape with a diameter of about 0.2 micrometers. They have a bounding membrane surrounding stacks of lamellar lipids and an array of hydrolytic enzymes. At the boundary between the viable portion of the epidermis and the stratum corneum, the bounding membrane of the lamellar granule fuses into the cell plasma membrane, and the contents are extruded into the intercellular space. Hydrolytic enzyme action converts glucosylceramides and sphingomyelin into ceramides. Phosphoglycerides serve as precursors to free fatty acids and the fatty acids in cholesterol esters. These are the lipids that pass into the intercellular spaces of the stratum corneum.

One of the lamellar-granule associated glucosylceramides is an unusual lipid containing 30- through 34-carbon ω-hydroxyacids amide-linked to long-chain bases with linoleate ester-linked to the ω-hydroxyl group and glucose β-glycosidically-linked to the primary hydroxyl group of the base [31–33]. Much of this lipid is in the bounding membrane of the lamellar granule. This unusual lipid serves as the precursor to ω-hydroxyceramides which become ester-linked to acidic groups on the outer surface of the cornified envelope [34, 35]. The ω-hydroxyceramides that become covalently bound to the outer surface of the cornified envelope in human stratum corneum are shown in Figure 11.3.

Free long-chain bases identified in stratum corneum include sphingosines, dihydrosphingosines and 6-hydroxysphingosines [36, 37]. Interestingly, although phytosphingosine is present in some of the ceramides,

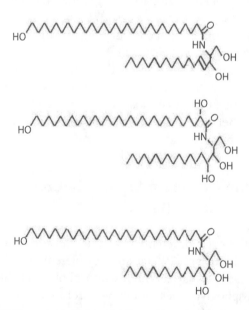

Figure 11.3 Chemical structures of the ω-hydroxyceramides that become covalently bound to the cornified envelope.

free phytosphingosine has not been detected. Ceramidase activities capable of liberating long-chain bases from the ceramides have been reported [38].

Several pieces of evidence indicate that the covalently bound ω-hydroxyceramides in the stratum corneum may be a preferred ceramidase substrates [Wertz, unpublished observations]. First, when young pigs are placed on a diet in which hydrogenated coconut oil is the only fat, essential fatty acid deficiency accompanied by progressive increase in transepidermal water loss develops. The increase in transepidermal water loss (TEWL) reflects the fact that without a source of linoleic acid the linoleate-containing acylceramide, ceramide EOS, cannot be synthesized, and this lipid is essential for barrier function of the skin. This decrease in barrier function is accompanied by a reduction in the amount of covalently bound ω-hydroxyceramide, with a concomitant increase in covalently bound ω-hydroxyacid as shown in Figure 11.4. This is what would be expected if, as barrier function is decreased, ceramidase acts on the covalently bound ω-hydroxyceramide to liberate free sphingosines and dihydrosphingosines leaving behind the covalently bound ω-hydroxyacid. Secondly, in both psoriatic scale and atopic dermatitis, where barrier function is compromised, the proportion of covalently bound ω-hydroxyacid relative to covalently bound ω-hydroxyceramide is elevated compared to normal healthy control stratum corneum [Wertz, unpublished observations].

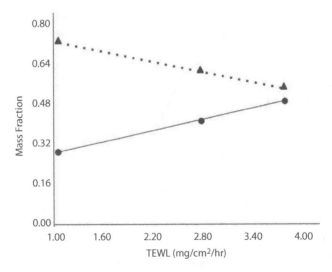

Figure 11.4 Decline in covalently bound ω-hydroxyceramide with concomitant increase in covalently bound ω-hydroxyacid as essential fatty acid deficiency develops in young pigs. Transepidermal water loss increases as essential fatty acid deficiency develops. ▲ = ω-hydroxyceramide; ● = ω-hydroxyacid.

11.4 Antimicrobial Activity of Fatty Acids

A study published by Burtenshaw in 1938 demonstrated that the skin had self-disinfecting properties [39]. In this study, aqueous suspensions of *S. aureus* or *Streptococcus pyogenes* were applied to the skin and dried. After some time, material was collected from the skin surface. The total number of bacteria was determined, and viability was determined by growing the cells on agar plates. It was clear that the skin surface had antimicrobial activity. It was postulated that the low pH of sweat may be an important factor.

In 1942, Burtenshaw published the first demonstration that lipids collected from the skin surface had antibacterial activity [40]. The skin surface was extracted with ethyl ether or with saline. The extracts were filtered and dried. Aqueous suspensions of the residues were tested against several strains of *S. aureus, S. pyogenes* and several other bacteria. The ether extracts proved to be antimicrobial, while the saline extracts were inactive. This clearly suggested an antimicrobial lipid. Although the composition of skin surface lipids was not completely known at this time, it was postulated that fatty acids derived from sebum could be the active component. Accordingly, Burtenshaw tested some available fatty acids including some short-chain fatty acids known to be present in human sweat (acetic acid, propionic acid, caproic acid, caprylic acid, citric acid. ascorbic acid and uric acid) and total fatty acids from hydrolyzed butter (butyric acid, caproic acid, caprylic acid, capric acid, lauric acid, palmitic acid, stearic acid, oleic acid, linoleic acid). Capric acid (C10:0), lauric acid (C12:), stearic acid (C18:0) and oleic acid (C18:1Δ9) were individually tested. None of the sweat organic acids had any activity. Total fatty acids from hydrolyzed butter as well as each of the individual butter fatty acids tested showed activity. Potency of the individual fatty acids was not ranked. Although the individual fatty acids tested and found to have antibacterial activity are now all known to be present in human sebum, there are other unique fatty acids in human sebum that have only recently been tested for antibacterial activity. In addition, a more recent study demonstrated that lauric acid killed *S. aureus*, while capric acid and stearic acid were bacteriostatic. Myristic acid and palmitic acid were also bacteriostatic. Oleic acid was not tested in this study [19].

A note of interest is that Burtenshaw did his work on the antimicrobial skin lipids in facilities at St. Mary's Hospital provided to him by Alexander Fleming. Fleming had discovered penicillin in 1928. By 1942, efforts were under way to produce penicillin on a large scale, and the first patient was treated. By D-day enough penicillin was available to treat the allied troops.

The main motivation for the sebaceous fatty acid analysis of Weitkamp, Smiljanic and Rothman [17] was an observation made by Rothman in his clinical practice. He saw many infants with a fungal infection of the scalp called *tinea capitis* or, more commonly, "cradle cap". This could be treated by occlusion, but it tended to recur until the child reached puberty, when it disappeared and did not return. Rothman speculated that because sebum secretion increases dramatically at the onset of puberty that a sebaceous component likely had antifungal activity against the causative agent, *Microsporum audouinii*. When the fatty acids isolated from hair clippings were tested for activity against this yeast the 7-, 9-, 11-, and 13-carbon fatty acids were active [41]. Other fatty acids were not active. So the short-chain odd-carbon fatty acids, each of which was less than 0.05% of the total fatty acid mass, proved to provide protection against fungal infection.

This finding was reminiscent of undecylenic acid, an 11-carbon fatty acid with a double bond between the last two carbons, identified as a component of human sweat. Undecylenic acid also proved to have activity against certain fungi [42], and is the active ingredient in over-the counter medications for treating athlete's foot and other fungal infections of the skin and nails. The short-chain saturated fatty acids from human sebum have not been similarly commercialized, at least in part because the C7:0 and C9:0 have strong and unpleasant odors. The C11:0 and C13:0 entities could have been exploited, but difficulty of production has likely precluded this.

According to the sebaceous fatty acid analyses of James and Wheatley [20], lauric acid constituted 3% of the fatty acids by weight. This has been shown to be a uniquely potent antimicrobial agent against bacteria, especially Gram-positive bacteria and yeasts but not Gram-negative bacteria [43, 44]. Susceptible organisms included *Pneumococcus spp. Streptococcus spp, Corynebacterium spp, Nocardia asteroides, Candida spp, S. aureus* and *S. epidermidis*. Some activity was seen with other saturated fatty acids, but minimum inhibitory concentrations for lauric acid were considerably lower in this study.

In a more recent study, lauric acid and sapienic acid had potent bactericidal activity against *S. aureus* [19]. Under the conditions used in this study, octanoic acid, decanoic acid, myristic acid and palmitic acid had degrees of bacteriostatic activity, but were not bactericidal. Stearic acid was inactive.

In other recent studies, both lauric acid and sapienic acid were active against a range of Gram-positive bacteria including *S. aureus, Streptococcus sanguinis, Streptococcus mitis, Corynebacterium bovis, Corynebacterium striatum* and *Corynebacterium jeikeium* [45]. Neither fatty acid was active against the Gram-negative *Escherichia coli, Pseudomonas aeruginosa* or *Serratia marcescens*, but both were active against the Gram-negative periodontal pathogen *Fusobacterium nucleatum*. Sapienic acid and lauric acid also has antimicrobial activity against the periodontal pathogen *Porphyromonas gingivalis* [46].

Some *Staphylococcus spp.* other than *S. aureus* and some *Corynebacterium spp.* are among the commensals normally found on human skin [47]. *Corynebacterium spp.* are more abundant in the moist regions and are associated with formation of malodorous compounds. Antimicrobial fatty acids and long-chain bases as well as undecylenic acid from sweat may all contribute to controlling the growth of these bacterial species. The activity profiles of lauric acid and sapienic acid against selected bacteria are summarized in Table 11.1.

S. aureus is a transient organism on human skin, but it can cause infections. Up to 30% of the human population are asymptomatic carriers of *S. aureus* in the nasal cavity, and this can be a source of *S. aureus* skin infections [48]. Due to this potential pool of *S. aureus*, the nasal cavity is routinely swabbed with mupirocin prior to surgery to minimize chances of post-operative skin infection. Among prepubertal children, impetigo caused by *S. aureus* is the most common skin infection [49]. The low levels of lauric acid and sapienic acid due to minimal sebum synthesis may contribute to susceptibility of this population.

Atopic dermatitis is an increasingly common skin disease seen in children. In this condition, skin infections are common. Most atopics carry nasal *S. aureus* and the atopic skin becomes colonized by *S. aureus* [50]. In atopic dermatitis, the composition of ceramides in the stratum corneum is altered, and the total ceramide content is diminished compared to normal stratum corneum [51, 52]. One reason for this alteration of stratum corneum ceramides is the expression of an enzyme, glucosylceramide sphingomyelin deacylase, which cleaves the amide linkage of sphingomyelin and glucosylceramides. This ultimately results in a reduced level of free sphingosine in the stratum corneum [53, 54]. It has been suggested that this reduced level of free long-chain base contributes to the susceptibility of this population to colonization by *S. aureus*. It has also been shown that the non-lesional skin surface in atopic dermatitis has a reduced level of sapienic acid compared to normal control skin [55]. There was a strong inverse correlation between the numbers of *S. aureus* colonizing normal or atopic skin and the level of sapienic acid, suggesting that sapienic acid protects against *S. aureus* colonization.

If low levels of lauric acid and sapienic acid contribute to the susceptibility of prepubertal children to skin infections, it might be expected

Table 11.1 Activity of lipids against selected bacteria.

Gram-positive bacteria	Lauric acid	Sapienic acid	Long-chain bases
Staphylococcus aureus	+	+	+
Staphylococcus epidermidis	+	+	nd
Streptococcus pyogenes	+	+	+
Streptococcus sanguinis	+	+	+
Streptococcus mitis	+	+	+
Corynebacterium bovis	+	+	+
Corynebacterium striatum	+	+	+
Corynebacterium jeikeium	+	+	+
Gram-negative bacteria			
Escherichia coli	–	–	+
Fusobacterium nucleatum	+	+	+
Porphyromonas gingivalis	+	+	+
Pseudomonas aeruginosa	–	–	–
Serratia marcescens	–	–	–

Based on [36–39, 51, 52]; + = active; – = inactive; nd = not done Dihydrosphingosine and phytosphingosine had activity profiles similar to sphingosine.

that elderly people would display similar susceptibility. In fact, the elderly are more susceptible to a variety of bacterial and fungal skin infections compared to younger adults [49]. Two skin conditions that are more common in elderly people are dry skin and seborrheic dermatitis, neither of which is related to the rate of sebum secretion [13]. Although the sebum secretion rate in elderly people is reduced compared to young adults it does not differ between people with either condition and people with normal skin. Dry skin itches, which leads to scratching. This can breach the stratum corneum, thereby creating openings for bacterial entry and contributing to a higher skin infection incidence in the elderly.

Among the most common bacterial skin infections in the elderly are cellulitis, impetigo, folliculitis, boils and secondary infections of skin abrasions or wounds, and *S. aureus* is the primary causative or contributing organism in each of these conditions [56]. Cellulitis is caused mainly by *Staphylococcus spp.*, usually *S. aureus*, and/or *Streptococcus spp.* Other bacteria that may be involved include *Pseudomonas spp.*, *Serratia spp.*, *Proteus mirabilis*, *Escherichia coli* and *Klebsiella spp.*. The other mentioned infections are mainly attributable to *S. aureus*. Secondary infections come about when the stratum corneum is compromised allowing *S. aureus* to invade. The most common fungal infections found in the elderly are tinea pedis and onychomycosis [49]. The causative agents are *Trichophyton rubrum*, *Trichophyton mentagrophytes* and *Epidermophyton floccosum*.

11.5   Antimicrobial Activity of Long-Chain Bases

In 1989, Bibel *et al.* reported that stratum corneum polar lipid fractions had antimicrobial activity against a range of microorganisms including *S. pyogenes*, *S. aureus*, *S. epidermidis*, *Micrococcus sp.* and *Candida albicans* [57]. Bibel, Aly and Shinefield later demonstrated that sphingosine and dihydrosphingosine had potent activity against *S. aureus*, while other pure phospholipids and sphingolipids were inactive [58]. The range of microorganisms susceptible to the long-chain bases was subsequently expanded to include *T. mentagrophytes*, *Trichophyton tonsurans*, *E. floccosum*, *S. sanguinis*, *S. mitis*, *C. bovis*, *C. striatum*, *C. jeikeium*, *E. coli* and *F. nucleatum* [46, 59]. The activity of free long-chain bases against selected bacteria is summarized in Table 11.1.

Free sphingoid bases are also potent inhibitors of protein kinase C [60]. The generation of free sphingoid bases in the stratum corneum may provide, in addition to antimicrobial activity, a feedback mechanism through inhibition of protein kinase c that modulates cell proliferation and differentiation in the epidermis [61]. It has also been suggested that exogenous sphingosine could possibly be useful in treatment of hyperproliferative conditions [61].

Although the concentration of sphingosine has been measured in normal human epidermis and in epidermis from several skin diseases, no study has been performed to determine if the concentration varies with anatomic site. Samples of human foot callus contained about 5 mg of free long-chain base per g of dry tissue in one study [36]. In another study, leg stratum corneum was found to contain 2 mg sphingosine per gram of stratum corneum, suggesting regional variation in sphingosine concentration [62].

Subjects with erythrodermic ichthyoses showed significantly lower levels of stratum corneum sphingosine (0.2–0.4 mg sphingosine/g stratum corneum). Subjects with non-erythrodermic ichthyoses did not differ significantly from controls in their sphingosine content.

11.6   Conclusion

The human skin surface is colonized by C. *acnes, Corynebacterium spp., Staphylococcal spp.* other than *S. aureus, Malassezia spp.* and other minor species. The density and composition of microorganisms varies regionally according to variations in the skin surface environment. Sebaceous fatty acids, mainly the short odd-carbon species (C7:0, C9:0, C11:0 and C13:0), lauric acid (C12:0) and sapienic acid (C16:0Δ6) provide differential antimicrobial activity against a wide range of potentially pathogenic Gram-positive bacteria and some yeasts. The long-chain bases have a broader range of activity against bacteria and yeast. It is an interesting possibility that application of formulations containing sapienic acid and/or lauric acid could be used to prevent or treat skin infections in the elderly or other populations susceptible to skin infections. Further work is needed to determine the distribution of long-chain bases in different regions of skin and to better our understanding of the roles of these sphingoid bases in innate immunity.

Future studies should determine the anatomic distribution and effects of age on the long-chain bases at the human skin surface. Existing *in vitro* results as well as observation on *S. aureus,* sapienic acid and sphingosine suggest that supplementation of the skin surface with such lipids could protentiall prevent or treat skin infections. Clinical trials should be set up to explore this possibility.

References

1. Kligman, A.M., Leyden, J.J., McGinley, K.J., Bacteriology. *J. Invest. Dermatol.*, 67, 160, 1976.
2. Byrd, A.L., Belkaid, Y., Sefre, J.A., The human skin microbiome. *Nat. Rev. Microbiol.*, 16, 143, 2018.
3. Graham, P.L., Lin, S.X., Larson, E.L.A., Population-based survey of *Staphylococcus aureus* colonization. *Ann. Intern. Med.*, 59, 126, 2006.
4. Peacock, S.J., Justice, A., Griffiths, D., de Silva, G.D., Kantzanou, M.N., Crook, D., Sleeman, K., Day, N.P., Determinants of acquisition and carriage of *Staphylococcus aureus* in infancy. *J. Clin. Microbiol.*, 41, 5718, 2003.

5. Noble, W.C., Valkenburg, H.A., Wolters, C.H., Carriage of *Staphylococcus aureus in* random samples of a normal population. *J. Hyg. (London)*, 65, 567, 1967.

6. Gorwitz, R.J., Kruszon-Moran, D., McAllister, S.K., McQuillan, G., McDougal, L.K., Fosheim, G.E., Jensen, B.J., Killgore, G., Tenover, F.C., Kuehnert, M.J., Changes in the prevalence of nasal colonization with *Staphylococcus aureus* in the United States, 2001-2004. *J. Infect. Dis.*, 197, 1226, 2008.

7. Gonzalez, B.E., Martinez-Aguilar, G., Hulten, K.G., Hammerman, W.A., Coss-Bu, J., Avalos-Mishaan, A., Mason, E.O., Kaplan, S.L., Severe staphylococcal sepsis in adolescents in the era of community-acquired methicillin-resistant *Staphylococcus aureus*. *Pediatrics*, 115, 642, 2005.

8. Safdar, N. and Golub, J.E., The risk of infection after nasal colonization with *Staphylococcus aureus*. *Am. J. Med.*, 121, 310, 2008.

9. Werthelm, H.F.L., Melles, D.C., Vos, M.C., van Leeuwen, W., van Belkum, A., Verbrugh, H.A., Nouwen, J.L., The role of nasal cariage in *Staphylococcus aureus* infections. *Lancet Infect. Dis.*, 5, 751, 2005.

10. Strauss, J.S., The sebaceous glands: Twenty-five years of progress. *J. Invest. Dermatol.*, 67, 90, 1976.

11. Agache, P., Blanc, D., Barrand, C., Laurent, R., Sebum levels during the first year of life. *Br. J. Dermatol.*, 103, 643, 1980.

12. Pochi, P.E., Strauss, J.S., Downing, D.T., Age-related changes in sebaceous gland activity. *J. Invest. Dermatol.*, 73, 108, 1979.

13. Downing, D.T., Stewart, M.E., Strauss, J.S., Changes in sebum secretion and sebaceous glands. *Clin. Geriatric Med.*, 5, 109, 1989.

14. Nicolaides, N. and Rothman, S., Studies on the chemical composition of human hair fat. I. The squalene-cholesterol relationship in children and adults. *J. Invest. Dermatol.*, 19, 389, 1952.

15. Nicolaides, N. and Rothman, S., Studies on the chemical composition of human hair fat. II. The overall composition with regard to age, sex and race. *J. Invest. Dermatol.*, 21, 9, 1953.

16. Nicolaides, N. and Wells, G.C., On the biogenesis of free fatty acids in human skin surface fat. *J. Invest. Dermatol.*, 29, 423, 1957.

17. Downing, D.T., Strauss, J.S., Pochi, P.E., Variability in the chemical composition of human skin surface lipids. *J. Invest. Dermatol.*, 53, 322, 1969.

18. Weitkamp, A.W., Smiljanic, A.M., Rothman, S., The free fatty acids of human hair fat. *J. Am. Chem. Soc.*, 69, 1936, 1947.

19. Drake, D.R., Brogden, K.A., Dawson, D.V., Wertz, P.W., Thematic review series: Skin lipids. Antimicrobial lipids at the skin surface. *J. Lipid Res.*, 49, 4, 2008.

20. James, A.T. and Wheatley, V.R., Studies of sebum. 6. The determination of component fatty acids of human forearm sebum by gas-liquid chromatography. *Biochem. J.*, 63, 269, 1956.

21. Haati, E., Major lipid constituents of human skin surface with special reference to gas chromatographic methods. *Scand. J. Clin. Invest.*, 13:Suppl, 59, 1961.

22. Nakamura, M., Kamatami, I., Higaki, S., Yamagishi, T., Identification of Propionibacterium acnes by polymerase chain reaction for amplification of 16S ribosomal RNA and lipase genes. *Anaerobe*, 9, 5, 2003.
23. DeAngelis, Y.M., Saunders, C.W., Johnstone, K.R., Reeder, N.L., Coleman, C.G., Kaczvinsky, J.R., Jr., Gale, C., Walter, R., Mekel, M., Lacey, M.P., Keough, T.W., Fieno, A., Grant, R.A., Begley, B., Sun, Y., Fuentes, G., Youngguist, R.S., Xu, J., Dawson, T.L., Jr., Isolation and expression of a Malassezia globosa lipase gene, LP1. *J. Invest. Dermatol.*, 127, 2138, 2007.
24. Wang, Y., Huang, S., Kuo, S., Shu, M., Tapia, C.P., Yu, J., Two, A., Zhang, H., Gallo, R.L., Huang, C.M., Propionic acid and its esterified derivative suppress the growth of methicillin-resistant *Staphylococcus aureus* USA300. *Benef. Microbes*, 5, 161, 2014.
25. Li, H., Goh, B.N., Teh, W.K., Jiang, Z., Goh, J.P.Z., Goh, A., Wu, G., Hoon, S.S., Raida, M., Camattari, A., Yang, L., O'Donoghue, A.J., Dawson, T.L., Jr., Skin commensal Malassezia globosa secreted protease attenuates *Staphylococcus aureus* biofilm formation. *J. Invest. Dermatol.*, 138, 1137, 2018.
26. Dreno, B., Pecastaings, S., Corvec, S., Veraldi, S., Khammari, A., Roques, C., Cutibacterium acnes (Propionabacterium acnes) and acne vulgaris: A brief look at the latest updates. *J. Euro. Acad. Dermatol. Venereol.*, 32, suppl2:5, 2018.
27. O'Neill, A.M. and Gallo, R.L., Host-microbiome interactions and recent progress into understanding the biology of acne vulgaris. *Microbiome*, 6, 177, 2018.
28. Merey, Y., Gencalp, D., Guran, M., Putting it all together to understand the role of Malassezia spp. in dandruff etiology. *Mycopathologia*, 183, 893, 2018, https://doi.org/10.1007/s11046-018-0283-4.
29. Presland, R.B. and Dale, B.A., Epithelial structural proteins of the skin and oral cavity: Function in health and disease. *Crit. Rev. Oral Biol. Med.*, 11, 383, 2000.
30. Wertz, P., Epidermal lamellar granules. *Skin Pharmacol. Physiol.*, 31, 262, 2018.
31. Wertz, P.W. and Downing, D.T., Acylglucosylceramide of pig epidermis: Structure determination. *J. Lipid Res.*, 24, 753, 1983.
32. Abraham, W., Wertz, P.W., Downing, D.T., Linoleate-rich acylglucosylceramide from pig epidermis: Structure determination by proton magnetic resonance. *J. Lipid Res.*, 26, 761, 1985.
33. Bowser, P.A., Nugteren, D.H., White, R.J., Houtsmuller, U.M., Prottey, C., Identification, isolation and characterization of epidermal lipids containing linoleic acid. *Biochim. Biophys. Acta*, 834, 419, 1985.
34. Wertz, P.W. and Downing, D.T., Covalently bound ω-hydroxyacylsphingosines in the stratum corneum. *Biochim. Biophys. Acta*, 917, 108, 1987.
35. Swartzendruber, D.C., Wertz, P.W., Madison, K.C., Downing, D.T., Evidence that the corneocyte has a chemically bound lipid envelope. *J. Invest. Dermatol.*, 88, 709, 1987.
36. Wertz, P.W. and Downing, D.T., Free sphingosine in human epidermis. *J. Invest. Dermatol.*, 94, 159, 1990.

37. Stewert, M.E. and Downing, D.T., Free sphingosines of human skin include 6-hydroxysphingosine and unusually long-chain dihydrosphingosines. *J. Invest. Dermatol.*, 105, 613, 1995.

38. Wertz, P.W. and Downing, D.T., Ceramidase activity in porcine epidermis. *FEBS Lett.*, 268, 110–112, 1990.

39. Burtenshaw, J.M.L., The mortality of haemolytic Streptococcus on the skin and on other surfaces. *J. Hygiene, Cambridge*, 38, 575, 1938.

40. Burtenshaw, J.M.L., The mechanism of self-disinfection of the human skin and its appendages. *J. Hyg. (London)*, 42, 161, 1942.

41. Rothman, S., Smiljanic, A.M., Weitkamp, A.W., Mechanism of spontaneous cure in puberty of ringworm of the scalp. *Science*, 104, 201, 1946.

42. Shipiro, A.L. and Rothman, S., Undecylenic acid in the treatment of dermatomycosis. *Arch. Dermatol. Syphilol.*, 52, 166, 1945.

43. Kabara, J.J., Swieczkowski, D.M., Conley, A.J., Truant, J.P., Fatty acids and derivatives as antimicrobial agents. *Antimicrob. Agents Chemother.*, 2, 23, 1972.

44. Kabara, J.J. and Vrable, R., Antimicrobial lipids: natural and synthetic fatty acids and monoglycerides. *Lipids*, 12, 753, 1977.

45. Fischer, C.L., Drake, D.R., Dawson, D.V., Blanchette, D.R., Brogden, K.A., Wertz, P.W., Antibacterial activity of sphingoid bases and fatty acids against Gram-positive and Gram-negative bacteria. *Antimicrob. Agents Chemother.*, 56, 1157, 2012.

46. Fischer, C.L., Walters, K.S., Drake, D.R., Dawson, D.V., Blanchette, D.R., Brogden, K.A., Wertz, P.W., Oral mucosal lipids are antibacterial against Porphyromonas gingivalis, induce ultrastructural damage, and alter bacterial lipid and protein compositions. *Int. J. Oral Sci.*, 5, 130, 2013.

47. Byrd, A.L., Belkaid, Y., Segre, J.A., The human skin microbiome. *Nat. Rev. Microbiol.*, 16, 143, 2018.

48. Sakr, A., Bregeon, F., Mege, J.L., Rolain, J.M., Blin, O., *Staphylococcus aureus* nasal colonization: An update on mechanisms, epidemiology, risk factors, and subsequent infections. *Front. Microbiol.*, 9, 2419, 2018.

49. Darmstadt, G.L. and Lane, A.T., Impetigo: An overview. *Pediatric. Dermatol.*, 11, 293, 1994.

50. Wrobel, J., Tomcjak, H., Jenerowicz, D., Czamecka-Operacz, M., Skin and nasal vestibule colonization by *Staphylococcus aureus* and its susceptibility to drugs in atopic dermatitis patients. *Ann. Agric. Environ. Med.*, 25, 334, 2018.

51. Di Nardo, A., Wertz, P., Giannetti, A., Seidenari, S., Ceramide and cholesterol composition of the skin of patients with atopic dermatitis. *Acta Derm. Venereol.*, 78, 27, 1998.

52. Imokawa, G., Abe, A., Jin, K., Higaki, Y., Kawashima, M., Hidano, A., Decreased level of ceramides in stratum corneum of atopic dermatitis: An etiologic factor in atopic skin? *J. Invest. Dermatol.*, 96, 523, 1991.

53. Higuchi, K., Hara, J., Okamoto, R., Kawashima, M., Imokawa, G., The skin of atopic dermatitis patients contains a novel enzyme, glucosylceramide sphingomyelin deacylase, which cleaves the N-acyl linkage of sphingomyelin and glucosylceramide. *Biochem. J.*, 350 pt3, 747, 2000.

54. Arikawa, J., Ishibashi, M., Kawashima, M., Takagi, Y., Ichikawa, Y., Imokawa, G., Decreased levels of sphingosine, a natural antimicrobial agent, may be associated with vulnerability of the stratum corneum from patients with atopic dermatitis to colonization by *Staphylococcus aureus*. *J. Invest. Dermatol.*, 119, 433, 2002.

55. Takigawa, H., Nakagawa, H., Kuzukawa, M., Mori, H., Imowawa, G., Deficient production of hexadecenoic acid in the skin is associated in part with vulnerability of atopic dermatitis patients to colonization by *Staphylococcus aureus*. *Dermatology*, 211, 240, 2005.

56. Ribeiro de Castro, M.C. and Ramos-e-Silva, M., Cutaneous infections in the mature patient. *Clin. Dermatol.*, 36, 188, 2018.

57. Bibel, D.J., Miller, S.J., Brown, B.E., Pandey, B.B., Elias, P.M., Shinefield, H.R., Aly, R., Antimicrobial activity of stratum corneum lipids from normal and essential fatty acid deficient mice. *J. Invest. Dermatol.*, 92, 632, 1989.

58. Bibel, D.J., Aly, R., Shinefield, H.R., Antimicrobial activity of sphingosines. *J. Invest. Dermatol.*, 98, 269, 1992.

59. Bibel, D.J., Aly, R., Shah, S., Shinefield, H.R., Sphingosines: Antimicrobial barriers of the skin. *Acta Derm. Venereol.*, 73, 407, 1993.

60. Hannun, Y.A., Loomis, C.R., Merrill, A.H., Bell, R.M., Sphingosine inhibition of protein kinase C and of phorbol dibutyrate binding *in vitro* and in human platelets. *J. Biol. Chem.*, 261, 12604, 1986.

61. Hannun, Y.A. and Bell, R.M., Functions of sphingolipids and sphingolipid breakdown products in cellular regulation. *Science*, 243, 500, 1989.

62. Paige, D.G., Morse-Fisher, N., Harper, J.I., The quantification of free sphingosine in the stratum corneum of patients with hereditary ichthyosis. *Brit. J. Dermatol.*, 129, 380, 1993.

12

Innate Immunity in Epidermis

Miroslav Blumenberg

The R. O. Perelman Department of Dermatology, NYU School of Medicine,
NYU Langone Medical Center, New York, USA

Abstract

Here we present the current understanding of the innate immunity systems in human skin. The innate immune system acts as a physical and chemical barrier to environmental harmful agents; it recognizes microbial patterns or tissue damage and produces defensive antimicrobial proteins. The innate immune system also initiates production of specific signals that activate inflammation and other cellular protective mechanisms, recruits specialized white blood cells that can identify and remove foreign material present, activates the complement system and initiates the adaptive immune responses by antigen presentation to the immune B and T cells, causing their activation. As a novel concept, we suggest that the skin-resident commensal microorganisms constitute a crucial, active component of the skin innate immunity and fully participate in protecting the organism from pathogens.

Keywords: Antigen presenting cells, antimicrobial proteins cytokines, commensalism microbiome

12.1 Introduction

Whereas the adaptive immunity is a protection from infectious agents characterized by immunological memory acquired after exposure to specific

---

Email: Miroslav.Blumenberg@nyulangone.org

Nava Dayan (ed.) *Skin Microbiome Handbook: From Basic Research to Product Development,*
(237–260) © 2020 Scrivener Publishing LLC

antigens, and executed by B- and T- lymphocytes, the innate immunity is the immediate protection system already present in the organism, active even without previous exposure to the injuring agent. The innate immunity must provide urgent protection immediately upon encountering a microbe, inside the period of several days necessary for the adaptive immunity develops and begins to function. Moreover, innate immunity responses are not specific to a particular pathogen but must react to a very broad range of potential harmful microorganisms, as well as to tissue damage. The innate immune responses are activated by common molecular patterns present on microbes or in damaged tissue.

Consistent with the wide variety of potential dangers, the innate immunity must perform a variety of protective action. The major functions of the innate immune system include:

1. To act as a physical and chemical barrier to infectious agents.
2. To recognize microbial patterns or tissue damage.
3. To produce defensive antimicrobial proteins.
4. To generate cytokines, specific signals that activate inflammation and other cellular protective mechanisms.
5. To use specialized white blood cells to identify and remove foreign material present.
6. To activate the complement system.
7. To signal and initiate the adaptive immune responses by antigen presentation to the immune B and T cells, causing their activation.

Potential pathogens are first encountered by epithelia through touch, ingestion and inhalation; this means that the integument, digestive tract and respiratory airway are the sentinels ready to activate their innate immune responses. Arguably, human skin, acting as the interface between the host and the environment, is our organ most exposed to microbes from the environment and accordingly contains many components of innate immunity.

12.2   Skin Acts as an Anatomical Physical and Chemical Barrier to Infectious Agents

The exterior epithelial surface of skin, stratum corneum, forms a formidable physical barrier impermeable to most infectious agents. Human stratum corneum has a characteristic structure comprising protein and lipids. The protein derives from terminally differentiated keratinocytes, cells full of proteins such as keratins and cornified envelope components. Importantly, the epidermal transglutaminases can covalently and nonspecifically crosslink these proteins, i.e., crosslink any keratinocyte protein to all others. This creates a large macromolecular jumble substantially resistant to proteolysis and nonenzymatic degradation. It is also quite resistant to microbial penetration [1]. The cornified layer proteins are immersed in a lipid milieu with its own antimicrobial effects; these are described in detail in this volume by Dr. P. Wertz *et al.*

The living cells below the stratum corneum are connected by desmosomes and tight junctions. Desmosomes are mechanically strong cell-to-cell adhesion structures, connected intracellularly to the cytoskeleton. Such arrangement provides powerful mechanical resilience to the epidermis. The tight junctions, on the other hand, provide a watertight physical seal between cells, thus preventing the paracellular access of microorganisms to the host [2].

The skin has a slightly acidic surface, ranging between pH 4.0 to 6.5, optimally ~ 5.5. The "acid mantle," is derived from free fatty acids excreted by the sebaceous glands, and mixed with lactic and amino acids from sweat. The acidic pH of the epidermis is not favorable for most microbes and constitutes another element of the barrier [3].

An important aspect of the epidermal barrier is its desquamation, the constant shedding of skin outermost layer, which helps remove microbes that have adhered to the epithelial surfaces. Lysosomal and extracellular proteolytic enzymes are responsible for the desquamation [4].

Certain inflammatory skin diseases, such as psoriasis and atopic dermatitis, characterized by barrier disruption, are associated with characteristic changes in the skin microbiome [5].

12.3   Epidermal Cells Recognize Conserved Features of Pathogens, as well as the Indicators of Tissue Damage

The skin innate immunity must recognize pathogens on its surface. To accomplish this, skin uses receptors for pathogen-associated molecular patterns, PAMPs. These are molecular motifs found on various classes of microbes, such as lipopolysaccharides (LPS), lipoteichoic acid, bacterial endotoxins, flagellin, peptidoglycans and glycoconjugates [6]. Viral and prokaryotic DNA and RNA can also activate pattern recognition receptors, PRRs. Arguably, the most studied PRRs belong to the Toll-like receptor family, TLRs [7]. Humans have at least ten TLRs, some on the cell surface, others in the cytoplasm, which respond to different PAMPs. This allows innate immune cells to determine generally what type of infection is occurring, e.g. bacterial, viral, or fungal. TLRs are abundant on the surface of macrophages and neutrophils, as well as on the keratinocytes. The intracellular signal transduction pathways of TLRs activate downstream transcription factors, such as NF-κB protein, which induce the transcription of genes responsible for initiating inflammatory responses, promote phagocytosis by cells such as neutrophils and macrophages, as well as help induce adaptive immune responses (see below). Activation of TLRs leads to production and secretion of downstream signals, signaling molecules such as prostaglandins as well as cytokines which coordinate the recruitment and activation of additional immune responses

Intracellular sensors of PAMPs include NOD-like receptors (NLRs), which synchronize responses with TLRs. NLRs are important for the formation of the inflammasome, a multiprotein assembly responsible for the maturation and secretion of pro-inflammatory cytokines IL-1β and IL-18 [8].

Tissue damage can also activate danger-associated molecular patterns, DAMPs, also known as alarmins. DAMPs can be nuclear or cytosolic and, when released from the cell or exposed on its surface in response to following tissue injury, they initiate noninfectious inflammatory responses [6].

12.4   Defensive Antimicrobial Proteins AMPs

AMPs or defensins are short proteins, peptides, less than 50 amino acids in length found in all animals and plants [9]. They are generally positively charged, and have a hydrophobic or an amphipathic domain in their folded structures. They exhibit a broad spectrum of antibiotic activities, able to kill or inactivate bacteria, fungi, some parasites and even certain enveloped viruses. It is thought that their hydrophobic or amphipathic domains insert into the membrane of their targets, disrupting membrane integrity. AMPs are widely expressed and can be constitutive or quickly mobilized at epithelial surfaces. Because of the relatively nonspecific nature of their action, it is relatively rare that the microbes acquire resistance to the defensin, although some microbes have developed mechanisms to inactivate or withstand AMPs. Neutrophils use defensins to kill phagocytosed pathogens (see below). In addition to their antibiotic role, AMPs often have additional functions in regulating host defenses, innate and acquired. Several bioinformatics databases compile antimicrobial peptides data, such as ADAM (A Database of Anti-Microbial peptides) and CAMP (Collection of sequences and structures of antimicrobial peptides) [10].

In humans, two classes of defensins can be found: α-defensins and β-defensins [11–13]. The genes for all six a-defensins, DEFAs, are found linked on chromosome 8p23. Four DEFAs have been isolated from neutrophils; all are expressed as pre-propeptides with no antimicrobial activity. The C-terminal antimicrobial part of the peptide can be released by metalloproteinases. In skin, these are found in the dermis and their role in innate immunity is unclear (Table 12.1).

The genes for three b-defensins, DEFB1-3, are also clustered on chromosomal region 8p23. Three other b-defensin genes were discovered in this region DEFBD4-6 [14], but these seem not expressed in skin. DEFB1 and 2 show microbicidal activity against Gram-negative bacteria, whereas DEFB3 is a broad spectrum antibiotic effective against many pathogenic bacteria and yeasts. Besides their antimicrobial activity, defensins stimulate cell proliferation [15], induce expression of cytokine and adhesion molecules [16] and are chemoattractant for immune cells [17].

Cathelicidin LL-37 is a 37 amino acid long peptide with antimicrobial activity; it is derived proteolytically from the human CAP18 protein [18]. LL-37 is expressed in leukocytes and in keratinocytes when induced by inflammatory or infectious stimuli. Besides having antimicrobial activity, LL-37 binds and neutralizes LPS, is chemotactic for some lymphocytes, causes degranulation of mast cells and stimulates wound healing [19].

Table 12.1 The sequences of human AMPs are between 30 and 47 amino acids long.

a-defensins		
HNP-1	ACYCRIPACIAGERRYGTCIYQGRLWAFCC	30 aa
HNP-4	VCSCRLVFCRRTELRVGNCLIGGVSFTYCCTRVD	34 aa
HD-5	ARATCYCRTGRCATRESLSGVCEISGRLYRLCCR	34 aa
HD-6	RAFTCHCRRS-CYSTEYSYGTCTVMGN-HRFCCL	32 aa
b-defensins		
HBD-1	DHYNCVSSGGQCLYSACPIFTKIQGTCYRGKAKCCK	36 aa
HBD-2	DPVTCLKSGAICHPVFCPRRYKQIGTCGLPGTKCCKKP	38 aa
HBD-3	QKYYCRVRGGRCAVLSCLPKEEQIGKCSTRGR KCCRKK	39 aa
HBD-4	LDRICGYGTARCRKKCRSQEYRIGRCPNTYAC CLRKPWDESLLNRTK	47 aa
Cathelicidin		
LL-37	LLGDFFRKSKEKIGKEFKRIVQRIKDFLRNLVPRTES	37 aa

Dermcidin is a broad spectrum antimicrobial with no homology to other known antimicrobial peptides [20, 21]. It is specifically and constitutively produced by the eccrine sweat glands and secreted into the sweat. A processed 47–amino acid C-terminal peptide of dermcidin has antimicrobial activity against bacteria and fungi, and may be helpful in limiting infection bacterial in the first few hours following infection. This means that sweat also plays a role in the innate immunity by producing dermcidin.

12.5   Cytokines, Specific Signals that Activate Inflammation and Further Cellular Protective Mechanisms

Cytokines are also small proteins (~5–20 kDa), secreted by cells to carry out in cell-to-cell signaling [22]. Cytokines can be involved in autocrine, paracrine and endocrine signaling, generally as immunomodulating agents. Cytokines cannot cross cell membranes; instead they act through cognate receptors on cell surfaces. Cytokines can be, loosely, classified according to their effects on the target cells as chemokines, interferons, interleukins, lymphokines, and growth factors. Cytokines are produced by a broad range of immune cells, such as macrophages, mast cells, B and T lymphocytes, but also by nonimmune cell types, such as keratinocytes, fibroblasts, endothelial cells and others. They can affect the maturation, responsiveness, growth, and silencing of particular cell populations. Cytokines interact in complex ways, can trigger the release of other cytokines, and either enhance or inhibit the action of other cytokines.

Binding of a cytokine to its matching cell-surface receptor initiates a cascade of intracellular signaling, including up or downregulation of transcription factors, and release of secondary signals. Cytokines produced by resident activated macrophages are chemoattractants for neutrophils, the first cells recruited in large numbers to the site of the new infection. Subsequently, other cytokines attract monocytes and dendritic cells [22].

Just as with AMPs, some pathogens have developed mechanisms to resist the inflammatory response. For example, some viruses encode potent cytokine antagonists, often modified forms of cytokine receptors, acquired by the viral genome from the host to bind the cytokines blocking their activity [23]. Dysregulation of cytokine production or responses can lead to pathological inflammation, tissue damage and even sepsis [24].

Inflammation is one of the first responses of the immune system to infection or irritation [25]. Cytokines produced by macrophages and other resident cells of the innate immune system initiate the inflammatory response. Some cytokines are pro-inflammatory, some are anti-inflammatory. The inflammatory response in skin is characterized by redness, swelling, pain, increased local temperature and possibly disruption of the local barrier. Signals produced during inflammation, such as histamine, leukotrienes, prostaglandins, bradykinin and serotonin, cause local vasodilation and attract phagocytes, especially neutrophils. Neutrophils then trigger other parts of the immune system by releasing cytokines that summon additional leukocytes and lymphocytes.

12.6   Specialized White Blood Cells Identify and Remove Pathogens

As a result of acute inflammation, innate immune effector cells such as neutrophils and macrophages are recruited to the site of infection in the skin. These cells rapidly phagocytose any bacteria present, which they then destroy, as well as the damaged cellular debris. They generally identify that the phagocytosed material, e.g., a bacterium, rather than a virus, based on which pattern recognition receptors are activated. This rapid response allows the innate immune system to maintain a control over the infection even before initiation of the adaptive immune response.

Most innate immune white blood cells cannot divide or reproduce, but are the maturation products of multipotent hematopoietic stem cells present in the bone marrow. The innate leukocytes include a) mast cells, b) natural killer cells, c) eosinophils and basophils and the phagocytic cells such as d) macrophages, e) neutrophils, and f) dendritic cells.

a. Mast cells are a type of innate immune cell with the primary role in providing first-line surveillance and defense against pathogenic microbes, but also in regulating inflammatory reactions and in shaping innate and adaptive immune responses. When activated, mast cells rapidly release into their environment preformed characteristic granules rich in histamine and heparin. They also rapidly release cytokines and hormonal mediators. Subsequent delayed release of multiple cytokines from mast cells induces activation of adaptive immunity, regulates responses to tissue injury and, eventually, resolution of inflammation. The capacity to recognize and to react to danger and the ability to cross-talk with other immunocompetent cells make mast cells a unique effector cell of innate responses and a main bridge between innate and adaptive immunity [26, 27].

b. Natural killer cells, NK cells, do not directly attack invading microbes, but destroy compromised host cells, such as virus-infected cells by inducing the infected cell to apoptose [28]. They recognize such cells by a abnormally low levels of MHC I cell-surface marker; healthy cells are not recognized and attacked by NK cells because they are protected by the intact MHC self-antigens. Interferons enhance the activity of NK cells.

c. Eosinophils and basophils are cells related to neutrophils (see below). Upon activation, basophils release histamine, important in the defense against parasites. When activated, eosinophils secrete several highly toxic proteins and free radicals. These are highly effective in killing pathogens, but may damage tissue causing an allergic reaction. The function of eosinophils is tightly regulated to prevent excessive tissue destruction [29].

Phagocytes are immune cells that engulf, or 'phagocytose', pathogens. A phagocyte extends portions of its plasma membrane, wrapping it until the pathogen is enveloped completely inside the cell, within a phagosome. Phagosomes merge with lysosomes, which contain catabolic enzymes that kill and digest the invader. The phagocytes themselves search for pathogens, but also react to molecular signals produced by other cells, the cytokines. The phagocytic cells of the innate immune system include macrophages, neutrophils, and dendritic cells.

d. Macrophages express a variety of cell-surface receptors, such as TLRs, that enable them to recognize and engulf pathogens. Binding to any of these receptors induces cytoskeletal rearrangement, causing the phagocyte's plasma membrane to envelope the pathogen, engulf it into a membrane-enclosed phagosome. Then, the phagosome is acidified and fused with lysosomes, which contain lysozyme and hydrolases that degrade bacterial cell walls and proteins. Lysosomes also contain defensins (see above). Phagocytes assemble an NADPH oxidase complex on their membrane causing production reactive oxygen compounds, including superoxide, hypochlorite, hydrogen peroxide, hydroxyl radicals, and nitric oxide NO; this production results in a transient increase in oxygen consumption by the cells, called the respiratory burst. Activation of macrophages also stimulates them to produce chemokines, with which they summon other innate immunity cells to the site of infection [30].

e. Neutrophils have distinctive lobed nuclei and in their cytoplasm have granules that contain a variety of toxic substances that kill or inhibit bacteria and fungi. Neutrophils are the most abundant type of phagocyte, normally representing 50-60% of the total circulating leukocytes, and are usually the first cells to arrive at the site of an infection. Neutrophils, like macrophages, also attack pathogens by activating a respiratory burst and they contain large amounts of AMPs to help in pathogen destruction [31].

f. Dendritic cells, DCs, are resident phagocytes in tissues that are in contact with the external environment, so named for abundant dendrites that cover a large area probing for foreign antigens. In the epidermis they are called Langerhans cells [32]. They are present in all epidermal layers, prominently in the stratum spinosum. Langerhans cell, like dendritic cells in other tissues, actively capture, uptake and process antigens. The dendritic cells carry the antigens from the invading pathogens to nearby lymph nodes, where they present the antigens to lymphocytes. Once in secondary lymphoid tissue, Langerhans cells interact with naive T-cells, educating them about the presence of the antigen. This is important for activating the adaptive immune system. Therefore Langerhans cells serve as a crucial link between the innate and adaptive immune systems.

γδ T cells are a sub-population of dendritic cells within the epidermis [33]. They have a distinctive T-cell receptor on their surface. γδ T cells exhibit characteristics that place them at the interface between innate and adaptive immunity. On one hand, large number of γδ T cells respond within hours to common molecules produced by microbes, on the other hand they rearrange T-cell receptor genes to produce junctional diversity and develop a memory phenotype. γδ T cells were shown to facilitate wound healing in human skin.

12.7   Complement System

The complement system is a biochemical cascade of the immune system of about 20 interacting soluble proteins that circulate in the blood and extracellular fluid. Complement has been associated with several skin diseases, such as psoriasis, lupus erythematosus, and bullous dermatoses and recurrent cutaneous infections, where complement has a destructive, detrimental effect; potentially, these could be treat these diseases with complement inhibitors [34, 35].

12.8   Innate Immune System Activates the Adaptive Immune System

One of essential functions of the innate immunity system is to activate and instruct the adaptive immune system to fight invading pathogens [36]. Antigen-presenting cells, APCs, fragment and process antigens and present them to the T-cells. T cells, using their T cell receptors, recognize antigen fragments displayed on cell surfaces, bound to the major histocompatibility complex (MHC). There are two types of MHC molecules MHC-I and MHC-II, and correspondingly, two categories of antigen-presenting cells: professional and non-professional [37]. Professional antigen-presenting cells express MHC class II molecules, along with co-stimulatory molecules, whereas the non-professional APCs express MHC class I molecules. The tasks of both cytotoxic and helper T cells is dependent on APCs; this accounts for the subsequent specificity of adaptive immune responses. Skin contains both professional APCs including macrophages and dendritic cells, and non-professional APCs, including keratinocytes [38, 39].

Dendritic cells are necessary for activating naive T cells and can present antigen to both helper and cytotoxic T cells. Dendritic cells also function in peripheral tolerance, alleviating some auto-immune disorders.

Macrophages can be stimulated by interferon gamma to express MHC class II and co-stimulatory B7 molecules, and then present phagocytosed peptide fragments to helper T cells. After dendritic cells phagocytose a pathogen, the internalized antigen is digested into smaller peptides and the cells migrate to the draining lymph nodes, where they can interact with T cells.

All nucleated cell types are potentially non-professional antigen presenting cells to display endogenous peptides on the cell membrane. Typically, non-professional APCs do not express MHC class II molecules, however, keratinocytes, especially after IFNg stimulation, produce copious amounts of MHC class II protein. Therefore, epidermal keratinocytes function as non-professional APCs and are important in stimulating T cell proliferation and activation. This activating function is in addition to the role of skin professional epidermal APCs, the Langerhans cells and macrophages [40, 41].

Importantly, keratinocytes, as non-professional antigen-presenting cells, can support superantigen-induced proliferation of resting T cells even *via* indirect, non-contact mechanism. Exosomes are small membrane vesicles that can transfer antigens to recipient cells. Exosomes produced by keratinocytes contain MHC I and II, interact with T cells and, following interferon γ stimulation, can induce the proliferation of CD4+ and CD8+ T cells [42].

12.9 Antiviral Defenses

Viral components, such as viral dsRNA, are recognized by Toll-like receptors and MDA5 and RIG-I receptors [7]. These pathways converge in inducing the host cell to produce and secrete interferons α and β. In turn, these interferons then induce expression of many antiviral proteins that play a role in antiviral host defenses. For example, IFNs stimulate the activation of a protein kinase that inactivates the protein synthesis initiation factor eIF-2, thereby shutting down most protein synthesis in the infected host cell. In addition, skin cells can also detect the presence of viral dsRNA and, in attempt to eliminate it, degrade the dsRNA into small, about 20–25 bp fragments. These fragments form heteroduplexes host cell RNAs, resulting in the destruction of the host RNA. These mechanisms deny the viruses a healthy host cell in which viruses can replicate [43].

12.10 Innate Immunity Memory?

The innate immune system can adapt after former insults. Protection against reinfection has been reported even in plants and invertebrates, organisms that do not have adaptive immunity [44]. The innate immunity can be modified by previous encounters with pathogens, which has been termed "trained immunity" or" innate immune memory." There is a cross-protection from infections with different pathogens. Trained immunity involves epigenetic reprogramming, sustained changes in gene expression and cell physiology without permanent genetic changes essential for adaptive immunity [45, 46]. Trained immunity involves, on one hand specific cell types, myeloid, natural killer, and innate lymphoid cells, and on the hand recognition and effector molecules already encoded in the germline e.g. cytokines and pattern recognition receptors, that are not rearranged in response to pathogens. Increased responsiveness to secondary stimuli is not pathogen specific and depends on transcriptional regulation and epigenetic reprogramming [47, 48]. Short-lived trained immunity for weeks-to-months, rather than years characteristic of acquired immunity.

The innate immunity memory must be distinguished from the effects of tissue-resident memory T cell; these are part of the adaptive immunity with rearranged DNA.

12.11 Cutaneous Microbiome: A Newly Surfaced Contributor to Innate Immunity

The pioneering work from the Blaser lab and the Segre lab identified a very large number of previously uncharacterized microbes on our skin [49–51]. It became obvious that the epidermis is teeming with many members of three phyla Actinobacteria, Firmicutes, and Proteobacteria. These species are chiefly nonpathogenic, either commensal or actually beneficial. For example, the commensals on skin generate a skin-specific immune composition, separate from the humoral immunity [52].

The interactions among microbes on our skin are directly protective, the commensals competing and combating with the potential pathogens. Therefore, the cutaneous microbiome represents an important and insufficiently explored component of the innate immunity of skin.

Works by Gallo and his coworkers and other groups described several mechanisms by which our commensal microbes protect us from pathogens [53–55]. For example, a biosynthetic gene cluster in Cutibacterium acnes (formerly Propionibacterium acnes) produces a new thiopeptide antibiotic, cutimycin. Cutimycin regulates resistance against Staphylococcus species. Variety of mechanisms comprises epigenetic changes in the epidermis, production of antibiotics and antimicrobial peptides, production of specific metabolites by fermentation, inhibition of biofilm production, etc. [56–58]. These reactions can be harnessed to boost the effects of the commensals against the pathogens [59].

a. Short-chain fatty acids & lipids. One of the efficient mechanisms by which skin commensals protect from pathogens is by producing short-chain fatty acids, SCFAs, such as acetate, propionate, and butyrate. For example, the glycerol fermentation by skin commensal Propionibacterium acnes (P. acnes), suppressed growth of USA300, the most prevalent community-acquired MRSA). The growth suppression of USA300 resulted from direct antimicrobial activity of propionic acid, independent from acidifying of the medium. Propionic acid exhibited a broad-spectrum antimicrobial activity, e.g., against Escherichia coli and Candida albicans. Moreover, the commensal (but not pathogenic) *Staphylococcus aureus* strains are selectively competent to achieve glycerol fermentation to produce short-chain fatty acids [60–62]. The expression levels of six metabolic enzymes, including glycerol-3-phosphate dehydrogenase and phosphoglycerate mutase, in commensal *S. aureus* are more than three-fold higher than in the pathogenic strain USA300. The commensal *S. aureus* effectively suppressed the growth of pathogenic MRSA *in vitro* and *in vivo*. Furthermore, commensal *S. aureus* provided immune protection against pathogenic skin infection with *Staphylococcus aureus*. Excessive use of antibiotics may affect the skin commensals that fight pathogen infection. Long-chain polyunsaturated fatty acids can also provide protection against Propionibacterium acnes and *Staphylococcus aureus* [63, 64]. Generally, these compounds were bactericidal for *S. aureus* but growth inhibitory for P. acnes. The ability of skin lipids to provide a permeability barrier and to have antibacterial, antifungal, and antiviral activity is described elsewhere in this volume Wertz PW.

b. Competition for Fe++ ions. Iron, Fe, is essential element for all life and despite being quite abundant on the Earth, its bioavailability is limited by the very low solubility of the Fe^{3+} ion. Microbes release siderophores (Greek:

"iron carrier") to scavenge iron from the environment. Siderophores are high-affinity iron-chelating compounds secreted by bacteria and fungi and serve to transport iron across cell membranes by active transport mechanisms [65]. In mammals, iron is tightly bound to proteins such as hemoglobin, transferrin, lactoferrin and ferritin. Consequently, there are great evolutionary pressures on pathogenic bacteria to secure sufficient iron. Iron limitation induces expression of genes involved in microbe siderophore production and uptake. The siderophores are secreted into the extracellular environment, where they sequester and solubilize the iron. Specific receptors on the cell membranes of bacteria recognize siderophores and the Fe-loaded siderophore complex is actively transported into the cell. Once in the cytoplasm of the cell, the $Fe3+$-siderophore complex is often reduced to $Fe2+$, releasing the necessary iron [65]. While the bitter microbial competition for iron is evident, it is commonsensical that microbes on skin also compete for other nutrients, lipids, amino acids etc. This is an underexplored area of research, it may provide a new set of armaments to keep skin homeostasis.

c. The hygiene factor. Bacteria thrive on the human skin; human skin flourishes in symbiosis with its microbiome. What, then, is the role of hygiene, washing the bacteria off our skin? Groundbreaking change in preventing nosocomial infections by simple hand-washing is a well-known and enormous benefit of medical practice [66]. However, since the microbiome, contributing to innate defense of the skin, is essential for maintaining skin homeostasis and health, perhaps skin hand-washing may be harmful by altering the microbiome. Typically, the microbiome on the human palmar surfaces harbors more than 150 unique species-level bacterial phylotypes, and a total of 4,742 unique phylotypes was identified across all of the hands examined on the hands of 51 healthy young adult volunteers [67]. Palms of the dominant and non-dominant hands of the same individual shared only 17% of the phylotypes, whereas different individuals shared usually only 13%. Women had higher phylotype diversity than men, but a major effect on the plantar microbiome was dependent on the time since last hand washing [67]. Washing human forearms caused a small but significant decrease in the level of antimicrobial peptide Cathelicidin LL-37 on the skin surface. Nevertheless, no significant change in the bacterial community was detected after hand-washing. Addition of antimicrobials to soap did slow the subsequent growth of pathogenic Group A Streptococci [68].

These studies confirm the importance of hand-washing in preventing infections. However, the mechanism of the prevention may not be the commonly assumed one, i.e., reducing the total load of bacteria on skin. The mechanism perhaps, is to 'reboot' the skin microbiome: washing diminishes the quantity of both commensal and pathogenic bacteria, but the commensals are better at re-establishing their number and dominance over the pathogens. Commensals are 'housetrained' to live on human skin, the host supports their proliferation, and commensals, in turn, protect the skin from the pathogens. Thus, the cutaneous microbiome represents an important component of the innate immunity of skin. The detailed knowledge of the interactions among the components of the skin microbiome deserves serious research efforts and leads to better understanding and, potentially, better, focused and individualized treatments of skin infections.

12.12 Conclusion

The most striking feature of the human cutaneous innate immunity system is its diversity and breadth of reach. This system must be ready to deal with an amazing variety of potential hazards, from physical and mechanical, via chemical, to biological. The biological agents include bacteria, the most closely studied component, but also fungi, viruses, multicellular eukaryotes etc. All are potentially harmful and must be dealt with. Consequently, the innate immunity system comprises a large variety of agents, methods, pathways and structures to protect the underlying organism from invading microorganisms. Importantly, specifically in humans, the epidermis is the outermost protective barrier, a role occupied by fur in other mammals. Hence the extraordinary resources employed by the human cutaneous innate immunity system.

The skin innate immunity system includes a chemical and physical barrier, specific recognition of microbes, antimicrobial proteins, proinflammatory and immunomodulating signaling, recruitment of leukocytes, activation of the adaptive immunity, complement activation and antiviral defenses. These systems act independently, but they also interact and cross-modulate in very complex ways.

Interestingly, human skin has conscripted certain microbes to fight other, pathogenic microbes, as a crucial component of innate immunity. This aspect has recently garnered much attention and remains largely unexplored.

12.13 Future Perspectives

There is still much unknown about the innate immunity system of human skin. This review focused on the antibacterial protection; antifungal and antiviral defense, while as important, have not received as much research attention, a shortcoming that will soon be overcome, hopefully. Specifically for the human cutaneous viruses, it is often hard to distinguish infection from just passive, transient presence on skin. Antiviral processes also need much more deep study. Even in the bacteriome, the interactions among residents are difficult to unravel. We can expect much deeper and more detailed analysis of the human skin innate immunity system (Table 12.2).

In the future, we can expect the increased understanding to lead to novel, exciting and powerful therapies. Topical treatment specifically targeting MRSA with a fragment of an antimicrobial peptide is already in the works [69]. Other components of the innate immunity will be harnessed for specific treatment of infections and, why not, other types of skin conditions. Innate immunity modulation may be harnessed, as well as against aging, for UV protection and in cosmetic industry. The range of possibilities is thrilling.

Table 12.2 Innate immunity pathways.

Pathway	Cellular components	Subcellular components	Activators	Reference
Physical and chemical barrier	Keratinocytes, stratum corneum	Lipids, transglutaminases	Probiotics, e.g., Lactococci, Bifidobacteria	[70, 71]
Recognizing microbial or tissue damage patterns	Keratonocytes, leukocytes	TLRs, NLRs, alarmins	Flagellins, lipopolysacharides, lipopeptides, CpG, RNA	[72]
Antimicrobial proteins, AMPs	Keratonocytes, leukocytes	a- and b-defensins, cathelicidins	Constitutive	[73]
Activation of inflammation	Leukocytes	Interleukins and interferons	Cytokines and chemokines	[74]
Specialized white blood cells	Mast cells, NK cells, macrophages, dendritic cells etc.	–		[75–77]
The adaptive immune system	B and T Lymphocytes	Antigens, receptors	IgE, activation of TLRs and NLRs, venoms, cytokines	[78]
Cutaneous microbiota	S. epidemidis, others	AMPs, SCFAs, siderophores	Antigen presenting cells	[79]

References

1. Eyerich, S., Eyerich, K., Traidl-Hoffmann, C., Biedermann, T., Cutaneous Barriers and Skin Immunity: Differentiating A Connected Network. *Trends Immunol.*, 39, 4, 315–327, 2018.

2. Yokouchi, M. and Kubo, A., Maintenance of tight junction barrier integrity in cell turnover and skin diseases. *Exp. Dermatol.*, 27, 8, 876–883, 2018.

3. Elias, P.M., The how, why and clinical importance of stratum corneum acidification. *Exp. Dermatol.*, 26, 11, 999–1003, 2017.

4. Elias, P.M., Epidermal lipids, barrier function, and desquamation. *J. Invest Dermatol.*, 80 Suppl, 44s–49s, 1983.

5. Sanchez, D.A., Nosanchuk, J.D., Friedman, A.J., The skin microbiome: Is there a role in the pathogenesis of atopic dermatitis and psoriasis? *J. Drugs Dermatol.*, 14, 2, 127–30, 2015.

6. Bianchi, M.E., DAMPs, PAMPs and alarmins: All we need to know about danger. *J. Leukoc. Biol.*, 81, 1, 1–5, 2007.

7. Vidya, M.K., Kumar, V.G., Sejian, V., B.agath, M., Krishnan, G., Bhatta, R., Toll-like receptors: Significance, ligands, signaling pathways, and functions in mammals. *Int. Rev. Immunol.*, 37, 1, 20–36, 2018.

8. Kim, Y.K., Shin, J.S., Nahm, M.H., NOD-Like Receptors in Infection, Immunity, and Diseases. *Yonsei. Med. J.*, 57, 1, 5–14, 2016.

9. Lee, H.T., Lee, C.C., Yang, J.R., Lai, J.Z., Chang, K.Y., A large-scale structural classification of antimicrobial peptides. *BioMed Res. Int.*, 2015, 475062, 2015.

10. Waghu, F.H., Gopi, L., Barai, R.S., Ramteke, P., Nizami, B., Idicula-Thomas, S., CAMP: Collection of sequences and structures of antimicrobial peptides. *Nucleic Acids Res.*, 42, Database issue, D1154–8, 2014.

11. De Smet, K. and Contreras, R., Human antimicrobial peptides: defensins, cathelicidins and histatins. *Biotechnol. Lett.*, 27, 18, 1337–47, 2005.

12. Niyonsaba, F., Kiatsurayanon, C., Chieosilapatham, P., Ogawa, H., Friends or Foes? Host defense (antimicrobial) peptides and proteins in human skin diseases. *Exp. Dermatol.*, 26, 11, 989–998, 2017.

13. Lai, Y. and Gallo, R.L., AMPed up immunity: How antimicrobial peptides have multiple roles in immune defense. *Trends Immunol.*, 30, 3, 131–41, 2009.

14. Yamaguchi, Y., Nagase, T., Makita, R., Fukuhara, S., Tomita, T., Tominaga, T., Kurihara, H., Ouchi, Y., Identification of multiple novel epididymis-specific beta-defensin isoforms in humans and mice. *J. Immunol.*, 169, 5, 2516–23, 2002.

15. Murphy, C.J.1., BA, Foster, MJ, Mannis, ME, Selsted, Reid, T.W., Defensins are mitogenic for epithelial cells and fibroblasts. *J. Cell Physiol.*, 155, 2, 408–13, 1993.

16. Chaly, Y.V., Paleolog, E.M., Kolesnikova, T.S., Tikhonov, I.I., Petratchenko, E.V., Voitenok, N.N., Neutrophil alpha-defensin human neutrophil peptide

modulates cytokine production in human monocytes and adhesion molecule expression in endothelial cells. *Eur. Cytokine Netw.*, 11, 2, 257–66, 2000.

17. Territo, M.C., Ganz, T., Selsted, M.E., Lehrer, R., Monocyte-chemotactic activity of defensins from human neutrophils. *J. Clin. Invest.*, 84, 6, 2017–20, 1989.

18. Gudmundsson, G.H., Agerberth, B., Odeberg, J., Bergman, T., Olsson, B., Salcedo, R., The human gene FALL39 and processing of the cathelin precursor to the antibacterial peptide LL-37 in granulocytes. *Eur. J. Biochem.*, 238, 2, 325–32, 1996.

19. Zanetti, M., Cathelicidins, multifunctional peptides of the innate immunity. *J. Leukoc. Biol.*, 75, 1, 39–48, 2004.

20. Schittek, B., Hipfel, R., Sauer, B., Bauer, J., Kalbacher, H., Stevanovic, S., Schirle, M., Schroeder, K., Blin, N., Meier, F., Rassner, G., Garbe, C., Dermcidin: A novel human antibiotic peptide secreted by sweat glands. *Nature Immunol.*, 2, 1133–1137, 2001.

21. Lai, Y.P., Peng, Y.F., Zuo, Y. *et al.*, Functional and structural characterization of recombinant dermicidin-1L, a human antimicrobial peptide. *Biochem. Biophys. Res. Commun.*, 328, 1, 243–50, 2005.

22. Liles, W.C. and Van Voorhis, W.C., Review: nomenclature and biologic significance of cytokines involved in inflammation and the host immune response. *J. Infect Dis.*, 172, 6, 1573–80, 1995.

23. Alcami, A., Viral mimicry of cytokines, chemokines and their receptors. *Nat. Rev. Immunol.*, 3, 1, 36–50, 2003.

24. Chousterman, B.G. and Swirski, F.K., Weber GF. Cytokine storm and sepsis disease pathogenesis. *Semin Immunopathol.*, 39, 5, 517–528, 2017.

25. Pasparakis, M., Haase, I., Nestle, F.O., Mechanisms regulating skin immunity and inflammation. *Nat. Rev. Immunol.*, 14, 5, 289–301, 2014.

26. Igawa, S. and Di Nardo, A., Skin microbiome and mast cells. *Transl. Res.*, 184, 68–76, 2017.

27. Cardamone, C., Parente, R., Feo, G.D., Triggiani, M., Mast cells as effector cells of innate immunity and regulators of adaptive immunity. *Immunol. Lett.*, 178, 10–4, 2016.

28. Awad, A., Yassine, H., Barrier, M., Vorng, H., Marquillies, P., Tsicopoulos, A., Duez C. Natural killer cells induce eosinophil activation and apoptosis. *PLoS One.*, 9, 4, e94492, 2014.

29. Willebrand, R. and Voehringer, D., Regulation of eosinophil development and survival. *Curr. Opin. Hematol.*, 24, 1, 9–15, 2017.

30. Gentek, R., Molawi, K., Sieweke, M.H., Tissue macrophage identity and self-renewal. *Immunol. Rev.*, 262, 1, 56–73, 2014.

31. Mantovani, A., Cassatella, M.A., Costantini, C., Jaillon, S., Neutrophils in the activation and regulation of innate and adaptive immunity. *Nat. Rev. Immunol.*, 2511, 8, 519–31, 2011.

32. Deckers, J., Hammad, H., Hoste, E., Langerhans Cells: Sensing the Environment in Health and Disease. *Front Immunol.*, 1, 9, 93, 2018.

33. Carding, S.R. and Egan, P.J., Gammadelta T cells: Functional plasticity and heterogeneity. *Nat. Rev. Immunol.*, 2, 5, 336–45, 2002.

34. Kotnik, V., Complement in skin diseases. *Acta Dermatovenerol Alp Pannonica Adriat*, 20, 1, 3–11, 2011.

35. Giang1, J., Seelen2, M.A.J., van Doorn3, M.B.A., Rissmann4, R., Prens3, E.P., Damman1, J., Complement Activation in Inflammatory Skin Diseases. *Front Immunol.*, 9, 639, 2018.

36. Withers, D.R., Innate lymphoid cell regulation of adaptive immunity. *Immunology*, 149, 2, 123–30, 2016.

37. Pollack, B.P., Sapkota, B., Cartee, T.V., Epidermal growth factor receptor inhibition augments the expression of MHC class I and II genes. *Clin. Cancer Res.*, 17, 13, 4400–13, 2011.

38. Kim, B.S., Miyagawa, F., Cho, Y.H., Bennett, C.L., Clausen, B.E., Katz, S.I., Keratinocytes function as accessory cells for presentation of endogenous antigen expressed in the epidermis. *J. Invest Dermatol.*, 129, 12, 2805–17, 2009.

39. Black, A.P., Ardern-Jones, M.R., Kasprowicz, V., Bowness, P., Jones, L., Bailey, A.S., Ogg, G.S., Human keratinocyte induction of rapid effector function in antigen-specific memory CD4+ and CD8+ T cells. *Eur. J. Immunol.*, 37, 6, 1485–93, 2007.

40. Tokura, Y., Yagi, J., O'Malley, M., Lewis, J.M., Takigawa, M., Edelson, R.L., Tigelaar, R.E., Superantigenic staphylococcal exotoxins induce T-cell proliferation in the presence of Langerhans cells or class II-bearing keratinocytes and stimulate keratinocytes to produce T-cell-activating cytokines. *J. Invest Dermatol.*, 102, 1, 31–8, 1994.

41. Nickoloff, B.J., Mitra, R.S., Green, J., Shimizu, Y., Thompson, C., Turka, L.A., Activated keratinocytes present bacterial-derived superantigens to T lymphocytes: Relevance to psoriasis. *J. Dermatol. Sci.*, 6, 2, 127–33, 1993.

42. Cai, X.W., Zhu, R., Ran, L., Li, Y.Q., Huang, K., Peng, J., He, W., Zhou, C.L., Wang, R.P., A novel noncontact communication between human keratinocytes and T cells: Exosomes derived from keratinocytes support superantigeninduced proliferation of resting T cells. *Mol. Med. Rep.*, 16, 5, 7032–7038, 2017.

43. Banno, T., Adachi, M., Mukkamala, L., Blumenberg, M., Unique keratinocyte-specific effects of interferon-gamma that protect skin from viruses, identified using transcriptional profiling. *Antivir Ther.*, 8, 6, 541–54, 2003.

44. Zipfel, C., Plant pattern-recognition receptors. *Trends Immunol.*, 35, 7, 345–51, 2014.

45. Netea, M.G., Joosten1, L.A.B., Latz 2,3,4, E., Mills 5, K.H.G., Natoli 6, G., Stunnenberg 7, H.G., O'Neill 5, L.A.J., Xavier 8,9, R.J., Trained immunity: A program of innate immune memory in health and disease. *Science*, 352, 6284, aaf1098, 2016.

46. Ho, A.W. and Kupper, T.S., T cells and the skin: From protective immunity to inflammatory skin disorders. *Nat. Rev. Immunol.*, 16, 490–502, 2019.

47. Jiang, X., Clark, R.A., Liu, L., Wagers, A.J., Fuhlbrigge, R.C., Kupper, T.S., Skin infection generates non-migratory memory CD8+ T(RM) cells providing global skin immunity. *Nature*, 483, 7388, 227–31, 2012.

48. Lau, C.M., Adams, N.M., Geary, C.D., Weizman, O.-E., Rapp, M., Pritykin, Y., Leslie, C.S., Sun, J.C., Epigenetic control of innate and adaptive immune memory. *Nature Immunol.*, 19, 963–972, 2018.

49. Gao, Z., Tseng, C.H., Pei, Z., Blaser, M.J., Molecular analysis of human forearm superficial skin bacterial biota. *Proc. Natl. Acad. Sci. U. S. A.*, 104, 8, 2927–32, 2007.

50. Grice, E.A., Kong, H.H., Renaud, G., Young, A.C., NISC Comparative Sequencing Program, GG, Bouffard, RW, Blakesley, TG, Wolfsberg, ML, Turner, Segre, J.A., A diversity profile of the human skin microbiota. *Genome Res.*, 18, 7, 1043–50, 2008.

51. Grice, E.A., Kong, H.H., Conlan, S., Deming, C.B., Davis, J., Young, A.C., NISC Comparative Sequencing Program, GG, Bouffard, RW, Blakesley, PR, Murray, ED, Green, ML, Turner, Segre, J.A., Topographical and temporal diversity of the human skin microbiome. *Science*, 324, 5931, 1190–2, 2009.

52. Naik, S., Bouladoux, N., Linehan, J.L., Han, S.J., Harrison, O.J., Wilhelm, C., Conlan, S., Himmelfarb, S., Byrd, A.L., Deming, C., Quinones, M., Brenchley, J.M., Kong, H.H., Tussiwand, R., Murphy, K.M., Merad, M., Segre, J.A., Belkaid, Y., Commensal-dendritic-cell interaction specifies a unique protective skin immune signature. *Nature*, 520, 7545, 104–8, 2015.

53. Nakatsuji, T., Chen, T.H., Narala, S., Chun, K.A., Two, A.M., Yun, T., Shafiq, F., Kotol, P.F., Bouslimani, A., Melnik, A.V., Latif, H., Kim, J.N., Lockhart, A., Artis, K., David, G., Taylor, P., Streib, J., Dorrestein, P.C., Grier, A., Gill, S.R., Zengler, K., Hata, T.R., Leung, D.Y., Gallo, R.L., Antimicrobials from human skin commensal bacteria protect against *Staphylococcus aureus* and are deficient in atopic dermatitis. *Sci. Transl. Med.*, 9, 378, eaah4680, 2017.

54. Wang, Y., Kuo, S., Shu, M., Yu, J., Huang, S., Dai, A., Two, A., Gallo, R.L., Huang, C.M., *Staphylococcus epidermidis* in the human skin microbiome mediates fermentation to inhibit the growth of Propionibacterium acnes: Implications of probiotics in acne vulgaris. *Appl. Microbiol. Biotechnol.*, 98, 1, 411–24, 2014.

55. Dorrestein, P.C., Gallo, R.L., Knight, R., Microbial Skin Inhabitants: Friends Forever. *Cell*, 165, 4, 771–2, 2016.

56. Williams, M.R., Costa, S.K., Zaramela, L.S., Khalil, S., Todd, D.A., Winter, H.L., Sanford, J.A., O'Neill, A.M., Liggins, M.C., Nakatsuji, T., Cech, N.B., Cheung, A.L., Zengler, K., Horswill, A.R., Gallo, R.L., Quorum sensing between bacterial species on the skin protects against epidermal injury in atopic dermatitis. *Sci. Transl. Med.*, 11, 490, eaat8329, 2019.

57. Claesen, J., Spagnolo, J.B., Flores Ramos, S., Kurita, K.L., Byrd, A.L., Aksenov, A.A., Melnik, A.V., Wong, W.R., Wang, S., Hernandez, R.D., Donia, M.S., Dorrestein, P.C., Kong, H.H., Segre, J.A., Linington, R.G., Fischbach, M.A.,

Lemon, K.P., Cutibacterium acnes antibiotic production shapes niche competition in the human skin microbiome. https://doi.org/10.1101/594010.

58. Sanford, J.A., Zhang, L.J., Williams, M.R., Gangoiti, J.A., Huang, C.M., Gallo, R.L., Inhibition of HDAC8 and HDAC9 by microbial short-chain fatty acids breaks immune tolerance of the epidermis to TLR ligands. *Sci. Immunol.*, 1, 4, eaah4609, 2016.

59. Kao, M.S., Huang, S., Chang, W.L., Hsieh, M.F., Huang, C.J., Gallo, R.L., Huang, C.M., Microbiome precision editing: Using PEG as a selective fermentation initiator against methicillin-resistant *Staphylococcus aureus*. *Biotechnol. J.*, 12, 4, 2017.

60. Yang, J.J., Chang, T.W., Jiang, Y., Kao, H.J., Chiou, B.H., Kao, M.S., Huang, C.M., Commensal *Staphylococcus aureus* Provokes Immunity to Protect against Skin Infection of Methicillin-Resistant *Staphylococcus aureus*. *Int. J. Mol. Sci.*, 19, 5, E1290, 2018.

61. Shu, M., Wang, Y., Yu, J., Kuo, S., Coda, A., Jiang, Y., Gallo, R.L., Huang, C.M., Fermentation of Propionibacterium acnes, a commensal bacterium in the human skin microbiome, as skin probiotics against methicillin-resistant *Staphylococcus aureus*. *PLoS One*, 8, 2, e55380, 2013.

62. Wang, Y., Dai, A., Huang, S., Kuo, S., Shu, M., Tapia, C.P., Yu, J., Two, A., Zhang, H., Gallo, R.L., Huang, C.M., Propionic acid and its esterified derivative suppress the growth of methicillin-resistant *Staphylococcus aureus* USA300. *Benef. Microbes.*, 5, 2, 161–8, 2014.

63. Desbois, A.P. and Lawlor, K.C., Antibacterial activity of long-chain polyunsaturated fatty acids against Propionibacterium acnes and *Staphylococcus aureus*. *Mar. Drugs*, 11, 11, 4544–57, 2013.

64. Wertz, P.W., Lipids and the Permeability and Antimicrobial Barriers of the Skin. *J. Lipids*, 2018, 5954034, 2018.

65. Ellermann, M. and Arthur, J.C., Siderophore-mediated iron acquisition and modulation of host-bacterial interactions. *Free Radic. Biol. Med.*, 105, 68–78, 2017.

66. Best, M. and Neuhauser, D., Ignaz Semmelweis and the birth of infection control. *Qual Saf Health Care*, 13, 3, 233–4, 2004.

67. Fierer, N., Hamady, M., Lauber, C.L., Knight, R., The influence of sex, handedness, and washing on the diversity of hand surface bacteria. *Proc. Natl. Acad. Sci. U. S. A*, 105, 46, 17994–9, 2008.

68. Two, A.M., Nakatsuji, T., Kotol, P.F., Arvanitidou, E., Du-Thumm, L., Hata, T.R., Gallo, R.L., The Cutaneous Microbiome and Aspects of Skin Antimicrobial Defense System Resist Acute Treatment with Topical Skin Cleansers. *J. Invest Dermatol.*, 136, 10, 1950–1954, 2016.

69. Nibbering, P.H., Göblyös, A., Adriaans, A.E., Cordfunke, R.A., Ravensbergen, B., Rietveld, M.H., Zwart, S., Commandeur, S., van Leeuwen, R., Haisma, E.M., Schimmel, K.J.M., Hartigh, J.D., Drijfhout, J.W., Ghalbzouri, A.E., Eradication of methicillin resistant *S. aureus* from human skin by the

novel LL-37-derived peptide P10 in four pharmaceutical ointments. *Int. J. Antimicrob. Agents*, 26, S0924–8579(19)30194-3, 2019.

70. Hausmann, C., Hertz-Kleptow, D., Zoschke, C., Wanjiku, B., Wentzien-Odenthal, A., Kerscher, M., Schäfer-Korting. Reconstructed Human Epidermis Predicts Barrier-Improving Effects of Lactococcus lactis Emulsion in Humans. *Skin Pharmacol Physiol.*, 32, 2, 72–80, 2019.

71. Guéniche, A., Bastien, P., Ovigne, J.M., Kermici, M., Courchay, G., Chevalier, V., Breton, L., Castiel-Higounenc, I., Bifidobacterium longum lysate, a new ingredient for reactive skin. *Exp. Dermatol.*, 19, 8, e1–e8, 2010.

72. Lim, K.H. and Staudt, L.M., Toll-like receptor signaling. *Cold Spring Harb Perspect Biol.*, 5, 1, a011247, 2013.

73. Oppenheim, J.J., Biragyn, A., Kwak, L.W., Yang, D., Roles of antimicrobial peptides such as defensins in innate and adaptive immunity. *Ann. Rheum Dis.*, 62 Suppl 2, ii17–21, 2003.

74. Yamanaka, K.I. and Mizutani, H., The role of cytokines/chemokines in the pathogenesis of atopic dermatitis. *Curr. Probl. Dermatol.*, 41, 80–92, 2011.

75. Draber, P., Halova, I., Polakovicova, I., Kawakami, T., Signal transduction and chemotaxis in mast cells. *Eur. J. Pharmacol.*, 778, 11–23, 2016.

76. Reber, L.L. and Frossard, N., Targeting mast cells in inflammatory diseases. *Pharmacol. Ther.*, 142, 3, 416–35, 2014.

77. Gordon, S. and Martinez, F.O., Alternative activation of macrophages: Mechanism and functions. *Immunity*, 32, 5, 593–604, 2010.

78. den Haan, J.M., Arens, R., van Zelm, M.C., The activation of the adaptive immune system: Cross-talk between antigen-presenting cells, T cells and B cells. *Immunol. Lett.*, 162, 2 Pt B, 103–12, 2014.

79. Granato, E.T., Meiller-Legrand, T.A., Foster, K.R., The Evolution and Ecology of Bacterial Warfare. *Curr. Biol.*, 29, 11, R521–R537, 2019.

Part 5
TESTING AND STUDY DESIGN

13

Next Generation Sequencing Reveals the Skin Microbiome

Niamh B O'Hara[1,2]

¹Jacobs Technion-Cornell Institute, Cornell Tech, New York, NY, USA
²Biotia, New York, NY, USA

Abstract

Skin health is often driven by the skin microbiome, however, clinicians still use culturing, limited technology from the 1800s, to characterize the microbiome and identify pathogens. This results in missed diagnoses and rampant overuse/misuse of antibiotics, which contributes to the growing global drug resistance crisis. The genomics revolution and computational advancements have provided the tools we need to understand the full microbial profile in order to understand and treat skin disease. This chapter focuses on current next-generation sequencing-based approaches to diagnose infectious disease in dermatology, among other fields. It discusses the astounding progress of metagenomics, recent work by my company Biotia, as well as the challenges we are facing, and the great promise ahead.

Keywords: Metagenomics, MRSA, VRSA, NGS

13.1 Introduction

Of late, I have personally encountered the confounding limitations of dermatological diagnostics. While it's literally my job to identify limitations in infectious disease diagnostics (I cofounded and run a precision infectious disease diagnostics company), I have hit the dermatological diagnostic wall from a new and desperate position. My husband has been having strange and recurrent swelling in his extremities that seem to start like hives but then progress to become infections. The differential diagnoses range from

Email: ohara@biotia.io

Nava Dayan (ed.) Skin Microbiome Handbook: From Basic Research to Product Development, (263–276) © 2020 Scrivener Publishing LLC

autoimmune disease to infection to allergic reaction. We have been in and out of a plethora of New York City urgent care centers, doctors' offices, and, most recently, the hospital as the swelling and redness started to snake up towards his heart. I found it wildly frustrating that the majority of doctors we have seen have simply referred us to someone else or said, "it's just very hard to diagnose skin conditions" and left it at that. Imagine if your mechanic just shrugged and sent you limping home with a flat tire. We are in desperate need of better technology to inform diagnostics and guide treatment.

In our recent trip to the hospital, the doctors put my husband on a succession of antibiotics culminating in intravenous vancomycin, previously considered a drug of last resort – *and they prescribed this drug without even testing for bacteria*. Treatment without diagnosis seems irrational when one considers the drug resistance crisis, but we have learned this practice is actually routine. The common line was: while it could be just an allergy, it might instead be methicillin-resistant *Staphylococcus aureus* (MRSA) and that MRSA, while previously hospital-acquired, is now often community-acquired. Therefore, it was considered safer to give him last-line antibiotics in case it was MRSA. These clinicians were justifying their actions and considering the worst-case scenario to protect my husband, which I appreciate, while simultaneously acting out the behavior that contributed to this drug resistance mess and could lead to a spread of a highly drug-resistant strain of vancomycin-resistant *Staphylococcus aureus* (VRSA). *Overuse and misuse of antibiotics in healthcare and agriculture is the very reason that MRSA is now so common – what happens if we lose vancomycin and other antimicrobials previously reserved as last-resort drugs?* My family is now waiting on blood culture results, from which they usually find nothing, and we won't even have that "nothing result" for a grueling five days.

We have arrived at the central problem: we have a profound need to identify pathogens and drug resistance before treating patients in order to prevent the rise in drug resistance. However, for the patient's safety, we often cannot wait until we get microbiology results before we start treating patients.

This experience is far too common and often deadly. On December 5th, 2003, Ricky Lannetti, a 21-year old football player at Lycoming College in Williamsport, was admitted to the hospital with flu-like symptoms; 12 hours later, he was dead. Ricky died while waiting for culture results that would identify the cause of his infection as MRSA and guide antimicrobial treatment. While waiting for culture results, his doctors put him on five different antibiotics, which were ineffective at stopping the spread of the pathogen from a skin infection [1]. Shockingly, drug resistance causes 700,000 deaths annually and the World Health Organization projects drug resistance-associated deaths to increase to 10M annually by 2050, far outpacing cancer [2].

Microbial species play a central role in skin health. Skin microbes are essential for modulation of many functions, including host immune response, physiology, and development. Dysbiosis of the microbiome is common and can result in infections [3]. One key bacteria driving skin infections is *Staphylococcus aureus*, or 'MRSA' when it is resistant to common beta-lactam antibiotics like methicillin. Because of widespread resistance and a lack of diagnostic advances, clinicians have changed their treatment behaviors to prescribe methicillin and other beta-lactams less and prescribe other drugs like trimethoprim-sulfamethoxazole (TMP/SMX; brand name: Bactrim) more [4]. However, microbial species are in a constant state of transition, evolving through migration, mutation, selection, and genetic drift to survive environmental challenges driven by the host and environment. Recently, the Atlantic Health System, the largest hospital system in New Jersey, has realized they may be witnessing the emergence of a new pattern: some of their MRSA samples now display resistance to trimethoprim-sulfamethoxazole (such as Bactrim), their safety drug. This is a phenomenon that wasn't observed a few years ago and indicates how quickly the efficacy of life-saving drugs can be threatened.

The characterization of the microbiome, its drug resistance profile, and its influence on health is a cutting-edge area of research. This chapter will focus on current approaches to diagnose infectious disease in dermatology among other fields, the astounding progress of metagenomics, recent work by my team and others, the challenges we are facing, and the great promise ahead.

13.2   Current Approaches to Test the Microbiome

Since the skin microbiome plays a central role in skin health, characterizing it, especially in the case of disease, is of critical importance. Shockingly, the current gold standard approach, culturing, relies on rudimentary technology from the 1800s (Figure 13.1). Culturing involves collecting a sample from a patient, growing it on media, identifying microbial species with the use of a microscope, and conducting additional tests to characterize it further. One example of an additional test is the Kirby Bauer test, which involves growing pathogens on agar with various antibiotic-soaked filter paper disks to test inhibition of growth of the pathogen near the antibiotic [5]. While culturing is a powerful diagnostic tool, it is slow, taking from days to weeks to grow the microbes. It is also prone to error and contamination, and limited because the vast majority of microbial species cannot be cultured [6]. Furthermore, culturing media differs from the body environment, therefore culturing actually alters the microbial profile.

	CURRENT METHOD	BiotiaDX
TECHNOLOGY	Culture/PCR	Sequencing & AI Software
SPECIES ID	Targeted, limited to what is on panel or can grow	Comprehensive, with 16,000 species in database including bacteria, fungi, viruses
DRUG RESISTANCE PROFILING	Limited and requires additional tests	Results microbial profile drug resistance, and virulence all provided rapidly in one single test
TURN AROUND TIME	2 days to weeks for culturing	~24 hours

Culturing: the current gold standard; technology from the 1800s, useful but slow labor intensive, limited

PCR: less accurate, recognizes limited targets, can't recognize new strains

Figure 13.1 Comparison of infectious disease diagnostic technology, including culturing, PCR-based tests, and BiotiaDX, our proprietary metagenomic diagnostic test.

Additional tests, which are increasing in popularity, include polymerase chain reaction (PCR)-based tests. This approach involves extracting the DNA from a sample and amplifying specific regions of interest using PCR. If a specific gene or loci is identified as being present, that may indicate the species of interest as being present as well. These test panels have their limitations because they need to be designed ahead of time to look for specific genetic markers. Additionally, in practice, clinicians need to have an idea of what they are looking for, and the microbes need to be genetically similar enough to the microbes used in designing the test. Unfortunately, this is often not the case because microbial populations are constantly evolving. This is also the reason for targeted PCR-based tests not recognizing novel, emerging threats, such as the emerging drug resistance health concern Atlantic Health is seeing.

13.3   The Genomics Revolution and Metagenomics

Fortunately for us in our battle against drug resistance, we are in the midst of a technological revolution: the genomics revolution. Over the last 20 years, we have developed the capabilities to sequence DNA quickly and affordably at the genomic and even population genomic scale. It cost a whopping $1B and a long 13 years to sequence the first human genome, completed in 2003 [7]. Since then, the cost of sequencing has dropped 10,000x! Sequencing is the fastest advancing technology in human history, growing at a rate even faster than that seen in the computing revolution described by Moore's law [8]. Companies are now working towards launching the $100 genome, while human genome sequence time has already decreased to about 24 hours [9].

A critical application of sequencing is in the field of metagenomics. Metagenomics is the sequencing of not just one single genome, but many mixed genomes, as one would find when exploring a soil or patient sample. These polymicrobial samples have traditionally been difficult to characterize. It is now possible to extract the DNA from a sample, such as a stool or skin sample, identify microbes from that sample *via* processing the DNA, and then sequence it to generate digital DNA sequence data. Due to computational advances, we can take those sequence data generated, analyze them, and compare them against a database of microbial DNA sequences. This allows for the identification of all the microbial species and strains in the sample, as well as any drug resistance and virulence markers (so long as they are in the database). This approach is comprehensive rather than limited/targeted like PCR, is fast (~24 hours), and far outpaces culturing in the number of species it can identify, working for everything in the ever-expanding database of over 16,000 species (Figure 13.1).

13.4   Metagenomics and the Skin Microbiome

Metagenomics has opened the door to address many important skin microbiome questions including more comprehensive characterization of the taxonomic diversity of this important environment, exploration of different microbial communities and how they affect health and disease and interaction with the host immune system (reviewed in [10]). Metagenomics allows for less biased identification of species than culturing (which favors growth of specific skin species over others) and enables higher resolution down to the species, and even strain, level to distinguish between more virulent strains and also characterize drug resistance.

While many studies have focused on the pathogenic profile of diseased skin, as discussed above, metagenomics also affords one the opportunity for a more comprehensive approach. A seminal study from 2016 used metagenomics to also profile the multitude of commensals, strains of *Cutibacterium acnes* (formerly *Propionibacterium acnes*), and metagenomic elements (e.g., virulence-associated factors and metabolic synthesis genes) to predict disease status through deep sequencing and constructing a quantitative prediction model [11]. The researchers used acne as a disease model and were able to predict disease status a high percentage of the time (~85%). This study also contributes to the weakening in the belief of a causal link between *C. acnes* and acne. In fact, they found a higher relative abundance of *C. acnes* and *Cutibacterium granulosum* in healthy patients, indicating the importance of these species in a healthy skin microbial community. Counter to the common approach for acne treatment of targeting *Cutibacterium (Propionibacterium)* spp., they suggested targeting specific problem strains and then supplementing with beneficial strains, as a probiotic for the skin. They also discussed exciting prospects of using *Cutibacterium (Propionibacterium)* phages as a therapeutic for acne, as has been done in Eastern Europe [12].

Metagenomic applications in skin research are one of the more active areas of metagenomic research, along with gut, oral, pulmonary, neurological, vaginal, and environmental applications. On a large scale, there is important work using metagenomics to characterize the skin microbiome of healthy individuals [13, 14], with the largest initiative to date being the Human Microbiome Project [15]. Characterization of healthy patients is essential, allowing us to build clinical reference ranges to facilitate clinical interpretation of metagenomic results. The HMP, along with other growing databases, will provide tools to accelerate additional advances in this field.

13.5   Our Work at Biotia

I run a startup, Biotia, launched from Jacobs Technion-Cornell Institute at Cornell Tech, that is bringing metagenomic technology into hospitals and health centers to rapidly profile the microbiome of the medical environment and patient samples to guide infection control and treatment. Our work at Biotia has connected us with many interesting centers: we have partnered with hospitals testing stool samples before fecal microbiota transplantation, we have tested and found the deadly, emerging, and drug-resistant fungus *Candida auris* in hospital environments, we have processed 1,000 patient urine samples in a Thailand hospital to develop a reliable approach for urine testing, and we conducted the first study using metagenomics in ambulances [16]. Randomly, we expect to receive 60 stool samples from horses next month.

Recently, when Atlantic Health System ran into challenges understanding the drug resistance they see emerging in New Jersey, they reached out to us. We have applied our technology to profile the metagenomics of their MRSA samples and characterize their drug resistance profiles. Finally, in early 2020, we plan to launch BiotiaDX, a precision infectious disease diagnostic product for clinicians (Figure 13.2). We will initially offer this diagnostic for urine and stool testing and continue to process other sample types, including skin, as a research-use-only product.

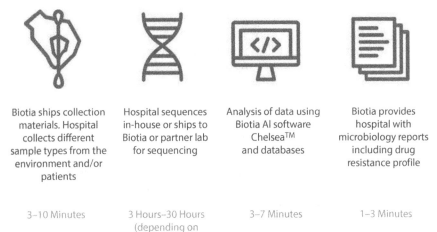

Biotia ships collection materials. Hospital collects different sample types from the environment and/or patients	Hospital sequences in-house or ships to Biotia or partner lab for sequencing	Analysis of data using Biotia AI software Chelsea™ and databases	Biotia provides hospital with microbiology reports including drug resistance profile
3–10 Minutes	3 Hours–30 Hours (depending on Sequencer)	3–7 Minutes	1–3 Minutes

Figure 13.2 BiotiaDX workflow.

13.6 Challenges and Solutions in Metagenomics

While the field of metagenomics has many strengths, we still face many challenges ranging from scientific to commercial. On the scientific side, there can be no adoption of new technology if there is no standardization. Results need to be reproducible over time, across space, and comparable. If a patient is being treated for an infection and tested at a hospital in New Jersey, and then retested a year later post-treatment at a hospital in California, the microbial profile results need to be reliable and comparable. Furthermore, without standardization, clinical metagenomics will never pass the regulatory hurdles required for full widespread adoption. To use metagenomics as a diagnostic test requires launching a laboratory-derived test (LDT) in a Clinical Laboratory Improvement Amendments (CLIA) lab, where samples need to be run in duplicate and duplicates need to yield the same results. Of course, there is always some error in any scientific test, therefore much of the current work is profiling and minimizing that error and determining thresholds to set to get reproducible results. Additionally, on the culture and adoption side, there are numerous regulatory hurdles, including CLIA and the more challenging FDA approval, which to date has not been granted for any metagenomic-based test to diagnose infectious disease. This technology is new, and hospitals and governmental agencies (e.g., CDC and WHO) tend to move very slowly on adoption, often waiting on regulatory approval.

An important issue specific to metagenomic testing is a high rate of false positives since some metagenomic tools will classify a species as being present because certain loci/genes are present. Because there is widespread genetic conservation, there are many shared loci between different species. Our team worked with our software to address this by requiring a minimum level of coverage across the species' genome, moving from a gene-centric to a genome centric view of metagenomics.

Collectively, scientists have sequenced and included in the RefSeq (NCBI) database a staggering 19M bacterial genomic accessions [17]. Research groups, including our team, are still transforming and annotating databases from a clinically relevant perspective. High-quality novel species and strains are constantly being added to public databases and being made available. But as fast as new strains are being added, new strains are evolving in a constant "arms race." Therefore, our work will never be done. The importance of a comprehensive genome cannot be overstated since we cannot reliably identify a species that is not in the reference database.

Additional challenges include differentiating between living and dead microbes. Because metagenomics uses the DNA, it also identifies dead microbes. Also, metagenomics faces the same challenge as other infectious disease diagnostic technologies, but perhaps to a greater extent due to its increased sensitivity: it is difficult to differentiate between colonization with a pathogen and an acute infection that requires treatment. With my team, we are using a machine learning-based approach to tackle this problem. As shown in Figure 13.3, metagenomics provides a wealth of data to mine to make sense of such questions, including profiling a healthy urine sample (top) and a sample for a patient with a UTI (bottom), and training the model to distinguish between healthy and unhealthy to be able to map new samples onto these two classes. Of course, this is a challenging problem that requires large datasets to train the AI.

There is a concerted effort to deal with these challenges. In regard to creating international standards and reproducibility, the International Metagenomics Microbiome Standards Alliance (IMMSA) is a group of researchers (including our cofounder Dr. Christopher E. Mason), from industry, academia, and government who are working on standardizing measurements in microbiome and metagenomics. There are studies that compare the precision and recall of a plethora of metagenomic tools available [18]. Additionally, there are companies that have built products to help reproducibility efforts. There are microbial-positive controls created with a known abundance of communities of microbes, sold as both cells and extracted DNA (ZymoBIOMICS, Zymo). These can be run along with negative controls on all sequence runs to test for contamination, reproducibility, and failed runs.

Urine Profile of Healthy Patient

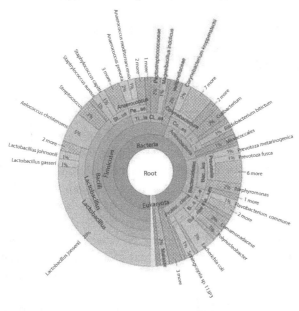

Urine Profile Indicating Infection

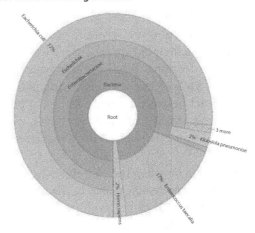

Figure 13.3 Examples of results for two urine samples using BiotiaDX, including a healthy sample with a diverse microbiome (top) and a sample from a patient with a UTI (bottom). This shows the characteristic reduction in microbial diversity with an overgrowth of *E. coli* and other pathogens.

13.7   The Microbial World is our Oyster

Despite these challenges (and others), with metagenomics, the microbial world is our oyster. We are now profiling the microbiome of whole cities. The PathoMap Project was launched in 2015 by our Biotia cofounder, Dr. Mason, as the first urban-scale microbiome initiative. PathoMap researchers sampled all subway stations in New York City and identified 1,688 taxa, including bacteria, viruses, archaea, and eukaryotes [19]. Shockingly, almost 1/2 of the DNA sequenced did not match any sequenced organism in the database, revealing the challenging work set out ahead of us. Importantly this study provided a baseline metagenomic map of New York City, which can be used for long-term surveillance and public health management. More recently, PathoMap has grown into another larger project, the MetaSub, project, in which I have been engaged, using metagenomics to profile the microbiome of more than 80 cities internationally. Through this expansion, we can address important global health concerns, including building a baseline to track emerging infectious threats and drug resistance patterns.

Another large-scale Biotia project was the first metagenomics study of pre-hospital settings. Working with Dr. Mason's lab at Weill Cornell, our team sampled 137 ambulances across the United States to characterize their microbial ecology. Many of the top microbial species identified are known skin-associated species, as well as species associated with hospital-acquired infections. We also found widespread drug resistance markers (in about 90% of the samples). Ambulances are an important first point-of-contact between patients and hospitals but have little regulation on cleaning and disinfection practices. Our findings warrant further testing and potentially instituting regulated cleaning and disinfection [16].

On a more outlandish side, The Extreme Microbiome Project (XMP) applies this technology in diverse places to characterize extremophiles and discover new organisms. They are profiling the microbiome of environments ranging from Alaskan permafrost to the Door to Hell, a gas crater in Turkmenistan that has been burning since 1971.

In the realm of important health advancements, metagenomics is being used to screen and guide Fecal MicrobiotaTransplants (FMT), an important treatment advancement for individuals suffering from gastrointestinal illnesses. FMT has been shown to have a striking 90% success rate for recurrent Clostridioides difficile infection [20], far better than antibiotics or other treatment options.

13.8 The Future of Metagenomics

The future of metagenomics is bright. We are seeing outstanding advancements in sequencing technology, including the establishment of a tiny mobile sequencer, Oxford Nanopore Minion, which allows for sequencing Ebola samples on the front lines of the outbreak in West Africa [21] all the way to sequencing in space aboard the space station [22].

We see concerted efforts to build comprehensive databases and make sense of all this data. Scientists are leveraging metagenomics and/or knowledge from metagenomics to build better probiotics (Seed Health), probiotic sprays for the skin (AOBiome), diagnose infectious disease to treat sepsis (Karius), and infections of the central nervous system (UCSF). Organizations are working on incorporating metagenomics to build better buildings to improve human health [Biology and the Built Environment (BIOBE)], to drill for oil and gas (a similarly named company, Biota), and to track production for factory manufacturing transparency, since every product carries the microbial signature of where it was made (Phylagen).

To understand the skin microbiome, we need to start with the ability to rapidly and reliably profile the microbial ecology of the skin. Metagenomics is an exciting new way to do just that. Recently, our team processed MRSA skin samples from Atlantic Health System. We found evidence for resistance to both methicillin and trimethoprim-sulfamethoxazole (Bactrim) in all the samples they sent us, confirming their worries about trimethoprim-sulfamethoxazole resistance. We also found evidence of co-resistance to other important drug classes, including Mupirocin, an important topical antibiotic used for decolonization before surgery. We found evidence of three clusters differentiated by their resistance profiles, suggesting three potential strains. Finally, we found discrepancies in the number of CDS regions, G+C content, and genome size from common MRSA strains available in the published literature. This suggests the potential of novel or uncharacterized MRSA strain(s) to be explored further. Metagenomics, as we can see, has the power to provide insight to characterize resistance and guide treatment. We hope to continue to build our databases to track emerging resistance and stay one step ahead of these evolving bugs to prolong the efficacy of essential antimicrobial treatments.

Acknowledgements

Contributions, edits, feedback and figures were kindly provided by Biotia team members and family including Dr. Chris Mason, Dr. Dorottya

Nagy-Szakal, Courteny Hager, Dr. Rachid Ounit, Dr. Raihan Faroqui, and Daniel Cassaro.

References

1. Pennington, B., *The Never-Ending Battle Against Sport's Hidden Foe*, The New York Times, 2017.
2. Walsh, F., *Superbugs to kill 'more than cancer' by 2050*, BBC News, 2014.
3. Kobayashi, T., Glatz, M., Horiuchi, K., Kawasaki, H., Akiyama, H., Kaplan, D., Kong, H., Amagai, M., Nagao, K., Dysbiosis and *Staphylococcus aureus* Colonization Drives Inflammation in Atopic Dermatitis. *Immunity*, 42, 4, 756–755, 2015.
4. Harris, A., *Patient education: Methicillin-resistant Staphylococcus aureus (MRSA) (Beyond the Basics)*, 2019, UpToDate.
5. Hudzicki, J., Kirby-Bauer Disk Diffusion Susceptibility. *Am. Soc. Microbiol.*, 2009. https://www.asmscience.org/content/education/protocol/protocol.3189
6. Stewart, E.J., Growing Unculturable Bacteria. *J. Bacteriol.*, 194, 6, 4151–4160, 2012.
7. Lewis, T., *Human Genome Project Marks 10th Anniversary*, 2013, Retrieved December 20, 2019, 2019. https://www.genome.gov/27555238/april-2013-the-10year-anniversary-of-the-human-genome-project-commemorating-and-reflecting
8. National Human Genome Research Institute, *DNA Sequencing Costs: Data*, 2019, Retrieved December 20, 2019, 2019. https://www.genome.gov/about-genomics/fact-sheets/DNA-Sequencing-Costs-Data
9. Brown, K.V., *A $100 Genome Within Reach, Illumina CEO Asks If World Is Ready*, Bloomberg, 2019.
10. Byrd, A.L., Belkaid, Y., Segre, J.A., The human skin microbiome. *Nat. Rev. Microbiol.*, 16, 3, 143–155, 2018.
11. Barnard, E., Shi, B., Kang, D., Craft, N., Li, H., The balance of metagenomic elements shapes the skin microbiome in acne and health. *Sci. Rep.*, 6, 1, 2016.
12. Sulakvelidze, A., Alavidze, Z., Morris, J.G., Jr., Bacteriophage Therapy. *Antimicrob. Agents Chemother.*, 45, 3, 649–659, 2001.
13. Mathieu, A., Delmont, T., Vogel, T., Robe, P., Nalin, R., Simonet, P., Life on human surfaces: Skin metagenomics. *PLoS One*, 8, 1, 2013.
14. Oh, J., Byrd, A.L., Deming, C., Conlan, S., Comparative Sequencing Program, N.I.S.C., Kong, H.H., Segre, J.A., Biogeography and individuality shape function in the human skin metagenome. *Nature*, 514, 649–659, 2014.
15. Human Microbiome Project Consortium, Structure, function and diversity of the healthy human microbiome. *Nature*, 486, 207–214, 2012.
16. O'Hara, N.B., Reed, H.J., Afshinnekoo, E., Harvin, D., Caplan, N., Rosen, G., Frye, B., Woloszynek, S., Ounit, R., Levy, S., Butler, E., Mason, C.E.,

Metagenomic characterization of ambulances across the USA. *Microbiome*, 5, 125, 11, 2017.

17. RefSeq (NCBI), 2019. RefSeq-release97.11042019.stats.txt. https://www. ncbi.nlm.nih.gov/books/NBK50679/#RefSeqFAQ.how_do_i_cite_the_ refseq_proje

18. McIntyre, A.B., Ounit, R., Afshinnekoo, E., Prill, R.J., Hénaff, E., Alexander, N., Minot, S.S., Danko, D., Foox, J., Ahsanuddin, S., Tighe, S., Hasan, N.A., Subramanian, P., Moffat, K., Levy, S., Lonardi, S., Greenfield, N., Colwell, R.R., Rosen, G.L., Mason, C.E., Comprehensive benchmarking and ensemble approaches for metagenomic classifiers. *Gen. Biol.*, 18, 182, 1, 2017.

19. Afshinnekoo, E., Meydan, C., Chowdhury, S., Jaroudi, D., Boyer, C., Bernstein, N., Maritz, J., Reeves, D., Gandara, J., Chhangawala, S., Ahsanuddin, S., Simmons, A., Nessel, T., Sundaresh, B., Pereira, E., Jorgensen, E., Kolokotronis, S., Kirchberger, N., Garcia, I., Gandara, D., Dhanraj, S., Nawrin, T., Saletore, Y., Alexander, N., Vijay, P., Hénaff, E., Zumbo, P., Walsh, M., O'Mullan, G., Tighe, S., Dudley, J., Dunaif, A., Ennis, S., O'Halloran, E., Magalhaes, T., Boone, B., Jones, A., Muth, T., Paolantonio, K., Alter, E., Schadt, E., Garbarino, J., Prill, R., Carlton, J., Levy, S., Mason, C., Geospatial Resolution of Human and Bacterial Diversity with City-Scale Metagenomics. *Cell Syst.*, 1, 1, 72–87, 2015.

20. Kassam, Z., Lee, C., Yuan, Y., Hunt, R., Fecal microbiota transplantation for Clostridium difficile infection: Systematic review and meta-analysis. *Am. J. Gastroenterol.*, 108, 4, 500–508, 2013.

21. Quick, J., Loman, N.J. *et al.*, Real-time, portable genome sequencing for Ebola surveillance. *Nature*, 530, 7589, 228–232, 2016.

22. Castro-Wallace, S.L. *et al.*, Nanopore DNA Sequencing and Genome Assembly on the International Space Station. *Sci. Rep.*, 7, 1, 2017.

14

Three-Dimensional Human Skin Models to Investigate Skin Innate and Immune-Mediated Responses to Microorganisms

Marisa Meloni* and Silvia Balzaretti

VitroScreen, In Vitro Research Laboratories, Milan, Italy

Abstract

This chapter presents the advantages, limitations and opportunities offered by an innovative *in Vitro* pre-clinical approach to the skin microbiome research based on 3D reconstructed skin models colonized with bacterial strains. 3D human tissues have been proven to be a valuable tool suitable for many different pre-clinical *in-vitro* studies for their large experimental flexibility and reproducibility. Reconstructed Living Human Skin models colonized with bacteria mimic the real site where the interaction skin-microbiome occurs and allow to identify the mechanisms by which individual bacterium and resident microbiome regulate skin response to the environment and, most importantly, the host response mediated by defense and adaptive mechanisms. The scientific community has just started scratching the surface of such powerful tool and more is still out there to be explored in order to improve the clinical relevance and predictive power of *in Vitro* pre-clinical models in dermatological and cosmetic research.

Keywords: Colonized 3D reconstructed human skin models, skin microbiota, atopic dermatitis, *S. aureus*, *S. epidermidis*

14.1 State-of-the-Art and Limits of Skin Microbiota Research

The skin is the largest external organ in the human body that is exposed to the external environment and therefore presents a defense barrier. Together with

---
Corresponding author: marisa.meloni@vitroscreen.com

Nava Dayan (ed.) *Skin Microbiome Handbook: From Basic Research to Product Development*, (277–288) © 2020 Scrivener Publishing LLC

its annexes (hair follicle, sebaceous glands and nails) it is also the natural habitat for a variety of microorganisms (bacteria, yeasts and molds). The colonization of the skin surface begins at birth, with, in normal delivery, the microbial population of the mother's birth canal transferred to the newborn. This particular environment allows for the different types of bacteria and yeast to grow in the restricted conditions of humidity, pH and nutritional availability. The different body districts have to be considered as the most diverse environments, and in fact there is a high variability of the microbial (both yeast and bacteria) species between skin parts on the body.

Skin microbiota plays an integral role in the maturation and homeostatic regulation of keratinocyte cells and host immune networks with systemic implications [1, 2]. The biodiversity of skin habitats is heavily influenced by the biodiversity of the ecosystems in which we live. Thus, factors which alter the establishment and health of the skin microbiome exhibit the potential to predispose the skin to cutaneous diseases [3].

In the last decades, in parallel with the research associated with the gut microbiome [4] the scientific community has raised its interest in investigating, describing and classifying the resident microbial population on the skin. A significant number of studies has analyzed the total composition of the skin microbiota with metagenomic approaches. The main findings can be summarized in a great microbiota variability both between the different body districts (skin humidity, concentration of sebaceous glands, exposure to environmental stressors) and a significant biological intersubject variability [5]. Also, factors specific to the host, such as age, location and sex, contribute to the variability. In fact, bacteria behave differently on the skin according to the host conditions and they can thus play different roles: commensal, opportunistic or severe pathogen. Skin is a renewable adaptive organ which is constantly redefined by the genetic and environmental interaction, therefore the individual's microbiome may adapt to changes during his/her lifetime. Considering that microbiota is also influenced by environmental cues to which it is directly exposed, also called "*exposome*" (which means the collection of external factors, UV, chemicals, toxicants, indoor and outdoor pollution in contact with the individual with an effect on health), it is challenging to fully explore and understand human skin microbiota. There is a consensus for the need to further identify the following phyla: Actinobacteria, Firmicutes, Bacteroidetes and Proteobacteria, as the most important bacteria colonizing the skin and its annexes. Since the microbiota certainly has a role both in health and pathologic conditions, the challenge today is identifying and clarifying the mechanisms and the underlaying interactions contributing to specific microbial activity; in particular, bacteria causing damage in specific conditions (opportunistic) and bacteria beneficial for skin homeostasis (commensal).

Nowadays, researchers have limited knowledge on skin functions and mechanisms related to a specific microbiota species; availability of numerous metagenomics data generated from numerous clinical studies on the skin microbiome underlines the presence of high variability in bacterial composition among subjects suffering the same skin pathology [1]. The achievement of a mechanistic understanding of the skin cells-microbiome communication and better understanding of the cause of the different skin conditions correlated to imbalance of the healthy microbiota can be considered the most important future challenge for skin microbiome research and experimental dermatology.

One key consideration is the dullness of research tools available for pre-clinical assessment. Several microbiological methods are commonly used to screen the effect of specific molecules on bacterial growth and physiology, allowing the rapid identification of actives with anti-microbial or prebiotic effects. However, these methods do not take into consideration the real site where the bacteria reside, that is the skin and the mucosae, an environment where the microbiota has different types of nutrients and is challenged by different types of stressful agents that can have a strong influence on their behavior. Moreover, the skin and the host immune systems have a strong influence on the residing bacteria as well.

14.2   Mechanism-Based Approach to Study Host Response to Associated Microbiome: 3D Skin Models

The skin and its microbiota have a strong symbiotic relationship in a continuous crosstalk, which influences both counterparts' behavior. Reconstructed human epidermis (RHE) colonized with bacteria mimics the real site where the skin-microbiome interaction occurs, allowing the assessment of microbiota's influence on skin health and appearance. The 3D models' relevance and predictivity versus *in-vivo* rely on the presence of an organized tissue with different living cell layers derived from human tissue. This *in-vitro* biological model allows the product effects assessment at conditions that mimic realistic exposure and clinically relevant doses.

The RHE is cultivated for 17 days from human keratinocytes isolated by healthy donors and reconstituted by airlifted culture on inserts of polycarbonate filter. In particular, the donor keratinocytes, cultivated in a chemically defined serum-free medium, rapidly proliferate and are seeded on the inert filter. The defined medium feeds the basal cells through the filter (airlifted culture), and after 14 days a stratified epidermis is formed. Morphologically, these tissues exhibit a well-stratified epithelium and cornified epidermis, with significantly improved barrier function and metabolic activity.

Despite the significant value of the *in-vitro* reconstructed system to pre-clinical evaluation and its relevance in studying biological cascades, it would be incorrect to claim that it can fully substitute clinical investigation on humans. The two approaches can be considered complementary; *in-vivo* clinical findings on humans are increasing in prevalence and they are based on large population panels; however, they still suffer from high biological variability that represents the major limitation of the *in-vivo* approach.

Furthermore, many of the clinical studies focus mainly on the identification and mapping of the bacterial population and not on the host response and mechanisms. Delving into the mode of action of the host represents the real advantage of *in-vitro* pre-clinical investigation on 3D human skin models.

Pre-clinical studies on 3D human skin models colonized with the most representative species inhabiting the skin and its annexes are a promising research field: they are contributing to the understanding of mechanisms that may represent a single element of skin microbiome and allow exploring these mechanisms on different models recapitulating a variety of skin conditions [6–8]. Examples for variations that can be applied to the model include healthy, fragile skin, various ethnic groups, inflamed, various age groups, exposed to stresses (UV, chemicals, drug, dehydrated, swollen).

The use of skin models may allow the quantification of the bacteria adhesion and invasion, and their viability over time by measuring complementary parameters: barrier function impairment, toxicity, morphological and biochemical changes, target gene expression regulation and in particular the innate response, as well as gaining insights into the role of their "secretome" (intended as all the molecules derived by primary or secondary metabolic pathways and secreted externally by the bacterium). Although yet to be standardized, monitoring the host response to specific bacteria strains in reproducible skin conditions represents a legitimate scientific approach and provides the R&D scientists with a robust tool for potential predictions and information that may be used in the development of a new generation of topical products; those that interact with skin microbiome, selecting the commensal and beneficial microbial population, limiting the growth of fastidious and opportunistic pathogen, as well as obtaining skin overall improvement through a microbiological rebalance.

14.3   Understanding *S. epidermidis* and *S. aureus* Behavior and Role on Reconstructed Human Epidermis (RHE)

The two staphylococcal species are mainly colonizing the outer layers of the epidermis [9]. Skin coagulase-negative staphylococci are major skin commensals of humans, and *S. epidermidis* is one of the most frequently isolated species from human epithelia with a ubiquitous presence on the skin.

The studies of specific markers of skin interaction with *Staphylococci* in 3D reconstructed epidermis have shown significant differences between *S. epidermidis* and *S. aureus*. *Staphylococcus aureus* is one of the most common contaminating bacteria able to easily form a biofilm on epidermal surface and it has been shown that its presence causes delays in the healing process [10]. This is due to innate resistance to antibiotics, disinfectants, and clearance by host defenses [11, 12].

The functional role of *S. epidermidis* has been elucidated as an immuno-modulatory and antimicrobial peptide synthesis stimulation, exerting a direct antagonistic effect against *S. aureus* and other pathogens. *S. epidermidis* under evolutionary pressure modified its cell wall external layers, in order to be recognized as safe by the host defense mechanisms, like Toll-like receptor-2 (TLR-2) [13].

In Figure 14.1 the different behavior of the 2 strains when in contact with the 3D RHE models (pigmented epidermis Photo type IV) is illustrated. *S. epidermidis* is evenly distributed on SC surface; on the contrary, *S. aureus* forms many bacterial clusters that appear to be ready to establish a "self-protecting" biofilm structure.

Colonization of reconstructed human epidermis, SkinEthic, with *S. epidermidis* ATCC 12228 strain for 24 h did not alter the skin morphology, and the immunofluorescence staining showed no significant differences of filaggrin (involved in epidermal homeostasis and modulation of water content) and involucrin inside the tissue (Figure 14.2a).

The innate immune system was stimulated by the *S. epidermidis* presence: β-defensin (DEFB4) gene was upregulated (Figure 14.2b).

In Figure 14.3b are reported (data not published) the results of the transcriptional activity of 2 genes relevant for innate immunity: TLR-2 and HBD2. The tissue is recognized as safe *S. epidermidis*: the TLR-2 in fact was not overexpressed (Figure 14.3b). *S. epidermidis* stimulates antimicrobial response of the skin and helps to increase defense protection and innate immune system (DEFB4). Eventually, it does not induce inflammation but stimulates skin defense (adaptive role).

COLONIZED RHPE IV

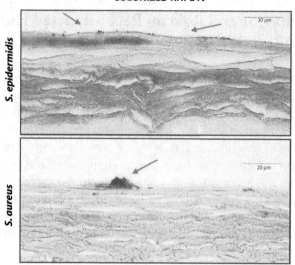

Figure 14.1 GRAM staining on reconstructed and pigmented human epidermis (RHPE IV) *S. aureus* and *S. epidermidis*: bacteria are stained in BLUE. 100x magnification: 2% of the entire RHE tissue diameter (0,78 cm) is visible in each picture.

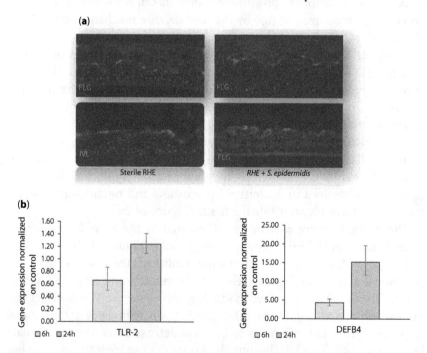

Figure 14.2 RHE colonized with *S. epidermidis*: immunofluorescence staining of FLG and IVL (a) and gene expression by qRT-PCR of TLR-2 and DEFB4 at 6 h and 24 h (b).

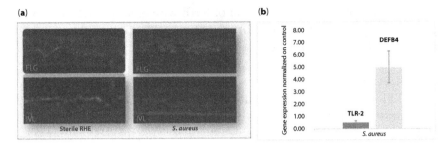

Figure 14.3 RHE colonized with *S. aureus*: immunofluorescence staining of FLG and IVL (a) and gene expression by qRT-PCR of TLR-2 and DEFB4 at 24 h (b).

Table 14.1 Relevant genes characterizing the RHE response to microbiota.

Gene	Biological role
TLR2	Pathogen antigens recognition and activation of innate immunity via stimulation of NF-κB.
HBD-2	Interaction with bacterial membrane, with consequent depolarization and cell lysis. It is also induced by skin wounding and inflammatory stimuli.
IL-8	Potent chemotactic and proinflammatory cytokine produced in the skin by a variety of cells in response to inflammatory stimuli. IL-8 attracts neutrophils to the site of skin infection for phagocytosis and killing of bacteria.
TNF-α	Pro-inflammatory cytokine which increases in the site of skin lesions in AD and psoriasis, triggering the acute immune response by inducing HBD and IL-13.
TSLP	Thymic stromal lymphopoietin links innate and adaptive immune responses through Toll-like receptors and Th2 cytokines. It is highly expressed in the skin of atopic dermatitis patients and associated with dendritic cell activation *in situ*.
FLG	Involved in the skin barrier function. Atopic dermatitis is associated to a reduced FLG and to a FLG gene mutation with heritable epithelial barrier defect, leading to reduced epidermal defense mechanisms to allergen and bacteria and to activation of Th2 lymphocyte responses with resultant chronic inflammation and autoimmune mechanisms.

On the contrary, the colonization of RHE with *S. aureus* ATCC 33591 causes a significant reduction of involucrin (Figure 14.3a), probably induced by the bacterial secretome (toxins, proteases).

The gene expression of TLR-2 was found as downregulated, eluding the epidermal innate immunity clearance mechanisms (Figure 14.3b). The DEFB4 is upregulated, because the bacterium is considered a threat by the host tissue and activates its defense mechanisms.

Table 14.1 shows the relevant genes characterizing the RHE response to microbiota and their biological meaning that can be explored.

14.4   Immuno-Competent Atopic Dermatitis Model

In the vicious circle of atopic dermatitis (AD), skin defense is reduced, favoring microbial colonization, which in turn might be responsible for the production of pro-inflammatory cytokines via the TLR-2 response. In more than 90% of patients, lesions are colonized by *S. aureus*, an opportunistic bacterium which can cause serious infections. Metagenomic studies of skin microbiota confirmed that during AD flare, a modification of the microbiota can be observed in favor of *S. aureus*. This might be due to the decrease of antimicrobial peptide but also to the alteration of the stratum corneum structure by facilitating adhesion.

Considering the complexity of AD and the ongoing research to unravel the mechanism of development of the pathology, it is currently difficult to evaluate new treatments aiming at improving atopic dermatitis phenotype or to treat it. Animal models can give precious insight but are limited by the fact that mice do not spontaneously develop AD, hence reducing the potential translation of results to humans. The developing technology of reconstructed epidermis allows the assessment of different compounds *in vitro* on tissues presenting similar characteristics to human skin, but also the investigation of biological mechanisms of human pathologies. AD is associated with reduced filaggrin production and to a FLG gene mutation with heritable epithelial barrier defect and resultant diminished epidermal defense mechanisms to allergens and microbes, followed by Th2 lymphocyte responses with resultant chronic inflammation, including autoimmune mechanisms. These lymphocytes release a series of cytokines—IL-4, IL-5, IL-13—and lead to elevated production of IgE, increasing inflammation in the skin, and aggravating the skin barrier defect in AD.

Microbiome changes in AD and novel approaches for treatment are further discussed in this book in Chapter 4.

The host response to skin microbiome on 3D skin models generally lacks the immune system. The contribution of the immune system is, however, essential and it is based on the recruitment of circulating monocytes in the dermal compartment and pushed to differentiate in macrophages.

A 3D skin model has been developed and validated by VitroScreen laboratory. The team successfully ideated and realized the atopic dermatitis (AD) model that takes into account the 3 main elements of AD: barrier impairment, *S. aureus* infection, and Th2-mediated immune response. The basal infiltration of immune cells in the RHE Cell Migration Model (RHE CMM Episkin), subjected to mechanical abrasion and colonized by *S. aureus,* induces a more realistic phenotype of atopic dermatitis by recapitulating the biological crosstalk and host response in a 3D environment.

The model can be used to test products as prevention or as treatment based on different mechanisms of actions (anti-inflammatory, antibacterial, anti-biofilm).

The immune response showed that the combination of THP-1 and *S. aureus* induced pro-inflammatory gene overexpression (the role of which is described in Table 14.1), as *in-vivo* TSLP is upregulated in an immune-competent AD model (results presented in Table 14.2).

Given the deep variability of the microbial population inhabiting the skin layers, it is fundamental to simplify the approach of investigation, to reduce the bias and to assess the precise role of any single actor (tissue, immune system, bacteria). For these reasons the pre-clinical phase is a relevant and helpful step before starting clinical trials.

Scientific knowledge of skin biology has been built up during decades, ignoring the contribution or the consequence of the microbiota community. The contribution of colonized RHE models in basic research and new approaches to skin protection and therapies to treat skin diseases appear encouraging.

Table 14.2 Gene expression (qRT-PCR results as reported as valid RQ values compared to negative control RQ=1) of atopic dermatitis gene signature in the 2 *in vitro* models: A) THP-1 cells in co-culture with RHE and B) THP-1 cells infiltrated in RHE-CMM model.

Model	HBD-2	IL-8	TLR-2	TNF-α	TSLP	FLG
A) RHE in co-cultured THP-1	4.4	8.2	1.1	6.8	3.49	0.75
B) RHE-CMM infiltrated THP-1	>100	85	13.3	13.5	20.8	0.4

14.5 Conclusion and Future Perspectives

Scientific knowledge of skin biology has been accumulating during decades, ignoring the contribution or the consequence of the microbiota community. The results of a combination model obtained on colonized RHE model appear encouraging as a robust and predictive pre-clinical tool and in basic research to better understand the microbiome role in influencing skin health and appearance. Clinical findings on humans are increasing and they are based on larger population panels; however, they focus mainly on the bacterial population and not the skin response. As a consequence, they suffer from high biological variability that still represents the major limitation of this approach.

Many questions are yet to be investigated. Those include:

- Where, how and how deep bacteria and yeast are localized in skin layers?
- What human cell type does the microbiome interact with?
- How does the gut-skin microbiota axis work? (Please refer to Chapter 2 on this topic).
- What is the interplay between the various types of organisms on and in the skin?
- Does the skin condition affect microbiota population or vice versa?
- What is a healthy skin microbiota?
- Is there any impact on skin appearance?
- What role does the single bacterium within the microbiota community have towards the host?
- How can metabolomics (on skin and bacteria) help to understand complexity of host-bacteria interaction?
- Does the microbiota affect skin responses to UV light?
- Last but not least, how to communicate microbiota's role to the layman consumer?

References

1. Grice, E.A. and Segre, J.A., The skin microbiome. *Nat. Rev. Microbiol.*, 9, 4, 244–53, 2011.
2. Prescott, S., Larcombe, D., Logan, A., West, C., Burks, W., Caraballo, L., Levin, M., Van Etten, E., Horwitz, P., Kozyrskyj, A., Campbell, D., The skin

microbiome: Impact of modern environments on skin ecology, barrier integrity, and systemic immune programming. *World Allergy Org. J.*, 10, 1, 29, 2017.

3. Sanford, J.A. and Gallo, R.L., Functions of the skin microbiota in health and disease. *Semin. Immunol.*, 30;25, 5, 370–7, 2014.

4. Gill, S.R., Pop, M., DeBoy, R.T., Eckburg, P.B., Turnbaugh, P.J., Samuel, B.S., Gordon, J., Relman, D., Fraser-Liggett, C., Nelson, K.E., Metagenomic analysis of the human distal gut microbiome. *Science*, 312, 5778, 1355–1359, 2006.

5. Costello, E., Lauber, C., Hamady, M., Fierer, N., Gordon, J., Knight, R., Bacterial community variation in human body habitats across space and time. *Science*, 18;326, 5960, 1694–7, 2009.

6. Lerebour, G., Cupferman, S., Bellon-Fontaine, M.N., Adhesion of *Staphylococcus aureus* and *Staphylococcus epidermidis* to the Episkin reconstructed epidermis model and to an inert 304 stainless steel substrate. *J. Appl. Microbiol.*, 97, 1, 7–16, 2004.

7. Cadau, S., Valla-Dury, L., Cenizo, V. *et al.*, Studying microbiote competition and skin interaction using organotypic 3d skin models. *Adv. Tissue Eng. Regen. Med. Open Access*, 2, 5, 233–234, 2017.

8. Rademacher, F., Simanski, M., Gläser, R., Harder, J., Skin microbiota and human 3D skin models. *Exp Dermatol.*, 27, 5, 489–494, 2018.

9. Otto, M., Staphylococcal Biofilms. *Curr. Top Microbiol. Immunol.*, 322, 207–28, 2008.

10. Schneider-Lindner, V., Delaney, J.A., Dial, S., Dascal, A., Suissa, S., Antimicrobial Drugs and Community-acquired Methicillin-Resistant *Staphylococcus aureus*, United Kingdom. *Emerg. Infect. Dis.*, 13, 7, 994–1000, 2007.

11. Holland, D.B., Bojar, R.A., Jeremy, A.H.T., Ingham, E., Keith, T., Holland, K.T., Microbial colonization of an *in vitro* model of a tissue engineered human skin equivalent- a novel approach. *FEMS Microbiol. Lett.*, 279, 110–11, 2008.

12. Archer, N., Mazaitis, M.J., Costerton, J.W., Leid, J.G., Powers, M.E., Shirtliff, M.E., *Staphylococcus aureus* biofilms: Properties, regulation, and roles in human disease. *Virulence*, 2:5, 445–459, 2011.

13. Stacy, A. and Belkaid, Y., Microbial guardians of skin health. *Science*, 18;363, 6424, 227–228, 2019.

15

Cutibacterium acnes (formerly *Propionibacterium acnes*) *In-Vivo* Reduction Assay: A Pre-Clinical Pharmacodynamic Assay for Evaluating Antimicrobial/Antibiotic Agents in Development for Acne Treatment

Stuart R. Lessin[1]* and James J. Leyden[1,2]

[1]*KGL Skin Study Center, Broomall, PA, USA*
[2]*Department of Dermatology, University of Pennsylvania, Philadelphia, PA*

Abstract

Cutibacterium acnes (formerly *Propionibacterium acnes*) is an anaerobic diphtheroid and a native constituent of the skin microbiome. The proliferation of *C. acnes* is involved in the pathogenesis of acne and contributes to its inflammatory characteristics. The pharmacodynamic effect of *C. acnes* reduction tracks with clinical efficacy of anti-acne treatments. A simple *in-vivo* assay can evaluate the effects of topical or systemic agents on *C. acnes* populations of the skin. Quantitative bacteriologic cultures are obtained from facial skin over two to six weeks from twenty-five healthy volunteers pre-screened for high levels of *C. acnes*. A split face design is employed and test product and vehicle control are applied under supervision. Historical data has demonstrated that a mean reduction of 1.0 to 2.0 logarithm colony forming units of *C. acnes* correlates with therapeutic effectiveness. This *in-vivo C. acnes* reduction assay is a valuable pre-clinical tool in assessing efficacy and tolerability of acne treatments early in commercial development and positive results can serve as a strong surrogate for success in 12-week Phase 3 acne clinical trials.

Keywords: Acne, *C. acnes*, antibiotic, antimicrobial

*Corresponding author: stuartlessin@kglssc.com

Nava Dayan (ed.) Skin Microbiome Handbook: From Basic Research to Product Development,
(289–302) © 2020 Scrivener Publishing LLC

15.1 Acne Pathogenesis and the Role of *Cutibacterium acnes* (formerly *Propionibacterium acnes*)

15.1.1 Introduction

Acne vulgaris is a disease of the pilosebaceous unit (sebaceous follicle) producing clinical manifestations of non-inflammatory (comedones) and inflammatory skin lesions (papules, pustules and cystic nodules) that can result in scarring of the face and upper trunk (Figure 15.1). Acne onset and persistence range for pre-teen years to young adulthood and can have severe adverse effects on psychosocial development and emotional and mental health [1, 2]. Affecting up to 85 percent of individuals worldwide, it contributes to the global burden of skin disease, ranking eighth in global prevalence with greater than 645 million affected [2, 3].

15.1.2 Pathogenesis

The pathogenesis of acne involves three interrelated processes that contribute to its clinical expression. The initial step is the enlargement of sebaceous glands and increased sebum production within the sebaceous follicle that is driven by hormonal stimulation from androgens. Puberty associated increases in circulating dehydroepiandrosterone (DHEA) and androstenedione are converted into testosterone and 5α-dihydroxytestosterone (DHT) in the skin and target sebaceous gland androgen receptors with high affinity [4]. The excessive sebum coupled with aberrant desquamation of epithelial cells within the follicular infundibulum creates a hyperkeratotic occlusion and formation of a microcomedone [5] that may evolve into either a comedone or an inflammatory lesion. The degree of inflammation is influenced by the presence of and interactions with *Cornibacterium acnes* (*C. acnes*).

15.1.3 The Role of *C. acnes* and its Microbiome

C. acnes is a commensal bacterium that is a part of the human skin microbiata. It is a gram-positive anaerobic dipheroid and proliferates in the cutaneous environment created by the mixture of excessive sebum and desquamated follicular cells [6]. Historically, it has been referred to as

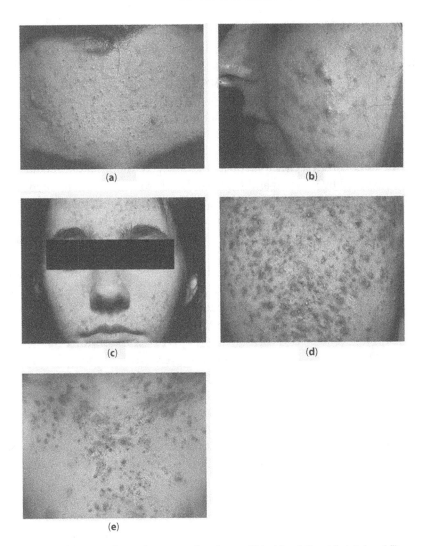

Figure 15.1 (a) Noninflammatory comedonal acne ("blackheads" and "whiteheads") on the forehand. (b) Inflammatory acne with papules on the face. (c) Widespread comedones and inflammatory lesions over most of the face. (d) Severe nodulocystic acne of the trunk. (e) Explosive inflammatory acne (acne fulminans) of the chest associated with ulcerative lesions and systemic signs and symptoms (fever, leukocytosis, and arthralgia). (Reprinted with permission from *The New England Journal of Medicine*, J.J. Leyden, Therapy for Acne Vulgaris, Vol. 336. Copyright © 1997 Massachusetts Medical Society).

Propionibacterium acnes (*P. acnes*); however, recent microbiome analysis utilizing 16S rRNA gene sequencing revealed significant diversity within the genus of *Propionibacterium*. It has been proposed that the taxonomy be reclassified to accurately reflect three distinct genera within the family of Propionibacteriaceae: *Acidipropionibacterium, Pseudopropionibacterium*, and *Cutibacterium* [7]. The term *Cutibacterium acnes* (*C. acnes*) is now used for the genus formerly known as *Propionibacterium* that still remains a part of the historic data linking it to acne and its pathogenesis. Initial acne studies demonstrated chemotactic factors and proinflammatory mediators were produced by *C. acnes* and supported their role as key components to acne-related inflammation [8–10]. Recent studies have delineated greater details into *C. acnes* induced inflammatory pathways and the complexity of the interaction of the cutaneous microbiome and host immune responses [11–14].

C. *acnes* has been shown to stimulate the secretion of mature interleukin-1β (IL-1β) from monocytes and sebocytes [11, 12]. The inflammatory cascade is initiated when *C. acnes* binds to Toll-like receptor (TLR)-2, receptors that signal through cytosolic nucleotide oligomerization domain-like receptor-3 (NLRP-3) that is part of a multiprotein complex involved in the activation of inflammatory responses termed the inflammasome. NLRP-3 initiates the oligomerization of the inflammasome components including caspace-1 that promote the maturation and secretion of proinflammatory cytokines IL-1β and interleukin-18 (IL-18) [11, 12]. Inflammation is amplified when the follicular epithelium is ruptured and leakage of *C. acnes* into the dermis contacts dermal macrophages with subsequent local release of bioactive IL-1β into a neutrophil-rich inflammatory microenvironment.

DNA-based microbiome analysis coupled with immunologic studies has further delineated the inflammatory acne microenvironment. Genome sequencing and ribotyping of *C. acnes* strains from microbiome analyses have found phylotypes IA-2 (ribotypes 4 and 5), 1B-1, and IC are associated with acne. In contrast, phylotypes IA-1, IA-2 (ribotype 1), IB-2, and IB-3 were found to be evenly distributed in patients with acne and individuals with healthy skin and phylotype II (ribotype 6) was found to be associated with healthy skin (Table 15.1) [13, 14]. These acne-prone and healthy skin phylotypes induce different T helper type 17 (Th17) cell responses. Acne-prone *C. acnes* induce the differentiation of interferon-gamma secreting Th17 cells compared to the induction of interleukin-10 (IL-10) secreting Th17 cells associated with healthy skin phylotypes [13, 14]. Furthermore, *C. acnes* strain specific IL-10+ IL-17+ producing cytotoxic CD4+ Th17 cell (Th17CTL) clones have been shown to encode gene products associated

Table 15.1 Skin phenotypes associated with *C. acnes* phylotypes [13, 14].

Skin phenotypes	*C. acnes* phylotypes
Acne prone skin	IA-2 (ribotypes 4 and 5), IB-1, IC
Acne prone skin and healthy skin	IA-1, IA-2 (ribotype 1), IB-2, IB-3*
Healthy skin	II (ribotype 6)

* Listed phylotypes found evenly distributed in patients with acne and individuals with healthy skin.

with cytotoxicity and eliminate *C. acnes* and other gram-positive and gram-negative bacteria [15].

These genotypic and immunophenotypic data provide intriguing new insights into the role of *C. acnes* in the pathogenesis of inflammatory acne, its interaction with the immune system, and its niche within the skin microbiome. Cutaneous microbiome/host interactions controlling inflammation initiation, transition from non-inflammatory lesions and chronicity remain to be defined. The importance of *C. acnes* as a focus of acne therapy will continue to grow as new *C. acnes* immunogenetic therapeutic targets are identified.

15.2 Current Therapies and Regulatory Approval

Antibiotics against *C. acnes* have long been a principle therapy in acne treatment. Both systemic (oral) and topical antibiotic formulations (single agent and combinations) have shown efficacy. These include tetracycline, minocycline, doxycycline, clindamycin, erythromycin along with benzoyl peroxide. Oral and topical retinoids, hormonal modulation in women (oral contraception and spironolactone) and energy based devices (laser, intense pulse light and photodynamic therapy) have expanded the therapeutic options for acne. Therapeutic benefits and toxicities, first line therapies, and treatment guidelines are presented elsewhere [16].

With the increase of new acne therapies coming to market, the criteria for United States Food and Drug Administration (U.S. FDA) approval have been codified. Investigator global assessments (IGA) and acne lesion counts are the primary clinical endpoints for efficacy and randomized, double-blind, clinical trials that include a placebo arm are required. Often two parallel phase 3 trails are required for a U.S. FDA new drug application

(NDA) [17], so the pathway for commercial development of new acne treatments is complex and expensive. The proficiency to assess new compounds' ability to target *C. acnes in-vivo* prior to phase testing, can provide essential information for prioritizing acne pharmaceutical development programs.

15.3   *In-Vivo C. acnes* Reduction Assay

An assay with the capacity to quickly quantify the reduction of the total *C. acnes* population on facial skin in a small group of healthy volunteers has the features of a highly useful screening method for assessing efficacy since the pharmacodynamic effect of *C. acnes* reduction tracks with clinical efficacy of anti-acne treatments [10, 18–23]. The *in-vivo C. acnes* reduction assay is a cultured-based analysis that was developed as a screening tool. It evaluates quantitative changes in the total population of *C. acnes* [10, 18–22] and has the capacity to track changes in antibiotic insensitive *C. acnes* populations [23]. It differs from DNA-based analysis in which bacterial DNA is extracted from specimens collected for the skin and subjected to either 16S rRNA gene-dependent amplicon-based sequencing or shotgun metagenomics sequencing. These microbiome analyses provide the capacity to identify and quantify all strains of microorganisms, metabolically active pathways, and generate taxonomic profiles [24, 25]. Culture-based analysis provides discrimination of viable bacteria and their minimal inhibitory concentrations (MIC) to antibiotics (Table 15.2).

Table 15.2 Comparison of *C. acnes* characterization methods.

Analytic characteristics	Culture-based analysis	DNA-based analysis
Strain quantification	+	+
Discrimination of viable bacteria	+	−
Antibiotic resistance	+	+
MIC determination	+	−
Phylotyping (16S rRNA gene analysis)	−	+

The assay's methodology is described as follows. It utilizes a split-face design and a subject sample size of at least 25 with supervised daily applications of a test product and vehicle control. Subjects are screened for the degree of follicular fluorescence detected by Wood's lamp (Ultra-violet Products, Inc. San Gabriel, CA) examination. *C. acnes* porphyrin production correlates with the level of the commensurate bacteria on the skin and the degree of facial follicular fluorescence is an estimated indication of *C. acnes* counts (Figure 15.2) [26]. Subjects who show a high degree of facial follicular fluorescence are selected for sample collection that are obtained at baseline and every 2 weeks for up to 6 weeks. Utilizing a swab-wash method [27, 28], *C. acnes* is cultured for the malar surfaces of each cheek. Each cheek is thoroughly cleansed with sterile gauze soaked with 0.1% Tween 80 to remove surface debris and bacteria and the malar surface areas to be cultured (4 cm²) are delineated by a sterile plastic template held firmly to the skin. The area is scrubbed with the cotton-tipped swab dipped into 2mL of wash solution for 30 seconds [28]. The swab is placed back into the 2mL of wash solution and wrung on the side of the tube before the site is scrubbed for a second time. After the second scrub, the cotton-tipped swab is wrung on the side of the tube and broken off into the 2mL of wash solution for processing. The current swab-wash method that samples the skin surface was recently compared to pore sampling methods including pore strips and cyanoacrylate glue follicular biopsy. All three methods were equally effective in their capacity to collect *C. acnes* from the

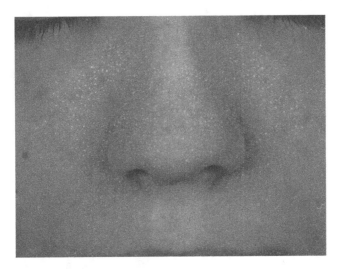

Figure 15.2 Wood's lamp demonstrating red-orange follicular fluorescence of *C. acnes* on the face.

skin and did not influence the capacity to characterize the abundance and diversity of *C. acnes* as determined by 16S rRNA gene and whole-genome metagenomic sequencing [29].

Each sample is processed by serial dilution using 0.05% Tween 80 (buffered with 0.075M phosphate buffer, pH 7.9) in four tenfold dilutions (Figure 15.3). Using a micropipettor, 0.05mL of each dilution is placed on a designated section of an agar plate containing Brucella agar supplemented with yeast extract, dextrose, and cysteine; five-drop dilutions per plate (Figure 15.4). Duplicate plates for each sample are allowed to dry, placed in an anaerobic jar with BBL Gas Pak Plus anaerobic system envelope and incubated anaerobically at 36.5-37.5°C for 7 days [22, 23].

Colony forming units (cfu) of *C. acnes* are counted manually at the dilution that contains between 10 and 100 cfu [21, 22]. Total densities of *C. acnes* are calculated and reported as log10 cfu per cm². Colony counts are assessed for uniformity of results and outliners (no or low growth) suggestive of growth-inhibiting technical factors are identified. Because growth inhibiting factors from inflammatory acne lesions can be trans-ferred to culture plates, normal volunteers are utilized in this assay. Repeat cultures are performed when possible; otherwise, these values are dropped from the final analysis.

A successful endpoint is a one or more log reduction of the mean *C. acnes* cfu count of the active test product from baseline that is statisti-cally significant when compared to the mean log reduction of the vehicle

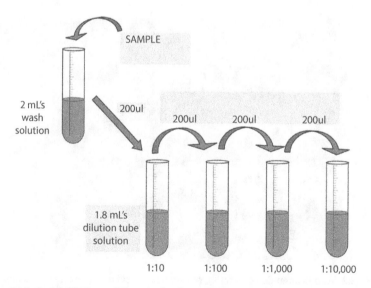

Figure 15.3 Serial dilutions of *C. acnes* for drop plating.

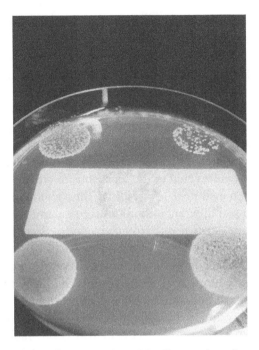

Figure 15.4 *C. acnes* colony forming units on Brucella agar plate after serial dilution and 7 day incubation.

control. The sample size of 25 provides statistical power to detect difference between the active and vehicle control at 4 weeks using a two-sided paired t-test (5% type I error) when there is ≥ 1 (SD ± 0.75) log reduction in the mean cfu count of the active that is 0.72 greater than the log reduction in the mean cfu count of the vehicle control.

The above method describes the evaluation of the total *C. acnes* population on the skin. In addition, antibiotic insensitive strains of *C. acnes* can be evaluated by using antibiotic incorporation plates to culture facial swabs. Minimal inhibitory concentrations (MICs) can be determined and the emergence of antibiotic insensitive *C. acnes* strains and the impact of treatment over time can be characterized [23].

15.4   Correlations of *C. acnes* Reduction and Clinical Efficacy

Both antibiotic and non-antibiotic antimicrobial therapies have been developed and approved for the treatment of acne. Their effectiveness and mechanisms of action may vary but they all demonstrate the importance of *C. acnes* as a therapeutic target.

Antibiotic treatment of acne works by two mechanisms: killing *C. acnes* and inhibition of *C. acnes* production of pro-inflammatory stimuli. The later is the rationale for the use of subantimicrobial doses of antibiotics in acne [10]. Regardless of mechanism, the challenge is to deliver antibiotics into the lipid rich environment of the microcomedone. The more lipid soluble the agent, the more effectively it is delivered to the target site. An antibiotic may demonstrate *C. acnes* killing with great sensitivity *in-vitro*; however, may not be delivered to the sebaceous microenvironment in sufficient levels to demonstrate *in-vivo* killing. Thus, an important measure of the relative efficacy of different antibiotics is to quantify the *in-vivo* effects of *C. acnes* reduction since the pharmacodynamic effect of *C. acnes* reduction tracks with clinical efficacy of anti-acne treatments. Table 15.3 lists the previously published data of the *in-vivo* C. acnes reduction assay for the most commonly used topical acne therapies including antibiotics and the antimicrobial benzoyl peroxide alone and in combination with erythromycin and clindamycin [10, 18–22]. The correlation between reduction of *C. acnes* counts and relevant clinical benefit is good. Table 15.4 lists that previously published data of systemic therapies [10, 18–22].

Table 15.3 *C. acnes* reduction from topical therapies [10, 18–22].

Drug	Log CFU week 4
2% Erythromycin gel	<1.0
2% Erythromycin solution	1.0–1.1
1% Clindamycin gel	0.5–1.2
Benzoyl peroxide 5%/3% erythromycin	2.0–2.2
Benzoyl peroxide 5%/clindamycin gel	3.0
Benzoyl peroxide gel	2.0
Benzoyl peroxide cleanser	1.2
Azelaic acid	<1.0
Tretinion	0.0
Alpha-hydroxy acids	0.0

CFU, colony forming units (cm²).

Table 15.4 *C. acnes* reduction from oral therapies [10, 18–22].

Drug	Log CFU week 4
Erythromycin	0.5
Trimethoprim-sulfamethoxazole	1.0
Tetracycline	1.0
Doxycycline	1.0–1.2
Minocycline	2.0–2.5
Isotretinion	3.0

CFU, colony forming units (per cm^2).

The less than one log reduction values reported for erythromycin and clindamycin reflect the well established emergence of antibiotic resistance to these antibiotics [10, 23]. Decades of antibiotic treatment of acne contributed to the clinical resistance of these antibiotic insensitive *C. acnes* strains [16]. Antibiotics work best in combinations with benzoyl peroxide and/or topical retinoids and can suppress and prevent the emergence of resistant strains [10, 22]. Benzoyl peroxide has no reported *C. acnes* resistance and demonstrated 1 to 3 log reduction in *C. acnes* counts as a single agent or in combination with erythromycin and clindamycin (Table 15.2). Tretinoin enhances penetration of antibiotics and perturbs the sebaceous microenvironment without any direct effect on reducing *C. acnes* counts (Table 15.2) [21]. Alpha-hydroxy acids, humectants, keratolytic and exfoliative agents do not reduce *C. acnes* counts as well. Their therapeutic effects lie in their comedolytic activity and penetration enhancement of antimicrobial agents [16]. It's interesting to note that azelaic acid, a non-antibiotic, did not demonstrate 1 log reduction at 4 weeks [19, 21] but did so only after 8-12 weeks of use [20], suggesting it's antimicrobial therapeutic effects are mediated through anti-inflammatory pathways. Our laboratory has assayed topical therapies that have failed to demonstrate a >1 log reduction of *C. acnes* colony counts. These include one nitrous oxide formulation, two minocycline gel formulations and four water soluble antimicrobial peptide formulations (unpublished data).

The *in-vivo C. acnes* reduction assay shows good correlation with clinical efficacy for systemic antibiotics with the degree of reduction of the *C. acnes* counts inversely correlated to the degree of antibiotic resistance. Isotretinoin's capacity to reduce sebum production and create what has been termed a "sebaceous drought" in the pilosebaceous unit [30] is another example of a non-antibiotic mechanism of *C. acnes* reduction [10]. Its 3 log reduction in *C. acnes* counts within 4-6 weeks correlates well with its powerful clinical efficacy [1, 2, 16].

15.5 Conclusion

The *in-vivo C. acnes* reduction assay is a simple and rapid method to assess an anti-acne treatment's ability to reduce *C. acnes* counts and can serve as a strong correlate for success in a standard 12 week acne clinical trial. This is particularly useful in the early, pre-clinical stages of commercial development of new acne therapies. With the characterization of antibiotic insensitive strains and pathogenic phylotypes of *C. acnes*, a new understanding into the complexity of *C. acnes'* niche in the skin microbiome has emerged and has corroborated its central role in the pathogenesis of inflammatory acne. This provides opportunities to identify new therapeutic targets and delineate novel antimicrobial therapies. The *in-vivo C. acnes* reduction assay is best utilized in the pre-clinical setting after *in vitro* testing has validated the anti-*C. acnes* activity of emerging therapies and prior to phase testing in clinical trials. It provides the capacity to evaluate new anti-acne treatments impact on the total population of *C. acnes*, antibiotic insensitive strains of *C. acnes* and compare *C. acnes* reduction levels to historic standards.

References

1. Leyden, J.J., Therapy for acne vulgaris. *N. Engl. J. Med.*, 336, 1156, 1997.
2. Zaenglein, A.L., Acne vulgaris. *N. Engl. J. Med.*, 379, 1343, 2018.
3. Hay, R.J., Johns, N.E., Williams, H.C. *et al.*, The global burden of skin disease in 2010: Analysis of the prevalence and impact of skin conditions. *J. Invest. Dermatol.*, 134, 1527, 2014.
4. Lai, J.J., Chang, P., Lai, K.P. *et al.*, The role of androgen and androgen receptor in the skin-related disorders. *Arch. Dermatol. Res.*, 304, 499, 2012.
5. Knutson, D.D., Ultrastructural observations in acne vulgaris: The normal sebaceous follicle and acne lesions. *J. Invest. Dermatol.*, 62, 288, 1974.
6. Leyden, J.J., McGinley, K.J., Mills, O.H., Jr., Kligman, A.M., *Propionibacterium* levels in patients with and without acne vulgaris. *J. Invest. Dermatol.*, 65, 382, 1975.
7. Scholz, C.F.P. and Kilian, M., The natural history of propionibacteria, and reclassification of selected species within the genus *Propionibacterium* to the proposed novel genera *Acidpropionibacterium* gen. nov., *Cutibacterium* gen.

nov. and *Pseudopropionibacterium* gen. nov. *Int. J. Syst. Evol. Microbiol.*, 66, 4422, 2016.

8. Webster, G.F. and Leyden, J.J., Characterization of serum-independent polymorphonuclear leukocyte chemotactic factors produced by Propionibacterium acnes. *Inflammation.*, 4, 261, 1980.

9. Vowels, B.R., Yang, S., Leyden, J.J., Induction of proinflammatory cytokines by a soluble factor of *Propionibacterium acnes:* Implications for chronic inflammatory acne. *Infect. Immun*, 63, 3158, 1995.

10. Leyden, J.J., The evolving role of *Propionibacterium acnes in* acne. *Semin. Cutaneous Med. Surg.*, 20, 139, 2001.

11. Qin, M., Pirouz, A., Kim, M.H., Krutzik, S.R., Garbán, H.J., Kim, J., *Propionibacterium acnes* induces IL-1β secretion *via* the NLRP3 inflammasome in human monocytes. *J. Invest. Dermatol.*, 134, 381, 2014. Erratum in: *J. Invest. Dermatol.*, 134, 1779 2014.

12. Li, Z.J., Choi, D.K., Sohn, K.C. *et al.*, *Propionibacterium acnes* activates the NLRP3 inflammasome in human sebocytes. *J. Invest. Dermatol.*, 134, 2747, 2014.

13. Yu, Y., Champer, J., Agak, G.W., Kao, S., Modlin, R.L., Kim, J., Different *Propionibacterium acnes* phylotypes induce distinct immune responses and express unique surface and secreted proteomes. *J. Invest. Dermatol.*, 136, 2221, 2016.

14. Agak, G.W., Kao, S., Ouyang, K. *et al.*, Phenotype and antimicrobial activity of Th17 cells induced by *Propionibacterium acnes* strains associated with healthy and acne skin. *J. Invest. Dermatol.*, 138, 316, 2017.

15. Agak, G., Ceja-Garcia, N., Dang, P. *et al.*, Antimicrobial Th17CTL targeting both gram-positive and gram-negative bacteria. *J. Invest. Dermatol.*, 139, S12 (abstract 70), 2019.

16. Thiboutot, D.M., Dréno, B., Abanmi, A. *et al.*, Practical management of acne for clinicians: An international consensus from the global alliance to improve outcomes in acne. *J. Am. Acad. Dermatol.*, 78, 2 Suppl 1, S1, 2018.

17. U.S. Department of Health and Human Services Food and Drug Administration Center for Drug Evaluation and Research, Acne Vulgaris: Establishing Effectiveness of Drugs Intended for Treatment Guidance for Industry. May 2018. https://www.fda.gov/downloads/Drugs/Guidances/UCM071292.pdf.

18. Leyden, J.J., Open-label evaluation of topical antimicrobial and anti-acne preparations for effectiveness versus *Propionibacterium acnes in vivo. Cutis*, 40, 8, 1992.

19. Cunliffe, W.J. and Holland, K.T., Clinical and laboratory studies on treatment with 20% azelaic acid cream for acne. *Acta Derm. Venereol. Suppl. (Stockh).*, 143, 31, 1989.

20. White, G.M., Acne therapy. *Adv. Dermatol.*, 14, 29, 1999.

21. Leyden, J.J., Current issues in antimicrobial therapy for the treatment of acne. *J. Eur. Acad. Dermatol. Venereol.*, 15, Suppl. 3, 51, 2001.

22. Leyden, J.J., Effect of topical benzoyl peroxide/clindamycin versus topical clindamycin and vehicle in reduction of *Propionibacterium Acnes. Cutis*, 69, 475, 2002.

23. Leyden, J.J., Preston, N., Osborn, C., Gottschalk, R.W., *In-vivo* effectiveness of adapalene 0.1%/benzoyl peroxide 2.5% gel on antibiotic-sensitive and resistant *Propionibacterium Acnes Clin. Aesthet. Dermatol.*, 4, 22, 2011.

24. Grogan, M.D., Bartow-McKenney, C., Flowers, L. *et al.*, Research techniques made simple: Profiling the skin microbiota. *J. Invest. Dermatol.*, 139, 747, 2019.

25. Kong, H.H., Andersson, B., Clavel, T. *et al.*, Performing skin microbiome research: A method to the madness. *J. Invest. Dermatol.*, 137, 561, 2016.

26. McGinley, K.J., Webster, G., Leyden, J.J., Facial follicular porphyrin fluorescence: Correlation with age and density of *Propionibacterium Acnes. Br. J. Dermatol.*, 102, 437, 1980.

27. Williamson, P. and Kligman, A.M., A new method for the quantitative investigation of cutaneous bacteria. *J. Invest. Dermatol.*, 45, 498, 1965.

28. Keyworth, N., Millar, M.R., Holland, K.T., Swab-wash method for quantification of cutaneous microflora. *J. Clin. Microbiol.*, 28, 941, 1993.

29. Hall, J.B., Cong, Z., Imamura-Kawasawa, Y. *et al.*, Isolation and identification of the follicular microbiome: Implications for acne research. *J. Invest. Dermatol.*, 138, 2033, 2018.

30. McKean, M., Oba, J., Ma, J. *et al.*, Skin ecology during sebaceous drought – how skin microbes respond to isotretinoin. *J. Invest. Dermatol.*, 139, 732, 2019.

Part 6

REGULATORY AND LEGAL ASPECTS FOR SKIN MICROBIOME RELATED PRODUCTS

16

Intellectual Property Tools for Protecting, Developing and Growing a Skin Microbiome Brand

Jeffrey K. Mills

Medler Ferro Woodhouse & Mills PLLC, McLean, VA

Abstract

As companies and researchers look to develop products for the skin microbiome, it is important to consider how to protect such innovation, as well as how to position these products in the marketplace. This chapter will provide an overview of the various kinds of intellectual property, including patents, trademarks, and trade secrets, and the requirements for each. It will also discuss how to utilize these "tools" to provide the developer of the technology with a market advantage.

Keywords: Intellectual property, patent, trademark, copyright, trade secret

16.1 Introduction

Research related to the skin microbiome presents a tremendous opportunity for developing new therapies and products designed to treat a vast number of diseases and disorders. With all rapidly growing areas of technology, navigating the landscape and potential competitors becomes increasingly difficult as new players, both large and small, enter the marketplace with goals of grabbing a piece of the pie.

This chapter will discuss how companies, institutions and researchers can utilize intellectual property to not only protect discoveries related to the skin microbiome, but also develop and grow a microbiome-focused

Email: jmills@medlerferro.com

Nava Dayan (ed.) Skin Microbiome Handbook: From Basic Research to Product Development, (305–320) © 2020 Scrivener Publishing LLC

brand. The following discussion is primarily limited to intellectual property in the United States (US), including the relevant US laws and rules.

16.2 The Tools of Intellectual Property

Intellectual property (IP) relates to the laws and regulations linked to creations of the mind. Like any other "property right," IP rights can be bought and sold, traded, rented (licensed) or even passed down to future generations via a will. The following provides a brief description of four of the most common types of intellectual property, their similarities and differences, and a discussion of some of the requirements for each. The discussion provided below does not include all of the elements necessary to maintain protection under each type of intellectual property, but provides a starting point for the outline that follows about how each can be used to build a portfolio for a skin microbiome brand.

16.2.1   Patents

Patents represent the most common intellectual property right, and often the most desired when developing a product and a brand. A patent provides a "right to exclude" someone from making, using, selling, or offering for sale, what is claimed in the patent. (*See* United States Patent Office Website (USPTO, www.uspto.gov) "Patents" Heading -- "Patent Basics"). Thus, the claims represent the most important part of the patent document, as they define the boundary, or the "fence," that surrounds the intellectual "property." It is important to remember, however, that a patent does not give the patent holder the right to practice what is claimed in the patent. It is still necessary to make sure that no other patents owned by third parties may be broader, and thus encompass making, using or selling a more expansive scope. As an analogy, owning a piece of land entitles the owner put up a fence and keep others out of the property. However, depending on local laws and ordinances, the owner may not be able to build a replica of the Eiffel Tower on the land. It is a similar analysis with patent law. Having a patent doesn't mean that the patent owner gets to make the product. It is very possible to obtain a patent that is new and not obvious, but that still may fall within the scope of another party's claims and thus be blocked from being made or used.

Patents have a number of requirements. In general, a patent must describe an invention in sufficient detail and tell someone working in the field how to make and use the invention, without having to undertake significant experimentation. (35 U.S.C. § 112(a)) (2012). In addition, the patent must be new and non-obvious. (35 U.S.C. §§ 102, 103) (2012). Recently, as will be discussed later in this chapter, a great deal of emphasis has been focused on determining whether or not certain subject matter is "patent eligible." (see 35 U.S.C. § 101) (2012).

In addition to obtaining patents for use as a defensive tool – that is to keep competitors out of a particular space; and as an offensive tool – to pursue potential infringers to recover lost profits; they can also be used as a way to generate money from licensing and other activities. Whether or not a company is making, using or selling a product that falls under the scope of a patent, other third parties may want to make it themselves. This requires the approval of the patent holder to market their own product. The result of this arrangement can be a licensing agreement where one company provides another group (potentially even a competitor) with the right to practice the invention without fear of being sued, in exchange for financial or other compensation. Licensing revenue from patents can often allow patent holders to obtain value for patents that they have no intention of ever practicing, or in situations where they may not be able to see the product come to market for various reasons (e.g., lack of funding, change of focus of the company).

Later in this chapter exemplary types of patents that can be obtained in the skin microbiome space will be discussed, and how each of them can be utilized, or leveraged, to help build a brand and/or a company.

16.2.2   Trademarks

While sometimes considered to take a back seat to patents in an intellectual property portfolio, trademarks can provide a significant advantage in both marketing and branding of a product or company. In addition, in areas such as consumer products, patent protection may not be viable due to the inability to show the product is "new and not obvious," but trademarks can still help a company secure a substantial market advantage.

Trademarks or Service Marks include any word, name, symbol, device, or combination, used to identify and distinguish the goods or services of one seller or provider from those of another. (See USPTO Website (www.uspto.gov) "Trademarks" Heading -- "Trademark Basics"). That is, a trademark indicates the source of a good or service. A trademark does not, and generally cannot, be descriptive of those goods or services. For example, while it is possible to obtain a trademark to the name of a brand of hand lotion, it is not possible to trademark the term "hand lotion" as that simply describes what the product is, and is a generic term for the good. Trademarks can be names, symbols, colors, even sounds.

In addition, trademarks must be "used in commerce." That is, they must be part of a product (either used on the packaging or product itself) or associated with the sale of the product to consumers. It is not possible to simply file a trademark for a product and then never use the name. This is significantly different from a patent, where it is not necessary to actually make or use anything that is covered by the patent. It is possible to simply hold on to the patent (and keep others out of the space if so desired). A company applying for a trademark must demonstrate that the mark is actually being used in commerce, in order to be granted the protection.

Upon a showing of the requirements necessary for registration, a trademarked name or symbol can be utilized in combination with the ® designation (indicating it is a trademark registered in the United States). Another common designation, ™, relates to trademarks that are not registered with the USPTO. Called "common law trademarks," these designations indicate that the trademark holder believes that the word or symbol identifies them as the source of a good or service. The ™ label can be utilized immediately upon association of the term or symbol with a good – it is not necessary to wait for registration with the USPTO. Often such common law trademarks are regional (e.g., a single state), rather than national, in coverage. While they are not as easy to enforce in a court of law, common law trademarks can be used in a similar way if others try to utilize a similar or confusing mark.

Another significant difference is that while patents are only enforceable for a period of 20 years, trademarks can be maintained forever, so long as there is continued of the mark in commerce, it continues signify the source of the goods (i.e., it hasn't become a generic term for a good), and the required fees are paid. Thus, trademarks can provide a significant branding tool for an extended period of time, providing advantages in both marketing and competitive positioning.

16.2.3 Copyrights

Copyrights represent the more "artistic" side of intellectual property, providing for the protection of original works of authorship fixed in a tangible medium of expression. Copyright covers both published and unpublished works. While most people recognize the standard forms that a copyright can take, i.e., written article or novel, song, painting or sculpture, copyright protection can also extend to things like photographs used on marketing materials, written descriptions or pamphlets related to products, and web-content. Copyright protects the specific form of the expression, not allowing for others to make a replica or exact copy of the work. In addition, copyright also protects the IP holder from others that attempt to use portions or parts of the work or create derivative works, depending on how closely they are related to the original creation.

As discussed above, patents and trademarks require approval from the USPTO to be enforceable. In contrast, the intellectual property rights associated with copyright affixes to the work immediately upon its creation. The advantage in "registering" a copyright with the United States Copyright Office (and obtaining the © designation) is that it is much easier to enforce against a potential infringer or competitor. In addition, while patents and trademarks can be very expensive to obtain (well into the thousands of dollars), copyright protection costs generally less than a few hundred dollars.

While copyrights do have a finite lifetime, it is far greater than the 20 years provided to a patent, and instead generally lasts 70 years beyond the life of the author. Thus, copyright can provide a significant advantage for a company and its brand for a long period.

16.2.4 Trade Secrets/Know-How

The final form of intellectual property that will be discussed in this chapter relates to what is known as "trade secrets" or sometimes "know-how."

Trade secrets are information that is generally not known to the public, and often relates to a recipe or formulation. However, trade secrets can also extend to business practices utilized by a company, including marketing strategies, client lists, etc. One of the most common trade secrets is the formula for COCA-COLA®, a recipe that has been maintained in secret for nearly 130 years.

Trade Secrets have three basic requirements. They must be something that provides a "business advantage;" they must be something that is not readily known; and preventative measures must be taken to keep this piece of information confidential. (*See* USPTO Website (www.uspto.gov) "Trade Secret Policy"). That is, employers must tell employees or others who have access to the information that this is a "trade secret" and that it should be kept confidential. If the trade secret is provided to others outside of a company without an indication of its confidentiality, then its designation as a trade secret can be lost. In addition, trade secrets are not useful for information that is easily reverse engineered. For example, if by simply looking at a product someone in the field could readily determine how it is put together or what it contains, then there is no value in keeping the information regarding it as a trade secret. In addition, trade secrets are often considered "mutually exclusive" to patents. As noted above, a patent must disclose in a very detailed manner how to make a use a patented product. It is not possible to also keep information secret that is deemed critical to how it is made – this is a violation of the requirement to disclose and fully enable an invention. This, often a decision must be made whether or not to file a patent on a process, or if it is better to simply keep the information secret.

Know-how is a form of trade secret. Know-how often relates to information or details known only to a few people in a company, or some unique aspect of a manufacturing process, that only those working with the product know. This can be as simple as the timing of a temperature shift when making a biologic product (e.g., an antibody or protein). Generally, such information is not patentable, but may be very significant to provide an optimal product. Thus, it can be maintained as a trade secret, or simply as "know-how," related to the process.

16.3   Building an Intellectual Property Portfolio for a Skin Microbiome Brand

Each of these forms of intellectual property has its own place in the toolbox for building, protecting, and maintaining a brand or product. With their own unique qualities and requirements, determining how to best use each of these tools can be a complex process. However, what to keep in mind is that collectively, they can provide unique advantages to a company, institution, or start-up effort.

It is important to look at intellectual *property* as intellectual *assets*, both individually and collectively. That is, "tangible" elements that can be enforced, bought and sold, rented, traded, and even passed down in a will. In many instances, intellectual property can make up most of, if not all of, the assets of a company. There are many start-ups that have little or no concrete assets (i.e., machinery, buildings or product), yet they have significant value as a result of the intellectual assets that they posses.

Described below are exemplary ways in which each of these forms of intellectual property can be used to develop a skin microbiome brand or product.

16.3.1   Patents to Define "The Fence"

A review of the number of patents and patent applications published in the last few years indicates an increasing trend in patent filings that include claims directed to the microbiome. (Data: Personal searches performed by

Author using PATBASE® database; MINESOFT® Global Patent Solutions (www.minesoft.com)). From 82 in 2015, up to 124 in 2016, and 213 in 2017, this nearly tripling in 3 years provides insight to the importance that various industries place on the growth of inventions and products in the microbiome space.

As discussed above, patents allow the asset owner to put up a fence around their property and keep others out of what is defined by the claims. When considering what types of claims to pursue in a patent portfolio, it is important to consider not only what a company is trying to make, use, or sell as a patent owner, but what competitors may be trying to do.

Perhaps the most common type of patent claims in the pharmaceutical space, including the skin microbiome, are those directed to a composition of matter, including a formulation. Traditionally, in the world of small molecule chemistry, patents were often directed to the compound itself, as well as various ways of formulating it (i.e., orally, topically). This claim type however takes a different form when considering the types of compounds being discovered and researched related to the skin microbiome.

In many cases, skin microbiome products are derived from, or related to, a natural product. For example, a collection of microbes, or a protein or selection of peptides unique to a particular bacterium. While such discoveries directly related to compounds or structures found in nature were traditionally patentable (i.e., an isolated polypeptide or an isolated nucleic acid molecule), following legal decisions from the United States Supreme Court beginning in 2013 (*Association for Molecular Pathology v. Myriad Genetics, Inc.*, 569 U.S. 576 (2013)), protecting these discoveries with a patent became increasingly difficulty. What the Supreme Court held in the *Myriad* case, essentially required a patent holder to show that his natural product was "markedly different" from that which is found in nature, in order for the discovery to be eligible for patenting. No longer was it enough for a patent claim to simply say that it was an "isolated" structure from nature (i.e., taken out of its natural surroundings). It had to be different from what is found in nature in some meaningful way. In general, decisions about whether or not a nucleic acid or protein sequence for a microbe, or collection of bacteria is "found in nature," come from reviews of relevant literature in the field. Courts and Patent Examiners rely on the information available to them from public sequence databases as well, such as the National Center for Biotechnology Information, Basic Local Alignment Search Tool (BLAST) (*see* NIH website, www.ncbi.nlm.nih.gov).

For inventions in the skin microbiome space, this now means that a protein or nucleic acid molecule must somehow be structurally or compositionally different than what is found in nature. It must contain, for example, a mutation or modification that isn't found in its natural setting. If the claim is directed to a collection of bacteria, those bacteria must not exist together in nature. Formulations of proteins or bacteria may still be eligible to receive a patent, but claims directed to such formulations generally must be more than simply adding known excipients to an isolated protein. A showing that the formulation provides added stability or enhanced efficacy to the biological material may be required in order to obtain a patent on the discovery.

Another area where recent changes in the laws related to "patent eligible subject matter" directly intersect with research in the skin microbiome, is with regard to personalized medicine. Discoveries related to how the skin microbiome reacts to the environment or drugs, or characteristics of a person's skin microbiome and the relationship to their overall health or disease state, all utilize information or correlations that are "natural processes." For example, the level of a certain bacteria as a function of skin health or age, or how a person's skin flora reacts to external stimuli, are all-natural processes. The use of information about these processes, once protectable in various diagnostic-type claims, in general is now much harder to protect via a patent.

Another decision from the Supreme Court in 2012 (*Mayo v. Prometheus*, 566 U.S. 66 (2012), just slightly before the *Myriad* case, stated that patents that simply claimed the "application" of a law of nature or a natural process, and didn't do more than what was "routine and conventional" when applying the natural process or law, were not considered eligible for patenting. Court cases subsequent to this change in the law have, in general, limited the ability to obtain patent claims that were traditionally in the area of personalized medicine. Thus, when considering how to patent inventions in this space, care must be taken to make sure that the claims are drafted to meet these new, and still developing, changes in the law.

In contrast to these areas, two other classes of U.S. patents that are still readily attainable in the skin microbiome space are methods of treatment and methods of preparation or synthesis. So long as a method of treatment claim includes an active "administering" or "treating" step, and does in fact require something to be given to a patient, these types of claims can still be obtained (or at least are eligible for patenting). Similarly, with regard to patent eligibility, a method of making a natural product, including synthesis or purification, can be still be protected.

Types of patents related to methods of treatment in the skin microbiome space are exemplified by U.S. Patent No. 10,017,731, owned by Aobiome LLC.

This patent claims a method of treating eczema comprising: administering, as a spray, aerosol or mist, a preparation comprising live ammonia oxidizing bacteria, to the skin of a subject. While "method of treatment" claims are generally directed to methods performed by a doctor or perhaps a pharmacist, they still do provide a mechanism for enforcement against competitors who make a similar product. So long as a competitor provides direction as to how to use its product, or tells a doctor (or even a patient) to use the product in a manner that falls within the scope of the claim, the patent may be able to be enforced against the competitor making the compound.

Patents claiming methods of preparation, synthesis, or purification can take many forms, including for example U.S. Patent No. 10,226,431, owned by Rebiotix, and directed to a method for manufacturing an oral microbiota restoration therapy (MRT) composition. The claimed method includes steps of manufacturing a drug substance comprising fecal-derived microbiota and a cryoprotectant, lyophilizing the mixture, processing of the mixture and encapsulation of the mixture. Method patents of these types can help stop competitors from practicing an optimized method, and can also be used to keep others out of a desired methodology. As discussed above, this includes patents that the company holding the patent may not even be practicing themselves.

With a patent or patents in hand, the next questions center around how to best utilize these intellectual assets to help protect and grow a company. Deciding how to proceed once a patent is obtained is a multi-layered strategy that requires looking both internally at a company's business goals, as well as the marketplace and how competitors are acting. The following provides a very brief overview of some of the considerations that go into these decisions.

16.3.1.1   Patents "As Sticks" - Enforcement of Infringement

Using a patent or an entire portfolio as a way to not only stop a competitor from practicing, but also to recover damages from their actions, is certainly one of the most common uses for these IP assets. Strategies for patent litigations require significant investments of not only money, but time, to consider how best to position the claims of the patents with regard to a company's own activities. In addition, consideration must be taken as to what a competitor is doing, or what it is believed they may do in the future. From a financial perspective, patent litigation can certainly provide a company with a significant windfall, depending on the stakes and market involved. However, undertaking a litigation is risky and comes with a significant upfront investment -- often on the order of hundreds of thousands to potentially millions of dollars. In addition, for global technologies, patent litigations can span multiple countries at the same time, pushing the costs exponentially higher.

Even if enforcement is not a desirable or feasible use of a patent or portfolio, simply having the patent can provide a significant deterrent to others from entering the field. In addition, the publication of the information in the patent can also provide a restriction to future competitors, as they will not be able to obtain a patent on the same subject matter. Thus, even if the patented technology is never enforced, a competitor may not consider it worthwhile to enter to patented landscape, as they know it is not possible to secure the space for themselves.

16.3.1.2   Patents "As Financial Boosts" – Licensing and Other Agreements

While there certainly are and will continue to be companies in the skin microbiome space that utilize patents for their enforcement purposes, perhaps a larger number will find use for them as ways to increase financial standing. Particularly in areas where technology is still in its early developmental stages, and many of the companies involved are smaller or even start-ups, use of patents for financial leverage is often the path selected.

Positioning patents for licensing or cross-licensing is perhaps one of the most common ways for a company to utilize these assets to obtain a financial advantage. Licensing arrangements can take various forms with regard to patents, including an arrangement where a single company has an "exclusive" license to practice under a patent, to arrangements where multiple companies may have "non-exclusive" agreements where each is able to practice in a particular medical field of use or geographic area. Cross-licensing arrangements can also be utilized where companies, including competitors, provide each other with access to their technologies. The ability to draft licensing agreements with very specific language and carve-outs can often result in an arrangement that provides significant benefits to both parties.

Certainly, in comparison to litigation, for smaller companies and start-ups, licensing and cross-licensing arrangements represent some of the most common uses for patents. These agreements in general also provide wider access for technologies, and in rapidly developing areas, provide a mechanism to increase access to new advances that may be developed outside of a company.

Another very common use of patents is as collateral for a bank loan. Like any other type of property, patents can be part of a security agreement that states that if the patent owner defaults on the loan, the lender then becomes the owner of the patent. This provides a very useful way to increase cash flow by utilizing an asset that might otherwise sit dormant.

A final use is simply to sell the patent or portfolio. Many times, the costs of obtaining a patent are far less than assembling the resources necessary to actually carry out the technology or make the product. It may be a better use of the asset to simply sell the patent to a third party and allow them to proceed in the field. As with licensing, agreements can be created that still may allow the selling party to practice in a particular area, even if they no longer control the assets.

16.3.2   Trademarks to Establish Brand Recognition

While trademarks may be viewed as less "powerful" than patents to protect a company's products and ideas, they can in fact be quite useful when considered as part of the overall strategy for a brand. As discussed above, trademarks, whether words, symbols, designs, or even colors, designate the source of a good or a service. Thus, they provide a vehicle to designate to the public that a single company is the primary source for a good, or the primary provider of a service, in a particular technological or commercial area.

Examining the various ways that research and development in the skin microbiome can manifest itself in products and services is somewhat akin to the traditional pharmaceutical space. However, with the increased importance of microbiome data and information in guiding treatment and diagnostics, this area also has characteristics similar to biologic service providers (e.g., gene sequencing companies).

Thus, much like traditional products in the pharma and dermatological space, trademarks can provide a mechanism to designate that a company is the source for the therapeutic or consumer good. Trademarks establish a link between quality and a product, which consumers will desire and seek-out, looking for a specific brand, coloration, name, tag-line, etc. For example, in the microbiome space, a number of companies have already established trademarked terms associated with their product lines.

For example, MOTHERDIRT® has a series of products designed to restore and balance the skin's Ammonia-Oxidizing Bacteria (AOB), each with it's unique trademarked name and coloration.

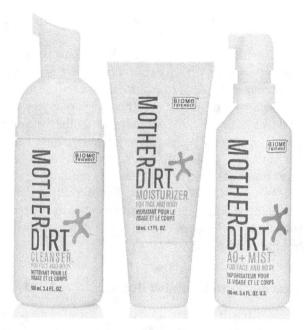

https://motherdirt.com/pages/science

By employing unique names, tag-lines, color schemes, etc., a company is able to ensure that consumers recognize their products when they see them. Consistency of the use of the branding also provides the public with a sense of a consistent product.

Other companies have used trademarks to signify they provide a unique or desired service to the microbiome space.

For example, COSMOSID® provides next generation sequencing and bioinformatics analysis to companies and institutions studying the human microbiome, including the bacterial make-up of the skin.

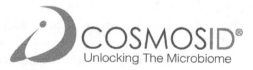

https://www.cosmosid.com/

The selection of a trademark for a skin microbiome company or product will often involve a discussion of the goal of the company, the type of clients or customers they are trying to attract, as well as the ability to actually use the trademark.

While considerations need to be taken to make sure that a trademark does not cause confusion with a similar mark, in general, finding a potential trademark that can be registered is a far less daunting task than trying to obtain a patent. In general, relatively minor changes to a trademark, including changing colors or word choice, can still maintain the desired impact on the consumer, but alleviate concerns that the registration will be refused. While a trademark can still be opposed by competitors if they believe that there is confusion with their own trademark, the overall cost of defending such a challenge is far less than trying to obtain and maintain a patent.

As with patents, trademarks can be used as "sticks" to enforce intellectual property and keep people out of using the same or similar trademark in order to try and confuse consumers. Like patents, obtaining numerous trademarks to the name of a company, a product, or service, as well as stylized or graphical representations of the brand name, all provide multiple layers of protection, and thus multiple avenues to ultimately enforce against a competitor.

Trademark licensing is also a mechanism to obtain value for these intellectual assets. Like patents, trademarks can be included in various deals and arrangements as part of one-way, or cross-licensing arrangements. For example, a trademark license can allow a distributor to indicate that they are an exclusive supplier of a product, or that another party's product includes a specific, trademarked component. In many cases, being able to say that a product includes a well-known ingredient or active agent can provide a significant sales advantage, even if it may not be possible to protect the product from copy-cats via patent protection.

As with patent portfolios, trademarks can be sold as an asset of a company, or used as loan collateral. In many instances, particularly if a company is being sold, patents and trademarks will often be packaged together as part of an intellectual asset portfolio.

16.3.3   Copyrights to Maintain Information

Copyrights in high technology fields such as skin microbiome research and products are often encountered in the relationship between the company and a technical journal, where the rights to the copyright of an article or abstract are signed over to the journal owner. In such instances, it is important to remember that the original author or the the company DOES NOT have the right to disseminate that article or paper once the copyright has been transferred to a journal. In many instances, the owner of the journal will allow certain limited rights to provide copies to colleagues, or will grant the rights to a broader distribution, if so desired. It is important to remember however, that most journals will not allow the sale or distribution of copies of the article for a fee. In addition, if the article is to be included on a website or as part of marketing material, the copyright agreement must be consulted to determine what rights have been maintained and which require permission first.

In general, copyrights often arise with company branding in terms of website design, photographs for marketing materials, or movies for promotional purposes. In general, such products are called "work-for-hire," which means that the company requesting the "work" should own the copyright to the product. It is very important to confirm this though in any agreement with a third party contractor. If such an agreement is not in place, or if the agreement allows the contractor to retain the copyright, there may be very limited rights in what can be done with that written or visual product.

In the context of the skin microbiome, another area that copyrights can come into play is in the text that accompanies a product, including methods for using the product, literature describing the product, or other materials that may be provided to the end user. In most cases, the copyright for these materials can be protected through registration. By doing so, this provides an additional layer of protection from competitors utilizing the same product literature or description. If it can be demonstrated that another company directly copied a copyright protected work, the activity can be stopped and potential monetary damages that it may have caused can be recovered. In addition, copyright can be used to stop other companies from including substantial portions of their protected work, for example in a competing marketing or advertising campaign.

16.3.4   Trade Secrets/Know-How to Keep A Competitive Edge

As noted earlier, trade secrets are information that is generally not known to the public, and often relates to a recipe or formulation, or can relate to a business practice utilized by a company. Similarly, know-how can relate to internal procedures or information that only those in a company are aware of – a secret or well-kept method of manufacturing or a unique way to carry out a procedure. All of these can provide advantages to a business and can the form the basis of trade-secret protection.

In research or non-profit institutional settings, maintaining protection of trade secrets may be difficult if not impossible, as the desire to publish and disseminate knowledge are cornerstones of such organizations. To the extent that collaborations occur between research groups and private companies, it is important that both sides understand what information may constitute trade secret (generally of the company) and make sure to maintain its confidentiality.

In the context of the skin microbiome, trade secrets can provide a distinct advantage over competitors. This is particularly relevant to companies working with methods of producing or purifying a microbiological product. As discussed in the section regarding patenting, such methods can certainly be protected via the claims of a patent. However, this assumes that the process is new and non-obvious in light of what was previously known. While such innovations can certainly occur, often the advantage gleaned from a production or purification process may simply be the result of a small change in the pH of a reaction, the temperature or time duration of a purification process, or a specific buffer utilized in a column filtration process. It may be very difficult to patent such "improvements," as they may be considered obvious changes of known processes. However, if they provide a company with a significant advantage over the competition, trade secret protection may provide a mechanism to prevent others from utilizing such modifications.

As discussed above, as of the writing of this chapter, it is not possible to patent "natural products" that do not differ from those found in nature. Thus, while patenting a microbiome-based product may not be possible, it can still be possible to protect information about the source, characteristics, etc., via trade secret protection. Thus, in instances where patent protection may not be possible, trade secrets provide a possible path for maintaining a business or technical advantage.

In order to protect such advantages, it is critically important that all persons involved with such a process or product are informed that the improvements are confidential, provide a manufacturing, technical, or business advantage, and are to only be shared with others that must know the trade secret. It is also important that a paper trail of these advantages and these discussions with employees about their importance is properly documented. Anyone who is involved with the process should sign documentation attesting to the importance of the trade secret, and the importance to actually keep it secret. Preparing such documentation is vital, and should include both internal and external legal teams to make sure that all steps are fully documented and carefully worded. It is also important that, once a trade secret policy is in place, the policy is adhered to and enforced. Having a document that says a secret cannot be shared outside of a certain circle of employees is only later enforceable if that policy was adhered to by all. If the policy is simply treated as a suggestion or a goal, it may not be possible to later enforce it if the secret is leaked or compromised.

While trade secrets do not protect from others "reverse engineering" or otherwise happening upon the discovery themselves, it does provide recourse for a company's own employees leaving and sharing this secret with a competitor. In addition, trade secrets can provide protection from competitors using improper tactics (i.e., bribing employees, stealing note-books, improperly listening in on discussions), to try and obtain infor-mation about the secrets. In industries like the skin microbiome that are developing quickly, there is also the possibility of rapid movement of employees, researchers and management teams, as companies look to position themselves to best serve the market. Trade secret protection is especially important in such fields, as it allows for maintaining the advan-tages that a company may have developed internally, even if those who developed them may move on to competitors.

As with all of the other intellectual property assets described in this chapter, trade secrets and know-how can also form the basis of a portfolio that can be licensed or sold to a third party. In the case of license agree-ments, care must be taken to not only identify trade secret information, but to make sure that the licensing party understands the confidential nature of the information and agrees to maintain its secrecy. In combination with patents and trademarks, trade secrets often form the bulk of the intellectual assets of a company and can provide great value in a number of settings.

16.4   Conclusion

The goal of this chapter was to provide an overview of the various types of intellectual property that are available to companies and researchers in the skin microbiome space. While patenting is often still the most powerful of the assets of an IP portfolio, because of the current challenges regarding patenting in areas where "natural products" and "natural processes" are critical, companies must often turn to other avenues to protect and grow their brand. The skin microbiome represents a rapidly developing field, reaching a diverse group of researchers, companies and impacting varied products. It will be important for those working in this area to protect their ideas even in view of the challenges currently facing products and pro-cesses so closely related to nature.

Trademarks, copyrights and trade secrets all represent additional types of protection that will see increased importance to skin microbiome com-panies to help them maintain business and technical advantages. Working with each of these types of assets, and understanding and leveraging their unique advantages, companies will be able to build strong brands, and pro-tect important information and product lines for years to come.

17

Regulatory Aspects of Probiotics and Other Microbial Products Intended for Skin Care: The European Approach

Atte von Wright

Professor Emeritus, University of Eastern Finland Institute of Public Health and Clinical Nutrition, Kuopio, Finland

Abstract

In the European Union there is a clear regulatory division between foods, pharmaceuticals, medical devices and cosmetics. Accordingly, probiotics or other microbial products intended for skin care could fall into very different regulatory categories depending on the type of the claim associated with the product and also of the type of administration (systemic or topical). Also, depending on the case, the authorization or notification of the product could happen either centrally or at the member state level. In cases requiring authorization at the EU level, special agencies, such as the European Food Safety Authority (EFSA) and the European Medicines Agency (EMA) have a central role in the evaluation of the products. If the claim refers to actual prevention, alleviation or cure of a disease, the product is either a pharmaceutical or a medical device depending, whether the effect is based on a physiological or immunological function or not (it should, moreover, be noted that live bacterial cells are not allowed in medical devices). If the product is consumed orally and the claim is associated with the reduction of a disease risk factor or with an enhanced physiological function, then the product could be classified as a functional or probiotic food or food supplement. In this case solid, documented scientific evidence of the effects should be available. Moreover, if the microbial used is not traditionally used in food applications (or does not have the Qualified Presumption of Safety status allowing a generic safety assessment), the product could be classified as a novel food, and would require a specific safety evaluation. If the product is applied topically as a purely cosmetic product, it should be notified at the member state level, its safety should be assessed by a

Email: atte.vonwright@biosafe.fi

Nava Dayan (ed.) Skin Microbiome Handbook: From Basic Research to Product Development, (321–342) © 2020 Scrivener Publishing LLC

qualified expert, and the truthfulness of any associated efficacy claim should be established. In practice topical products containing live or inactivated microorganisms with special claims related to skin care would probably fall within the borderline between cosmetics, medical devices and proper pharmaceuticals.

Keywords: The European Union (EU), directive, regulation, The European Food Safety Authority (EFSA), Qualified Presumption of Safety (QPS), novel foods, medical devices, pharmaceuticals

17.1   Introduction

The European Union (EU)—even after the eventual exit of the United Kingdom—is an association of 27 member states with a total population of approximately 450 million (www.europa.eu). The central aim of the EU is to ensure the free movement of people, capital and goods within this free market area. Harmonization of the legislation is an important part of this process. Accordingly, probiotics and other microbial products intended to promote the health and well-being of consumers are also subject to variable degrees of regulations at the EU level. Although probiotics have originally been understood as ingested live bacterial cultures enhancing the well-being of the host, the definition has been expanded to also cover topical applications. Probiotic skin care products could thus be classified as i) probiotic foods mediating their effects indirectly due to changes in the intestinal microbiota and its functions, ii) pharmaceuticals used either orally or topically, iii) as medical devices or iv) as topically used cosmetic products. Accordingly, they could fall into different regulatory categories and safety or efficacy requirements, depending on each particular case. In this chapter the regulatory requirements pertinent to each specific type of product are briefly reviewed.

17.2   The Governing Bodies and Decision-Making in the EU

The central players in the legislative process in the EU are the European Parliament, the European Commission and the Council of Ministers or the Council of the European Union.

The European Parliament is the only elected governing body in the EU. The members do not represent the member states from which they have been elected, but group themselves according to their political preferences along the spectrum of political views and ideologies present in the Parliament.

The European Commission can be considered as the government or the executive branch of the EU. Each member state has a commissioner or two. However, as is the case with the members of the Parliament, they are not representatives of their native countries, but are expected to focus on the general governance of the EU. Regarding the balance between the Parliament and the Commission it is important to note that only the Commission can initiate new legislation. In the Commission, several Directorates-General (DGs) run the executive functions and prepare the legislative initiatives. The central DG regarding food is the DG on Health and Food Safety (SANTE). For the political decision-making in matters related to food the SANTE Standing Committee on Plants, Animal, Food and Feed (PAFF), consisting of representatives of each member state, has a central role. In matters related to medicines and pharmaceutical products, the corresponding standing committee is Standing Committee on Medicinal Products for Human Use.

In questions related to risk assessment, the SANTE and Commission are assisted by independent special agencies, such as the European Food Safety Authority (EFSA) and the European Medicines Agency (EMA). In matters related to non-food consumer products, including cosmetics, the independent safety assessments are performed by the Scientific Committee on Consumer Safety (SCCS), while in matters related to the implementation of decision-making on cosmetics, the Standing Committee on Cosmetic Products has a role similar to PAFF in food-related matters.

The Council of the European Union consists of the responsible ministers of member states. It is the final decisive body of the EU. The legislation, initiated by the Commission and discussed by the Parliament will be finally approved in the Council. The decision of the Council requires the so-called qualified majority or the backing of 55% of the member states that together represent at least 65% of the total population.

17.2.1   The Legal Instruments of the EU

The two main types of union-wide legal documents in the EU are Directives and Regulations. Directives define measures that the member states have to incorporate into their national legislation within two years after the adoption of the Directive. In contrast, Regulations are automatically in force in all member states immediately after their promulgation. Thus, unlike the Directives, they are not considered as changes or expansions of national laws but independent acts. The general trend in the EU is to increasingly replace former Directives by Regulations.

17.3 Probiotic Foods and the European Regulations

There exists a very detailed regulatory framework for microbiological feed additives, including animal probiotics, in the EU. In contrast, human probiotics are specifically regulated only in three cases: i) if they are genetically modified microorganisms (GMMs), ii) if they are considered novel foods or iii) If they are associated with a health claim. In all these cases EFSA has a very central role as the principal risk assessment body providing the Commission with the assessment of safety—and in the case of health claims—also of the efficacy aspects of the products. The standard procedure in each of these cases is that an applicant, who wishes to get an authorization for a product falling under any of these different categories, prepares a dossier containing the necessary information according to the specific instructions outlined in the relevant legislation and in the specific guidance documents of EFSA. On the basis of this documentation EFSA prepares its opinion, formulated by its Scientific Panels consisting of independent experts. After receiving the opinion, the Commission makes a draft decision, which is then discussed in the PAFF Committee. The Committee decision requires the qualified majority as defined for the decision-making of the Council (see 17.2.). If the Committee agrees with the draft, the Commission can proceed with the authorization. If the qualified majority is not reached, the Council may decide on the draft decision, and if even the Council cannot reach an agreement, then the Commission has the final word.

The general scheme for decision-making outlined above is, of course, somewhat different for each category of the products due to product specific data requirements, which vary from case to case and from product to product. The general rules applied to microorganisms intentionally added to the food chain and the product category specific requirements are briefly described in the following sections.

17.3.1 The Safety Assessment of Microorganisms by EFSA, The QPS Concept

The starting point of the EFSA assessment of microorganisms is the proper characterization of the strain in question. The relevant EFSA document "Guidance on the Characterisation of Microorganisms Used as Feed Additives or as Production Organisms" entered into force in 2018 (EFSA 2017). The document combines several previous guidances and also introduces new elements, such as the requirement of whole genome sequencing

(WGS) for bacteria and yeasts and the bioinformatic analysis to check the presence of any genes of concern (antibiotic resistances, genes for toxins or virulence factors). Although the focus of the documents is on feed additive use, it has become the EFSA policy to apply the same requirements for all microorganisms submitted for evaluation, regardless of their end use. It should, however, be noted that the focus of EFSA is on orally consumed products only, and topically administered products are generally outside the remit of EFSA.

When it comes to safety assessment, feed additives in general are very strictly regulated in the EU according to principles of the Regulation (EC) No. 1831/2003 and the relevant EFSA guidance documents. The safety of additives, including animal probiotics, has to be demonstrated by relevant studies for the target animal, consumer, worker and the environment. In practice, this requirement introduced a discrepancy between the microorganisms intentionally added into foods, which ordinarily do not require even a notification, and microbiological feed additives subject to detailed safety studies. In order to clarify this situation, the concept of qualified presumption of safety (QPS) was introduced in 2007 [1].

The QPS concept is based on the assumption that for microorganisms that have a long history of safe use, there is only a limited need for safety studies, provided that certain qualifications are met. The basic requirement for a microorganism to be qualified as QPS is an unequivocal taxonomic identification. The second important EFSA qualification is the lack of transmissible antibiotic resistance markers. Additionally, there can also be some qualifications related to a specific taxonomic group (such as the lack of excessive production of bioactive lipopeptides by *Bacillus* strains).

The EFSA Panel on Biological Hazards (BIOHAZ) regularly reviews and updates the QPS list. The bacteria and yeasts qualified as QPS in the latest BIOHAZ opinion (EFSA 2018b) are listed in Table 17.1. It can be seen that among the bacteria the major lactobacilli, *Lactococcus lactis,* leuconostocs and pediococci, as well as *Streptococcus thermophilus* are included, but not, for example, enterococci. So far, no filamentous fungi are included in the QPS list.

The QPS status means that no specific safety assessments for humans, target animals (in the case of feed additives) or environment are required, although the proper characterization of the strain, as outlined in the EFSA 2017 guidance cited above, still applies, including the WGS analysis. Thus, the QPS approach really simplifies the safety assessment. Therefore, it is currently used as a reference point for the microbial safety evaluation across all the regulated microbiological products under the mandate of EFSA, thus having a relevance also in the assessment of human orally

326 SKIN MICROBIOME HANDBOOK

Table 17.1 The present list of QPS microorganisms.

Category	Genus	Species
Gram-positive non-spore-forming bacteria	*Bifidobacterium*	*adolescentis, animalis, bifidum, breve, longum*
	Carnobacterium	*divergens*
	Corynebacterium	*glutamicum*
	Lactobacillus	*acidophilus, amylolyticus, animalis, amylovorus, alimentarius, aviaries, brevis, buchneri, casei, cellobiosus, collinoides, coryniformis, crispatus, curvatus, delbrueckii, diolivorans, farciminis, fermentum, gallinarum, gasseri, helveticus, hilgardii, johnsonii, kefiranofaciens, kefiri, mucosae, panis, paracasei, paraplantarum, pentosus, plantarum, pontis, reuteri, rhamnosus, sakei, salivarius, sanfranciscensis*
	Lactococcus	*lactis*
	Leuconostoc	*citreum, lactis, mesenteroides, pseudomesenteroides*
	Microbacterium	*imperiale*
	Oenococcus	*oeni*
	Pasteuria	*nishizwae*
	Pediococcus	*acidilactici, dextrinicus, parvulus, pentosaceus*
	Propionibacterium	*freudenreichii, acidopropionicum*
	Streptococcus	*thermophilus*

(Continued)

Table 17.1 The present list of QPS microorganisms. (*Continued*)

Category	Genus	Species
Gram-positive spore-forming bacteria	*Bacillus*	*amyloliquefaciens, atrophaeus, clausii, coagulans, flexus, fusiformis, lentus, licheniformis, megaterium, mojavensis, pumilus, smithii, subtilis, vallismortis*
	Geobacillus	*stearothermophilus*
Yeasts	*Candida*	*cylindraceae*
	Debaryomyces	*hansenii*
	Hanseniaspora	*uvarum*
	Kluyveromyces	*lactis, marxianus*
	Komagatella	*pastoris*
	Lidneria	*jadinii*
	Ogataea	*angusta*
	Sacchramomyces	*bayanus, cerevisiae, pastorianus*
	Schizosaccharomyces	*pombe*
	Wickerhamomyces	*anomalus*
	Xanthophyllomyces	*dendrorhous*

administered probiotics, including those that might have beneficial effects on skin health as an efficacy claim.

17.3.1.1   The Safety Assessment of Non-QPS Microorganisms

For microorganisms that do not have the QPS status the EFSA guidance document (EFSA 2017) states: "For microorganisms and fermentation products, a basic set of toxicity studies should be provided consisting of genotoxicity/mutagenicity tests and a subchronic (90-day) oral toxicity study." The main intent is to eliminate the possibility of unknown metabolites that might cause safety concerns. From the toxicological point of view, the proposed procedure is somewhat problematic, because the genotoxicity studies on whole microbial cells do not make sense and neither are the repeated dose toxicity studies designed to address the specific questions on microbiological safety. In the case of enterococci, EFSA has taken a pragmatic approach by including a specific guidance in the document of EFSA 2018 focusing on the phenotypic genetic markers separating the virulent strains from the innocuous ones, instead of requiring the toxicological studies.

In practice, because the latest EFSA guidance documents require the whole genome sequences (WGS) of the microorganisms (at least bacteria and yeasts) to be assessed, it is to be expected that bioinformatic approaches will become more and more acceptable and even required in the final safety evaluation.

17.3.2   The Case of GMMs

The GMMs intended for food use would be evaluated according to Regulation EC No 1829/2003, and assessed by the Panel on Genetically Modified Organisms (GMO-Panel). EFSA has published a detailed guideline for the safety assessment (EFSA, 2011; [2]). The GMMs and the products derived or produced by them are divided into four categories, with each category having a somewhat different evaluation process.

- Category 1: Chemically defined purified compounds and their mixtures in which both GMMs and newly introduced genes have been removed (e.g., amino acids, vitamins);
- Category 2: Complex products in which both GMMs and newly introduced genes are no longer present (e.g., cell extracts, most enzyme preparations);
- Category 3: Products derived from GMMs in which GMMs capable of multiplication or of transferring genes are not present, but in which newly introduced genes are still present (e.g., heat-inactivated starter cultures);
- Category 4: Products consisting of or containing GMMs capable of multiplication or of transferring genes (e.g., live starter cultures for fermented foods and feed

Categories 3 and 4 are the regulatorily most complicated cases requiring safety assessment of the parental microorganism(s), the donor DNA and the final insert or plasmid in the recipient strain, evaluation of the ability of the GMM to survive in gastrointestinal conditions, eventual toxicity and allergenicity studies on the novel proteins synthetized (or even of the whole

GMM, if the compositional analysis indicates causes of concern), nutritional assessment, environmental impact assessment and post-marketing monitoring.

Up till now, no GMMs intended for food or feed use have been submitted for authorization, although several enzymes and amino acids produced by GMMs and belonging to Categories 1 and 2 have been assessed by EFSA.

17.3.3   Microorganisms as Novel Foods

The central legal document is Regulation (EU) 2015/2283 on Novel Foods. A novel food, according to paragraph 2 of Article 3 of the Regulation, means "any food that was not used for human consumption to a significant degree within the Union before 15 May 1997, irrespective of the dates of accession of Member States to the Union." Also, "foods consisting of, isolated from or produced from microorganisms, fungi or algae" (Article 3, paragraph 2) are mentioned as a special category of novel foods. Regarding traditional foods from third countries there is a specific notification procedure for them, outlined in Section II of the Regulation (articles 14–20).

The novel food authorization can start on the initiative of the Commission or following an application submitted in some member state. The Commission will then request the opinion of EFSA. In this case the relevant EFSA Panel is the Panel on Dietetic Products, Nutrition and Allergies (NDA panel). After the eventual authorization, the approved food is included in the Union list of novel foods.

Examples of authorized substances of microbial origin or novel microorganisms include dextran produced by *Leuconostoc mesenteroides*, vitamin K produced by *Bacillus subtilis* Natto, *Clostridium butyricum* as a food supplement, and *Bacteroides xylanosolvens* in fermented pasteurized milk products [3]. The particular *C. butyricum* strain has also been authorized as feed additive.

17.3.4   Human Probiotics and Functional Claims

A sharp distinction between food and medicines is characteristic of the EU legislation. Consequently, any health claims associated with a probiotic are strictly regulated, and this would apply also to probiotic foods intended to enhance or maintain the health of skin. Article 7 of Regulation (EU) No 1169/2011 specifically states: "food information shall not attribute to any food the property of preventing, treating or curing a human disease, nor refer to such properties." In the case of functional foods, such as probiotics, this sharp demarcation between nutritional and health-promoting properties becomes problematic. In order to address these difficulties, a specific Regulation (EC) 1924/2006 on nutrition and health claims was introduced.

The acceptable generic nutritional claims like "low energy," "low fat," "fat free," etc., are listed together with their definitions in Annex I of the Regulation.

Claims associated with health are divided into two categories, those that are not referring to the reduction of disease risk (Article 13), and those which specifically refer to the reduction of disease risk (Article 14). Note that even in the latter case the focus is on the reduction of disease risk, not on prevention or cure of an illness or disease. The cases covered by Article 13 are further divided into general function health claims and new function health claims, the latter based on new scientific evidence or having a proprietary interest. EFSA and its NDA panel have evaluated thousands of health claims related to Article 13 and submitted by member state competent authorities, and have provided a series of opinions about their acceptability. Further information is available on the EFSA website (https://www.efsa.europa.eu/en/topics/topic/nutrition-and-health-claims).

Both the new function health claims and the health claims associated with the reduction of disease risk require specific authorization, according to the procedure outlined in Section 17.3. Although several human probiotics have been assessed as products with new function health claims, no probiotic-associated claim has been accepted by EFSA. The main reasons have been deficient characterization of the strains, lack of sound human data showing a cause and effect, and poorly defined claims. Consequently, many probiotic products are sold without any health claims, either as foods or as food supplements. So far, no probiotic notification based specifically on beneficial cutaneous effects has apparently been submitted.

17.4   Probiotic Skin Care Products as Pharmaceuticals

The key legal documents dealing with the authorization of pharmaceutical products in the EU are i) Directive 2001/83/EC on the Community code relating to medicinal products for human use, and ii) Regulation (EC) No 726/2004 laying down Community procedures for the authorization and supervision of medicinal products for human and veterinary use and establishing a European Medicines Agency. In Directive 2001/83/EC the medicinal products are defined and classified, and the necessary quality, safety and efficacy criteria outlined as well as the national authorization procedures of the medicines in one or more EU countries. Regulation (EC) No 726/2004 further defines the cases in which the centralized authorization is required at Community level, establishing the role of the European Medicines Agency (EMA).

In Article 1 of Directive 2001/83/EC the medicinal products are defined as follows:

a. Any substance or combination of substances presented as having properties for treating or preventing disease in human beings; or

b. Any substance or combination of substances which may be used in or administered to human beings either with a view to restoring, correcting or modifying physiological functions by exerting a pharmacological, immunological or metabolic action, or to making a medical diagnosis.

Accordingly, any probiotic product, whether applied topically, orally or systematically, with an actual claim of preventing or curing a skin condition is a medicine. A borderline case might be a mechanism of action that would be based on the competitive exclusion of harmful bacteria or, for example, a pH effect in the skin microenvironment. In those cases, it could be argued that the action is not pharmacological, immunological or metabolic. These types of products might then be classified as medical devices (see Section 17.4.2).

17.4.1 The Authorization Procedure for Medicines

According to the present European legislation, there are two possibilities to get a medicine authorized in the EU, as indicated in Table 17.2.

Table 17.2 The options for the authorization of human medicines in the EU.

Authorising body	Procedure	Assessment of safety and efficacy	Applies to
Commission	Centralized	European Medicines Agency (EMA)	Whole EU
National competent authorities	National/mutual recognition/ decentralized	National competent authorities (in case of disagreement additional assessment by EMA)	The EU countries concerned

17.4.1.1 The Centralized Procedure

The products for which the centralized procedure and community level authorization are required, are defined in Annex 1 of Regulation (EC) No 726/2004. These include:

- Medicinal products developed by means of one of the following biotechnological processes:
  - Recombinant DNA technology,
  - Controlled expression of genes coding for biologically active proteins in prokaryotes and eukaryotes including transformed mammalian cells,
  - Hybridoma and monoclonal antibody methods.
- Advanced therapy medicinal products
- Medicinal products for human use containing a new active substance which, on the date of entry into force of this Regulation, was not authorized in the Community, for which the therapeutic indication is the treatment of any of the following diseases:
  - Acquired immune deficiency syndrome,
  - Cancer,
  - Neurodegenerative disorder,
  - Diabetes,
  - Auto-immune diseases and other immune dysfunctions,
  - Viral diseases.

Accordingly, a probiotic pharmaceutical product might conceivably become subject to a Community level authorization if it were a GMM or if it's considered as a new active, previously unauthorized substance and used to treat the conditions mentioned in the Annex. Actually, all of the diseases or pathological conditions listed could also result in skin disorders, and therefore this possibility is not just theoretical. Also, the so-called "orphan drugs," or drugs that remain undeveloped or untested or are otherwise neglected because of limited potential for commercial gain, should also be authorized at the Community level, and many probiotics might belong to this category.

In the centralized procedure, the EMA and its Committee for Medicinal Products for Human Use (CMHU) have a pivotal role. However, probiotics could also fall into the sphere of two other committees, Committee on Herbal Medicinal Products and—as indicated above—Committee for Orphan Medicinal Products. The applicant must submit the application with the supporting documentation directly to the agency, which will review the safety and efficacy data presented. Within 210 days after receiving the application, in case there has been no need for clarifications or extra studies ("clock stops"), EMA must formulate its opinion to the Commission, which will draft a decision within 15 days after receiving the document. This draft is then submitted to the Standing Committee on Medicinal Products for Human Use, where the member states are represented. The decision-making follows the procedure already referred to in Section 17.3. The time limit to reach the decision should be in total 67 days after the formulation of the EMA opinion.

Examples of probiotic products that have been assessed by EMA include Symbioflor 2, containing a specific strain of *Escherichia coli* and used to treat irritable bowel syndrome but not allowed for other intestinal disorders (https://www.ema.europa.eu/documents/referral/symbioflor-2-article-31-referral-ema-recommends-symbioflor-2-can-continue-be-used-irritable-bowel_en.pdf) and the granting of orphan drug status to a probiotic preparation containing *Lactobacillus acidophilus* and *Bifidobacterium bifidum* intended for the treatment of necrotizing colitis (https://www.ema.europa.eu/documents/orphan-designation/eu/3/13/1213-public-summary-opinion-orphan-designation-lactobacillus-acidophilus-bifidobacterium-bifidum_en.pdf). It should be noted that in the case of Symbioflor 2, the case involves an expert opinion on a product not centrally authorized but approved by national decisions in certain Member States (see Subsection 17.4.1.2.)

17.4.1.2   *National Authorizations and Authorizations by Mutual Recognition or Decentralized Procedures*

If there is no special requirement for a centralized authorization (as outlined above), the authorization is done on a national level following the principles laid down in Directive 2001/83/EC. For a product to be authorized in several member states there are two options; the mutual recognition procedure or the decentralized procedure.

In the mutual recognition procedure, the applicant, after having a medicinal product authorized in one Member State, requests the authorization to be expanded to one or more other Member States. These states then form a coordination group for the procedure. The applicant further asks the one Member State that granted the authorization to act as a reference Member State with a responsibility to prepare or update the required assessment report of the product. The aim is that all the concerned Member States acknowledge and recognize the authorization done by the reference

Member State. Symbioflor 2, previously mentioned in Subsection 17.4.1.1, is an example of a probiotic product authorized nationally in Germany, Austria and Hungary.

If the product has not been authorized in any Member State yet, the decentralized procedure, based on Directive 2004/27/EC amending Directive 2001/83/EC, is the option. Again, one country is selected as the reference Member State to carry out the evaluation of the product, the other Member States in the group accepting the outcome and eventual authorization recommended by the reference Member State.

In both mutual recognition procedure and in decentralized authorization the time limit to reach the decision is 210 days after the submission of a valid application. In case there are disagreements between the Member States involved, EMA and CMHU will arbitrate the situation.

17.4.2   Bacteria as Medical Devices

Medical devices are by definition medical products that do not achieve their principal intended action by pharmacological, immunological or metabolic means, in or on the human body. They do not have to be "devices" in the usual sense of the word, but even a topical ointment could be a medical device). The central piece of legislation on medical devices is Regulation (EU) 2017/245.

An important limitation introduced into the present Regulation regarding the use of microorganisms as a medical device or part thereof, is the rule outlined in Article 1, according to which "products that contain or consist of viable biological material or viable organisms, including living microorganisms, bacteria, fungi or viruses in order to achieve or support the intended purpose of the product" are excluded from the scope of the Regulation. Thus, any probiotics in medical devices should consist of non-viable cells or isolated cell fractions/components.

The notification of medical devices happens at the national level with the notified body nominated by each Member State having the central role. The medical devices have been further divided into four Classes (I, IIa, IIb and III), depending on the level of interaction with the human body. This means that the higher the number designated, the more significant is the interaction. According to the rules outlined in Annex VIII of the Regulation, topically applied probiotics could be classified either as IIa (if they are principally intended to manage the microenvironment of injured skin or mucous membrane) or IIb (if they are intended to be used principally for injuries to skin which have breached the dermis or mucous membrane).

The general requirement for a medical device is a unique device identifier (UDI, for example, in the form of a bar code) that unambiguously defines the product. The aspects to be included in the general Technical Documentation are outlined in Annex II of the Regulation, including data on the general safety and performance requirements. In a conformity assessment procedure both the production quality assurance and product verification are taken into account. The amount of the information and the role of the notified body depend on the classification of the device. It is specifically stated that "The conformity assessment procedure for class I devices should be carried out, as a general rule, under the sole responsibility of manufacturers in view of the low level of vulnerability associated with such devices. For class IIa, class IIb and class III devices, an appropriate level of involvement of a notified body should be compulsory." This means, for example, that the notified body should issue an EU-type examination certificate of the compliance of the product with conformity assessment.

The authorization of a probiotic or a beneficial microorganism as a medical device might be an option in certain cases. So far, no products for skin care apparently have been notified, but there are commercial examples of lactic acid bacterial vaginal suppositories classified as medical devices under previous legislation that allowed the use of bacterial cultures. Apparently, nowadays they should be authorized as pharmaceuticals.

17.5 Probiotics in Cosmetics

For cosmetic products no actual authorization either at the EU or Member State level is required. However, each member state must nominate a competent authority responsible for compliance with the regulation and the required notification procedure, the details of which are outlined in Regulation (EC) 1223/2009, including the requirement for safety assessment. The required safety report should be prepared by the notifier, as described below in Section 17.5.1. In case independent risk assessment is required, it is done by the SCCS Committee.

Cosmetic products are defined in Article 2 as follows: "'Cosmetic product' means any substance or mixture intended to be placed in contact with the external parts of the human body (epidermis, hair system, nails, lips and external genital organs) or with the teeth and the mucous membranes of the oral cavity with a view exclusively or mainly to cleaning them, perfuming them, changing their appearance, protecting them, keeping them in good condition or correcting body odors." Thus a beneficial microorganism or a product derived from them applied topically in the form of ointments, suspensions or solutions, powders, pastes, etc., for protective, hygienic or esthetic reasons but without any medical claims, would fall under this legislation.

The purely formal rules for placing a cosmetic product on the market are, briefly, the following. For each product, there has to be a natural or legal responsible person (most often the manufacturer or importer), who will answer for the compliance of the product with the EU legislation. The responsible person shall specifically take care that the safety assessment of the product has been properly done (Chapter III of the Regulation), and that the product information file, including the safety report, is prepared and kept abreast with the developments. Before placing the product on the market, the responsible person also submits a notification to the Commission, with the following product-specific information: i) the category of cosmetic product and its name or names, enabling its specific identification, ii) the name and address of the responsible person where the product information file is made readily accessible, iii) the country of origin in the case of import, iv) the Member State in which the cosmetic product is to be placed on the market, v) the contact details of a physical person to contact in the case of necessity, vi) the presence of substances in the form of nanomaterials and their identification including the chemical name (IUPAC) and other descriptors as specified in the Annexes of the Regulation, and the reasonably foreseeable exposure conditions, vii) the name and the Chemicals Abstracts Service (CAS) or EC number of substances classified as carcinogenic, mutagenic or toxic for reproduction (CMR), and viii) the frame formulation allowing for prompt and appropriate medical treatment in the event of difficulties. The responsible person should also inform the Commission immediately of any undesirable effects. Notifying the Commission of the original labeling of the product is also one of the duties of the Responsible person.

A list of ingredients is a mandatory part of the labeling of cosmetic products (Article 17 of the Regulation). The Commission shall compile a glossary of common ingredient names taking into account the International Nomenclature of Cosmetic Ingredients (INCI). However, this glossary should not be understood as a list of authorized substances (Article 33 of the Regulation).

17.5.1   Safety Aspects

Lists of the restricted or prohibited substances as well as positive lists of allowed chemicals (colorants, preservatives and UV filters) are given as specific Annexes of the Regulation (Annexes II, III, IV, V and VI).

A very significant aspect of the Regulation is a ban on animal testing in the safety assessment (Chapter VI), except in certain cases, in which a Member State can apply a derogation from this prohibition. This derogation can apply in situations when an ingredient is widely used, cannot be replaced and the possible threat to human health is substantiated.

In practice, the safety assessment of cosmetics is a part of the cosmetic product safety report. This report should follow the format laid out in Annex I of the Regulation. In Part A of the report, data are presented on the product composition, physicochemical characteristics, microbiological quality, impurities, expected uses, expected consumer exposure, toxicological profile of the substances, undesirable effects, and other relevant aspects. Part B contains the actual safety assessment. This should be done by an assessor, who is a recognized expert in the field (Article 10). Thus, in contrast to foods or pharmaceuticals, there are no detailed instructions for the tests that should be included in the assessments, which in practice are done on a case-by-case basis.

17.5.1.1 Microorganisms on Skin – Problems of Safety Evaluation

In contrast to microorganisms in food, there is no tradition of applying products containing live microorganisms on skin for cosmetic purposes. Thus, there is no body of knowledge associated with traditional safe uses that would allow a QPS-type approach to eventual probiotics developed for skin care. The traditional probiotic microorganisms, lactic acid bacteria and especially bifidobacteria, are not typical commensals on the skin, and there is no information on their survival or on their safety in the microenvironments of skin. Dermal yeasts can be quite numerous, but are mainly associated with fungal infections.

Consequently, many of the present cosmetic products that are advertised around the world with probiotic claims, are actually prebiotic and contain substrates that are supposed to enhance the natural skin microbiota. Others contain extracts of bacteria, or live bacteria isolated from unconventional sources. Many manufacturers do not specifically declare on the package what bacteria the product contains or if they are alive or dead. The claims associated with these products (alleviation of eczema, boosting the immunological functions, etc.) would, actually, be unlawful in the EU, because cosmetics are not supposed to have any pharmaceutical or metabolic functions.

Probiotic cosmetics could have great potential, but at present we do not know enough of the roles of the skin microbiota to be able to rationally select potential probiotic microorganisms suitable for either cosmetic or medical topical skin care. The successful microorganism should be safe, should be able to survive in the different matrices and in the presence of preservatives (at least, if viability is considered essential for the effects), should not affect the quality of the product by, for example, excessive lipase activity and, of course, have some beneficial effect. It may be inevitable that the probiotic cosmetics would, eventually, fall into the gray area between pharmaceuticals and proper cosmetics.

17.5.2 The Permissible Cosmetic Claims in the EU

The general principles of the permissible claims associated with cosmetic products are laid down in Commission Regulation (EU) No 655/2013. In the Annex of the Regulation, six criteria are listed that the marketing claims should comply with, namely i) legal compliance, ii) truthfulness, iii) evidential support, iv) honesty, v) fairness and vi) informed decision-making. Examples of the violations of these principles are also given. For example, a claim that the product has been authorized or approved would be misleading, because no authorization process for cosmetics exists. Presentation of an opinion as a verified claim would be a breach against truthfulness, while honesty requires that presentation of a product's performance shall not go beyond the available supporting evidence. Evidential support for the claim(s) should be self-evident, but might be difficult to obtain for a purely cosmetic probiotic product. Fairness means, among other things, that the competitors (or ingredients legally used) are not denigrated. Finally, the prerequisite for informed decision-making is that the claim is clear and understandable for an average end user.

17.6 Conclusions

In the EU the oral probiotics are extensively regulated in case a specific health claim is associated with them, and the same applies for any microorganism that is considered as a novel food or is genetically modified. So far, no probiotic-associated health claims have been accepted by EFSA, and no probiotic has been assessed for claims specifically associated with the maintenance of healthy skin, although probiotic products have been reported to have beneficial dermatological effects, such as alleviation of atopic eczema [4].

Probiotics with health claims could be authorized or notified also as pharmaceuticals, medicines or—if the microorganisms are not viable—as medical devices.

There is a lack of scientifically validated data on the efficacy and safety of topically applied probiotics as cosmetic products. This, together with the sharp demarcation between foods, drugs and cosmetics in the EU, makes both the development and notification of probiotic cosmetic products quite challenging.

In the decision tree outlined in Figure 17.1 the different regulatory options available in the EU for the authorization of probiotic skin care products are outlined. While interpreting the decision tree, it should be emphasized that the peculiar nature of the products might lead to case-by-case assessments that might land the eventual probiotic cosmetic products in the gray borderline area between the narrowly defined proper cosmetics and pharmaceuticals.

Probiotic skin care products are a very recent innovation, and their eventual introduction to the European market will, undoubtedly, provide both the authorities and industry useful precedent cases, which will clarify the present somewhat confusing regulatory situation.

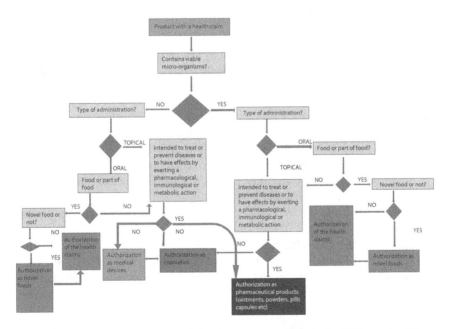

Figure 17.1 A Decision tree approach for the options available in the EU for authorizing a probiotic skin care product.

References

1. Leuschner, R.G.K., Tobin, P.R., Hugas, M., Cocconcelli, P. Sa., Richard-Forget, F., Klein, G., Licht, T.R., Nguyen-The, C., Querol, A., Richardson, M., Suarez, J.E., Thrane, U., Vlak, J.M., von Wright, A., Qualified Presumption of Safety (QPS): A generic risk assessment approach for biological agents notified to the European Food Safety Authority (EFSA). *Trends Food Sci. Technol.*, 21, 423–472, 2010.
2. Aguilera, J., Gomez, A.R., Olaru, I., Principles of the risk assessment of genetically modified microorganisms and their food products in the European Union. *Int. J. Food Microbiol.*, 167, 2–7, 2013.
3. Brodmann, T., Endo, A., Gueimonde, M., Vinderola, G., Kneifel, W., de Vos, W.M., Salminen, S., Gómez-Gallego, C., Safety of novel microbes for human consumption: Practical examples of assessment in the European Union. *Front. Microbiol.*, 8, 1725, 2017.
4. Zuccotti, G., Meneghin, F., Aceti, A., Barone, G., Calleagri, M.L., Di Mauro, A., Fanzini, M.P., Gori, D., Indrio, F., Maggio, L., Morelli, L., Corvaglia, L., Probiotics for prevention of atopic diseases in infants: Systematic review and meta-analysis. *Allergy*, 70, 1356–1371, 2015.

Legal Acts and Guidance Documents

Commission Regulation (EU) No 655/2013 of 10 July 2013 laying down common criteria for the justification of claims used in relation to cosmetic products. The Official Journal of the European Union L 190/131 – 190/134.

Directive 2001/83/EC of the European Parliament and of the Council of 6 November 2001 on the Community code relating to medicinal products for human use. The Official Journal of the European Union L311/67 – L311/128.

EFSA GMO Panel (EFSA Panel on Genetically Modified Organisms (GMO) 2011. Scientific Opinion on Guidance on the risk assessment of genetically modified microorganisms and their products intended for food and feed use. EFSA Journal 2011; 9(6):2193, 54 pp.

EFSA FEEDAP Panel (EFSA Panel on Products or Substances used in Animal Feed), 2017. Guidance on the assessment of the safety of feed additives for the consumer. EFSA Journal 2017;15(10):5022, 17 pp.

EFSA FEEDAP Panel (EFSA Panel on Additives and Products or Substances used in Animal Feed), 2018. Guidance on the characterisation of microorganisms used as feed additives or as production organisms. EFSA Journal 2018;16(3):5206, 24 pp.

EFSA BIOHAZ Panel (EFSA Panel on Biological Hazards), 2019. Statement on the update of the list of QPS-recommended biological agents intentionally added to food or feed as notified to EFSA 9: suitability of taxonomic units notified to EFSA until September 2019. EFSA Journal 2019;17(1):5555, 46 pp.

Regulation (EC) No 1831/2003 of the European Parliament and of the Council of 22 September 2003 on additives for use in animal nutrition. Official Journal of the European Union, L 268/29 – L 268/43.

Regulation (EC) No 1829/2003 of the European Parliament and of the Council of 22 September 2003 on genetically modified food and feed. Official Journal of the European Union L 268/1 – L268/23.

Regulation (EC) No 726/2004 of the European Parliament and of the Council of 31 March 2004 laying down Community procedures for the authorisation and supervision of medicinal products for human and veterinary use and establishing a European Medicines Agency. Official Journal of the European Union L 136/1 – L136/33.

Regulation (EC) No 1924/2006 of 20 December 2006 of the European Parliament and of the Council on nutrition and health claims made on foods. Official Journal of the European Union L404/9 – L404/29.

Regulation (EC) No 1223/2009 of the European Parliament and of the Council of 30 November 2009 on cosmetic products. The Official Journal of the European Union L 342/59 - L 342/209.

Regulation (EU) No 1169/2011 of the European Parliament and of the Council of 25 October 2011 on the provision of food information to consumers, amending Regulations (EC) No 1924/2006 and (EC) No 1925/2006 of the European Parliament and of the Council, and repealing Commission Directive 87/250/EEC, Council Directive 90/496/EEC, Commission Directive 1999/10/EC, Directive 2000/13/EC of the European Parliament and of the Council, Commission Directives 2002/67/EC and 2008/5/EC and Commission Regulation (EC) No 608/2004. Official Journal of the European Union L304/18 – L304/63.

Regulation (EU) No 2015/2283 of the European Parliament and of the Council of 25 November 2015 on novel foods, amending Regulation (EU) No 1169/2011 of the European Parliament and of the Council and repealing Regulation (EC) No 258/97 of the European Parliament and of the Council and Commission Regulation (EC) No 1852/2001. Official Journal of the European Union L327/1 – L327/22.

18

Regulation of Probiotic and Other Live Biologic Products: The United States Approach

Ronie M. Schmelz, Esq.

Tucker Ellis LLP, Los Angeles, California

Abstract

This chapter discusses the regulation of probiotic products in the United States. In the U.S், the intended use determines how a product is regulated. Products marketed to treat or prevent disease are regulated as drug or biologic products. Ingestible products, other than conventional foods, marketed to supplement the diet are regulated as dietary supplements while topical products that are designed to cleanse or beautify the body are regulated as cosmetics. The Federal Food and Drug Administration (FDA) is the primary agency responsible for regulating drugs, foods (including dietary supplements), and cosmetics. The Federal Trade Commission (FTC) shares jurisdiction with FDA and is the agency charged with ensuring that products are marketed truthfully and claims are properly substantiated. The myriad of U.S. regulations pursuant to which these agencies exercise their regulatory oversight of probiotic products is discussed below.

Keywords: Cosmetics, dietary supplements, drug, Federal Food, Drug, and Cosmetic Act (Act), Federal Trade Commission (FTC), food, Food and Drug Administration (FDA)

18.1 Introduction

The United States does not have a statutory or regulatory definition of "probiotics." According to the U.S. Food and Drug Administration (FDA)[1], probiotics, also known as "live biotherapeutic products" (LBP),

Email: ronie.schmelz@tuckerellis.com

Nava Dayan (ed.) *Skin Microbiome Handbook: From Basic Research to Product Development*, (343–376) © 2020 Scrivener Publishing LLC

refer to whole, live microorganisms that are ingested with the intention of providing a health benefit.[2] The extent and nature of U.S. regulation of probiotic products depends on how a product is used, or intended to be used, and is largely based on claims made about the product. For example, a product intended to, among other things, mitigate, treat, or prevent a disease is regulated as a drug or biological product, while an ingestible product that is not in conventional food form and is intended to supplement the diet may be regulated as a dietary supplement.[3] Topical products that do not claim to affect the structure or function of the human body may be categorized as cosmetics.

When examining product claims, U.S. regulators analyze claims on labels affixed to products, as well as statements made on product containers or wrappers, materials accompanying the product, and, under certain circumstances, product inserts, web sites, and other promotional materials. As discussed more fully below, the totality of claims made about a product informs its categorization, and the product categorization in turn determines the manner and extent to which the product is regulated.

The focus of this book is the skin microbiome and this chapter is aimed at reviewing key U.S. regulation of skin microbiome-related products. It is worth noting that at the time of publication the market for probiotic products is in its infancy and regulations are yet to be shaped to catch up with scientific advancements.

18.1.1   U.S. Legislative Landscape

The U.S. Food, Drug, and Cosmetic Act (Act) is a set of laws first passed in 1906 that give FDA the authority to oversee the safety and marketing of food (including dietary supplements), drugs (including LBPs and other biological products), cosmetics, and medical devices. The Act prohibits the misbranding[4] and adulteration[5] of food and drugs in the U.S., and has been amended numerous times to address public health concerns, tighten FDA control over regulated products, and enhance consumer protection. The Act was amended by the Dietary Supplement Health and Education Act of 1994 (DSHEA), which, among other things, defines and regulates dietary supplements and calls for adherence to good manufacturing practices established by FDA. The Act and DSHEA, as well as their implementing regulations, set forth a complex regulatory scheme governing the testing, marketing, labeling, and sale of regulated products, including, among other things, pre-market and licensing requirements for probiotics.

The Federal Trade Commission Act of 1914 as amended (FTC Act) gives the U.S. Federal Trade Commission (FTC) the power to, among other things, prevent unfair and deceptive advertising of consumer products.[6] An advertisement is considered misleading or deceptive if it contains a representation or omission of fact that is likely to mislead a consumer acting reasonably under the circumstances and the representation is material to the consumer's purchasing decision. Deceptive advertisements can include false claims, failure to disclose material facts, or make unsubstantiated claims. Although the level of substantiation required for product claims varies by product and advertising context, FTC has issued a guidance, entitled "Dietary Supplements: An Advertising Guide for Industry", that reflects FTC's thinking on the necessary level of substantiation required when advertising dietary supplements.[7]

The Fair Packaging and Labeling Act (FPLA) directs FDA and FTC to issue regulations governing the packaging and labeling of consumer products, including regulations respecting labeling of food, dietary supplements, cosmetics, and medical devices.[8] Among other things, labels must disclose a product's net contents, identity of commodity, and name and place of business of the product's manufacturer, packer, or distributor. The Nutrition Labeling and Education Act of 1990 (NLEA), which amended the Act, mandates that most food labels bear nutrient content information.[9] NLEA also authorizes use of nutrient content claims, health claims, qualified health claims, and structure/function claims for certain categories of products.[10] Marketing of products not properly labeled are considered adulterated or misbranded and subject to regulatory enforcement.

The U.S. Code of Federal Regulations (CFR) codifies the general and permanent rules published by U.S. regulatory agencies, including FDA. Title 21 of CFR sets forth the rules and regulations governing implementation and enforcement of the Act.

The Act sets forth varying degrees of regulatory oversight and statutory requirements for the marketing and sale of probiotic products, depending on how the product is intended to be used. The remainder of this chapter reviews the laws and regulations that attach to probiotic products sold as conventional foods, dietary supplements, drugs or biologics, and cosmetics.[11]

18.1.2   Foods[12]

Probiotics have traditionally appeared in foods, which along with cosmetics are the least regulated products in the U.S. The Act defines the term food as (1) articles used for food or drink for man or other animals, (2) chewing gum, and (3) articles used for components of any such article.[13] There are four additional regulatory categories of foods: food additives, color additives, substances generally recognized as safe (GRAS), and prior substances sanctioned by FDA or the U.S. Department of Agriculture (USDA) before 1958 for use in specific products. Probiotic ingredients intentionally added to a conventional food are likely classified as either an intentional food additive or GRAS substance.

The Act defines "food additive" broadly to mean "any substance the intended use of which results or may reasonably be expected to result, directly or indirectly, in its becoming a component or otherwise affecting the characteristics of food."[14] The definition expressly excludes substances approved by FDA or USDA before the food additive provision became law in 1958, as well as substances that are GRAS. Food additives that do not have a proven safety record as safe must obtain pre-market approval from FDA.

FDA has published a number of regulations in the CFR that detail allowed uses of microorganisms, most of which concern lactic acid-producing bacteria, flavor-producing bacteria, and glucose-fermenting bacteria used in the production of a variety of products. Examples of microorganisms approved by FDA (Table 18.1) pursuant to regulation include:

Table 18.1 FDA approved microorganisms.

Type of microorganism	Regulated uses in food
Harmless lactic acid-producing bacteria	Sour cream and acidified sour cream[15]; cheeses[16]; bread; rolls; and buns[17]
A characterizing bacterial culture that contains the lactic acid-producing bacteria *Lactobacillus bulgaricus* and *Streptococcus thermophiles*	Yogurt, low-fat and nonfat[18]
Harmless flavor-producing bacteria	Cheeses[19]
Glucose-forming bacteria	Dried egg whites[20]

If a food additive does not have a regulation authorizing its use, a manufacturer or other sponsor must seek pre-market approval from FDA, in the form of a food additive petition. The petition must include, among other information, the identity and composition of the additive, its proposed use in food, amount to be added to food, data establishing its intended effect, quantitative detection methods in foods, and full reports of toxicological and other safety studies. FDA reviews the petition to assess safety. If the Agency concludes the substance is safe, it publishes a regulation in the CFR describing the conditions under which the food additive may be used legally and authorizes its specific uses.[21]

Examples of authorized food additives (Table 18.2) derived from microorganisms include[22]:

Table 18.2 Authorized microorganism food additives.

Section in 21 CFR	Ingredient
§ 172.155	Natamycin derived from *Streptomyces natalensis* and *Streptomyces chattanoogensis*
§ 172.325	Baker's yeast protein derived from *Saccharomyces cerevisiae*
§ 172.695	XanthanGum derived from *Xanthomonas campestris*
§ 172.896	Dried yeasts, *Saccharomyces cerevisiae*, *Saccharomyces fragilis*, and dried torula yeast, *Candida utilis*
§ 173.160	*Candida guilliermondii* as the organism for fermentation production of citric acid
§ 173.280	A solvent extraction process for recovery of citric acid from *Aspergillus niger* fermentation liquor

Substances that achieve GRAS status are exempt from the pre-market approval requirements that apply to food additives.

To support GRAS determination, one must establish that scientists qualified by training and experience have access to pertinent, publicly available information, and, based on such information, agree that the intended use of the substance is safe for use. Companies can make self-determinations of GRAS status and keep their findings confidential. The Act also provides for an optional FDA GRAS notification process pursuant to which companies can submit documents to FDA supporting a GRAS determination, which is then made public and available on FDA's website.[23] Companies that elect to seek FDA confirmation of GRAS status must submit evidence sufficient to allow the Agency to assess the substance's safety, including information about general aspects of safety (e.g., exposure methods and methods of manufacturing), taxonomy, pathogenicity, potential toxin production, antibiotic resistance potential, safe history of use in food, and reports of adverse events. FDA responds to GRAS notices by issuing one of three letters: (1) a letter with no questions about the notifier's determination; (2) a letter stating the notice does not provide a basis for GRAS determination; or (3) a letter stating the notice was withdrawn at the request of the notifier.

FDA has affirmed GRAS status (Table 18.3) for a number of substances derived from microorganisms, including[24]:

Table 18.3 FDA affirmed gras microorganisms.

Section in 21 CFR	Ingredient or substance
§ 184.1005	Acetic acid may be produced by fermentation
§ 184.1115	Agar-agar, extracted from a number of related species of red algae class *Rhodophyceae*
§ 184.1372	Insoluble glucose isomerase enzyme preparations derived from recognized species of precisely classified, nonpathogenic, and nontoxicogenic microorganisms, including *Streptomyces rubiginosus*, *Actinoplane missouriensis*, *Streptomyces olivaceus*, *Streptomycers olivochromogenes*, and *Bacillus coagulans*, grown in a pure culture fermentation that produces no antibiotic
§ 184.1387	Lactase enzyme preparation from *Candida pseudotropicalis* for use in hydrolyzing lactose to glucose and galactose
§ 184.1695	Riboflavin biosynthesized by *Eremothecium ashbyii*
§ 184.1945	Vitamin B12 from *Streptomyces griseus*
§ 184.1985	Aminopeptidase enzyme preparation from *Lactococcus lactis* used as an optional ingredient for flavor development in the manufacture of cheddar cheese

FDA has also approved as GRAS the following substances from microorganisms for indirect use in food[25]:

Section in 21 CFR	Substance
§ 186.1275	Dextrans, made by fermentation of sucrose by *Leuconostoc mesenteroides* strain NRRL B-512(F)
§ 186.1839	Sorbose, made by oxidation of sorbitol by *Acetobacter xylinum* or by *Acetobacter suboxydans*

The following substances derived from microorganisms have been recognized as GRAS by FDA in Opinion Letters:

Enzyme
Carbohydrase, cellulose, glucose oxidase-cetalase, pectinase, and lipase from *Aspergillus niger*
Carbohydrase and protease from *Aspergillus oryzae*
Carbohydrase and protease from *Bacillus subtilis*
Invertase from edible baker's yeast or brewer's yeast (*Saccharomyces cerevisiae*)

FDA has also determined that the following compilation of foods that may contain or be derived from microorganisms may be consumed[26]:

Section in 21 CFR	Standardized food
§ 131.111	Acidified milk, with or without the addition of characterizing microbial organisms, and aroma – and flavor-producing microbial cultures. Conditions for their use are prescribed in the regulations.
§ 131.200	Yogurt made by the lactic acid-producing bacteria *Lactobacillus bulgaricus* and *Streptococcus thermophiles*
§ 131.106	Blue cheese, characterized by the presence of mold *Penicillium roquefortii*

Section in 21 CFR	Standardized food
§ 133.113	Cheddar cheese, subjected to the action of a lactic acid producing bacteria culture and clotting enzymes of animal, plant, or microbial origin used in the curing or flavor department
§ 136.110	Bread, rolls, and buns may contain as optional ingredients lactic acid-producing bacteria
§ 137.105	Flour may contain alpha-amylase obtained from the fungus *Apergillus oryzae*

18.1.2.1   Permissible Food Claims

Companies can add approved food additives to conventional foods and make the following claims without having to obtain pre-market approval from FDA, as long as they have proper substantiation for the claims: (1) structure/function; (2) health; (3) qualified health; and (4) nutrient content.

18.1.2.1.1   Structure/Function Claims

Structure/function claims, which are the most common claims made for marketing foods with probiotics, describe the role of a nutrient or dietary ingredient intended to affect the normal structure or function of the human body or characterize the action by which a nutrient or dietary ingredient maintains the structure or function of the body. Food structure/function claims must relate primarily to the product's taste, aroma, and nutritive value. Claims for conventional foods that veer away from the product's character as a food could be interpreted as a drug claim, which require pre-market approval from FDA. FDA acknowledges it is not always easy to differentiate between a proper structure/function claim and an impermissible drug claim, it provides the following examples for distinguishing the two:

Structure/function claim	Drug claim
Helps maintain joint health and flexibility	Reduces the pain and stiffness associated with arthritis
Provides relief of occasional constipation	Provides relief from chronic constipation

Structure/function claim	Drug claim
Helps maintain proper immune function	Stimulates the body's antiviral capacity
Use as part of a healthy diet to maintain healthy blood sugar levels	Helps maintain blood sugar levels in people with insulin dependency

Additional examples of appropriate structure/function claims for conventional foods include:

- Calcium builds strong bones
- Vitamin C helps maintain the body's natural defenses
- Fiber helps maintain digestive regularity
- Antioxidants maintain cell integrity.

Pictures, vignettes, and symbols used to market food may convert an otherwise proper structure/function claim into an impermissible drug claim. For example, depending on product labeling, use of a heart symbol may constitute an impermissible heart disease prevention claim.

There is no general rule for how many studies or what combination of studies are sufficient to substantiate general structure/function claims. FDA has, however, issued a draft guidance document[27] relating to substantiation of structure/function claims for infant formula expressing the Agency's view that "the replication of research results of independent, well-conducted studies make it more likely that the totality of scientific evidence will support the [structure/function] claim."[28] Although not binding, the draft guidance does help inform companies making structure/function claims for other conventional food products.

18.1.2.1.2   Health Claims

Health claims describe the link between a particular substance or nutrient in food and a particular disease.[29] An implied health claim includes statements, symbols, and other forms of communication that suggest a relationship between the presence or level of substance in a food and a disease.[30] NLEA permits both types of health claims on foods and dietary supplements if FDA determines there is evidence to support the claim, significant scientific agreement (SSA) among qualified experts about the claim, and the claim is truthful and not misleading.[31]

The Food and Drug Modernization Act of 1997 permits food manufacturers to make health claims if a scientific body of the U.S. government with official responsibility for public health protection and research directly related to human nutrition (e.g., National Institutes of Health or Center for Disease Control and Prevention), or the National Academy of Sciences has issued an authoritative statement about the relationship between a nutrient and the disease to which the claim refers.[32] Before making claims based on such authorities, a company must submit notification to FDA at least 120 days before the first introduction of the food with a label making the claim, during which time the Agency can prohibit the claim or require the company to modify the claim based on existing regulations.[33]

Permissible health claims must contain the elements of a substance and a disease or health-related condition, be limited to claims about disease risk reduction, not reference the diagnosis, cure, mitigation, or treatment of disease, and be approved by FDA before marketed. All health claims must be supported by SSA among qualified experts that the claim is supported by the totality of publicly available scientific evidence for a substance/disease relationship. In considering petitions for health claims, FDA considers the totality of available scientific evidence and evaluates the strength of scientific evidence by considering study types, methodological quality, the quantity of evidence for and against the claim, relevance to the U.S. population or target subgroup, replication of study results supporting the proposed claim, and the overall consistency of the evidence.[34]

Health claims that meet the SSA standard are authorized by publication of a final or interim rule in the CFR.[35] Once published, any product that meets the criteria established by FDA can be marketed with the approved health claim.

Examples of approved health claims include:

- Adequate calcium and vitamin D as part of a healthful diet, along with physical activity, may reduce the risk of osteoporosis in later life;
- Diets low in sodium may reduce the risk of high blood pressure, a disease associated with many factors;
- Diets low in saturated fat and cholesterol that include 25 grams of soy protein a day may reduce the risk of heart disease; and
- Adequate calcium throughout life may reduce the risk of osteoporosis.[36]

18.1.2.1.3   Qualified Health Claims

As with health claims, qualified health claims characterize a relationship between a substance and its ability to reduce the risk of a disease or health-related condition. Unlike health claims, however, the scientific evidence to support these claims falls below the highest SSA standard and may be supported by good to moderate levels of scientific agreement, low levels of scientific agreement, or very low levels of scientific agreement, all of which require a qualifier explaining the level of scientific evidence supporting the claim. FDA has established the following standardized language for qualified health claims:

- "…although there is scientific evidence supporting the claim, the evidence is not conclusive;"
- "Some scientific evidence suggests…however, FDA has determined the evidence is limited and not conclusive; and
- "Very limited and preliminary scientific research suggests… FDA concludes there is little scientific evidence to support this claim."[37]

Companies must petition FDA within 30 days of marketing a product with a qualified health claim, during which time FDA may or may not issue a letter of enforcement discretion specifying the nature of the qualified health claim FDA intends to consider in exercising its enforcement discretion for products marketed with the claim. Enforcement discretion letters signal that FDA does not intend to object to use of the qualified claim specified in the letter and any company meeting the claim criteria can make the claim.[38]

An example of an approved qualified health claim is "scientific evidence suggests, but does not prove, that whole grains (3 servings or 48 grams per day), as part of a low saturated fat, low cholesterol diet may reduce the risk of diabetes mellitus type 2."[39]

18.1.2.1.4   Nutrient Content Claims

The NLEA authorizes express and implied claims on food products intended for persons over two years old that directly or by implication characterize the level of a nutrient in a food.[40] Nutrient content claims can be express, relative, or implied. An express nutrient content claim is any direct statement about the level or range of a nutrient in a food, e.g., low sodium, contains 100 calories. A relative claim compares one food to another, e.g., 25% less sodium than other potato chips. Implied nutrient content claims describe the food or ingredient in a manner that suggests the nutrient is present or absent in a certain amount, e.g., "a good source of oat bran" or suggests that, because of the nutrient content, the product may be useful in maintaining a healthy diet and is made with an explicit statement about the nutrient, e.g., "healthy, contains 3 grams (g) of fat." Certain foods that contain nutrients in excess of FDA recognized reference amounts customarily consumed must include a disclaimer about the ingredient, e.g., "See nutrition information for sodium content."[41]

Most nutrient content claims are applied to nutrients or substances that have an established daily value. These claims are used to describe the percentage level of a dietary ingredient in a dietary supplement and may refer to dietary ingredients for which there is no established daily value, provided the claim is accompanied by a statement of the amount of the dietary ingredient per serving. Examples of such claims include "40% omega-3 fatty acids, 10 mg per capsule" and "twice the omega-3 fatty acids per capsule (80 mg) as in 100 mg of menhaden oil (40 mg)."[42] All nutrient content claims must be authorized by FDA and made in accordance with FDA's authorizing regulations.[43]

As of the date of publication, FDA has not established a daily value for probiotics, thereby precluding the making of any nutrient content claims for such products.

18.1.2.2   Additional Regulatory Considerations

Although foods do not require approval from FDA prior to being marketed, companies marketing foods in the U.S. must still satisfy a number of laws and regulations to ensure their products are not ordinarily injurious to health or adulterated. The standard for adulteration of food caused by naturally occurring substances is less rigorous than the standard for added substances. In both instances, a food is considered adulterated if it:

- Bears or contains any poisonous or deleterious substance which may render it injurious to health, but if the substance is a naturally occurring substance, the food is not considered adulterated if the quantity of the substance does not ordinarily render it injurious to health.
- Bears or contains:
  - any added poisonous or deleterious substance that is unsafe within the tolerance of poisonous ingredients;
  - pesticide residue; and/or
  - an unsafe food additive or new animal drug.

- Consists in whole or in part of any filthy, putrid, or decomposed substances, or is otherwise unfit for food.
- Is prepared, packed or held under unsanitary conditions.

Food manufacturers must also adhere to Good Manufacturing Practices (GMPs)[44], Hazard Analysis & Critical Control Points and Principles (HACCP)[45], ensure their products are labeled in accordance with existing regulations,[46] and comply with serious adverse events reporting requirements.

18.1.3   Dietary Supplements

On October 25, 1994, the U.S. Congress passed DSHEA, which amended the Act by adding, among other things, definitions for "dietary supplement" and "new dietary ingredient."

A "dietary supplement" is defined as a product (other than tobacco) intended to supplement the diet that bears or contains one or more of the following dietary ingredients: vitamin[47], mineral[48], herb or other botanical, amino acid, dietary substance[49] intended for use by man to supplement the diet by increasing the total dietary intake, or concentrate, metabolite[50], constituent[51], extract[52], or combination of any of the foregoing ingredients.[53] Dietary supplements do not include articles that were approved as a new drug or licensed as a biologic under section 351 of the Public Health Service (PHS).[54]

The Act specifically provides for dietary supplements to be in tablet, capsule, powder, softgel, gelcap, or liquid form.[55] The statute also permits dietary supplements in other forms as long as the product is intended for ingestion and is not represented as a conventional food or intended for use as a sole item of a meal or diet.[56] Although DSHEA does not require pre-market approval from FDA, manufacturers must ensure their products are safe for their intended use and report all serious adverse events to FDA.[57]

A bacterial microorganism is a dietary supplement if it is a dietary substance (intentional constituent in food) or otherwise falls within one of the categories listed in the definition of dietary supplement. For example, bacteria used to produce fermented foods that are consumed without a cooking or pasteurization step (e.g., lactic acid bacteria used to produce cheese or yogurt) could be a "dietary substance for use by man to supplement the diet by increasing the total dietary intake," which is one of the definitions of a dietary supplement. FDA does not have a separate regulatory category or definition for dietary ingredients consisting of live or viable microorganisms.[58]

A new dietary ingredient (NDI) is defined as an ingredient that was not marketed in the U.S. before DSHEA was passed on October 15, 1994.[59] NDIs must meet the statutory definition of a dietary ingredient.

There is no definitive list of ingredients marketed before passage of DSHEA, so it is up to the product manufacturer or distributor to determine whether the ingredient qualifies as an NDI. The Act provides that dietary supplements that contain NDIs shall be deemed adulterated unless they meet one of two requirements:

1. The dietary supplement contains only dietary ingredients which have been present in the food supply as an article used for food in a form in which the food has not been chemically altered; or
2. There is a history of use or other evidence of safety establishing that the dietary ingredient, when used as recommended, is reasonably expected to be safe and, at least 75 days before being introduced to market, the manufacturer or distributor of the dietary ingredient or dietary supplement provides FDA with information, including citation to any published articles, which is the basis upon which the manufacturer or distributor has concluded the dietary supplement containing an NDI reasonably expected to be safe.[60]

FDA has issued regulations to implement these pre-market notification requirements and guidance documents to assist companies in determining whether NDI notification is required and, if so, prepare such notifications.[61] FDA recommends that pre-market notifications relating to live microbial dietary ingredients[62] include the following information: strain, such as identification by internationally recognized third-party repositories (e.g., the American Type Culture Collection); and the relationship of the strain to the strain(s) of the same species used to establish the history of use or other evidence of safety for the NDI.[63]

Although dietary supplements do not require pre-market approval from FDA, only 75-day pre-market notification of the NDI, the Agency can take action to remove a product from the market if it finds it is adulterated (i.e., unsafe) or misbranded (i.e., the label is false or misleading).[64]

18.1.3.1   Permissible Dietary Supplement Claims

Dietary supplement manufacturers and distributors can make the following claims without the need to obtain pre-market approval from FDA, provided they possess proper substantiation for the claims: (1) structure/function; (2) health; (3) qualified health; and (4) nutrient content. The nature of these claims is discussed below.

18.1.3.1.1   Structure/Function

DSHEA explicitly authorizes structure/function claims for dietary supplements that describe the role of the supplement in the structure and function of human bodies.[65] Unlike food structure/function claims, which must focus on the nutritive value of a dietary ingredient, dietary supplements may focus on a product's non-nutritive and nutritive effects. Claims for dietary supplements cannot, however, explicitly or implicitly claim to prevent, treat, mitigate, cure, or diagnose a disease.

A dietary supplement structure/function claim may:

- Claim a benefit related to a classical nutrient deficiency disease (e.g., scurvy) and disclose the prevalence of such disease in the U.S.;
- Characterize the documented mechanism by which a nutrient or dietary ingredient acts to maintain the structure or function of the body; or
- Describe general well-being from consumption of a nutrient or dietary ingredient.[66]

Table 18.4 provides examples of appropriate dietary supplement structure/function claims, as contrasted to impermissible disease claims that can only attach to drug products:

Table 18.4 Dietary supplement v. drug structure/function claim.

Structure/function claim	Drug claim
Curbs appetite to help with weight loss	Aids weight loss to treat obesity
Supports immunity	Boosts the immune system against colds and flu
Helps maintain proper immune function	Stimulates the body's antiviral capacity
Maintains a healthy circulatory system	Prevents cardiovascular disease

As in the case of food labels, pictures, vignettes, and symbols on dietary supplements can convert an otherwise proper structure/function claim into an impermissible drug claim.

Marketers of dietary supplements must possess appropriate substantiation for their structure/function claims. DSHEA also imposes two additional requirements on dietary supplement companies: they must (1) notify FDA within 30 days of marketing a supplement with a structure/function claim[67]; and (2) include the following disclaimer on the dietary supplement label:

> "This statement has not been evaluated by the FDA. This product is not intended to diagnose, treat, cure, or prevent any disease."[68]

Manufacturers of dietary supplements that make structure/function claims, including claims relating to nutritional deficiency or general well-being, must possess substantiation that the claim is truthful and not misleading.[69] Although the Act does not define "substantiation," FDA has published a guidance on the extent and nature of substantiation manufacturers should have.[70]

In general, FDA recommends substantiation in the form of evidence derived from human studies that use widely accepted scientific methods and include background information, e.g., *in vitro* or animal studies, meta-analysis, and review articles.

FDA applies a standard of "competent and reliable scientific evidence" to substantiate claims about the benefit and safety of dietary supplements.[71] "Competent and reliable scientific evidence" has been defined as "tests, analyses, research, studies, or other evidence based on the expertise of professionals in the relevant area that has been conducted and evaluated in an objective manner by persons qualified to do so, using procedures generally accepted in the profession to yield accurate and reliable results."[72]

FDA recommends companies consider the following when determining whether they have "competent and reliable scientific evidence" to substantiate their claims:

1. The meaning of the claim(s) being made. Companies should consider all of the statements made about a product together; when a claim can have more than one reasonable meaning, companies should have substantiation for each interpretation.
2. The relationship of the evidence to the claim. Studies relied upon should identify the specific dietary supplement or

ingredient, serving size and conditions of use, and ensure the conditions used in the studies are similar to the labeling and proposed conditions of use for the dietary supplement for which the substantiation is submitted. Among other things, companies should consider similarities in formulation, serving size, route of administration, total length of exposure, and frequency of exposure. Studies should also clearly identify the endpoints used to substantiate the claimed effect and ensure they involve a population similar to that to which the dietary supplement is marketed. Foreign research may be sufficient to substantiate a claim as long as the design and implementation of the research are scientifically sound and the research pertains to the dietary supplement at issue.

3. The quality of the evidence. Scientific quality is based on several criteria including study population, study design and conduct (e.g., presence of a placebo control), data collection (e.g., dietary assessment method), statistical analysis, and outcome measures. FDA considers the "gold" standard to be randomized, double blind, placebo-controlled trial designs derived primarily from human studies, although the Agency will consider what experts in the relevant area of study consider competent and reliable evidence.

4. The totality of the evidence. There is no general rule for how many studies are sufficient to support a claim, but it is important to consider all relevant research, both favorable and unfavorable.[73]

18.1.3.1.2 Health Claims, Qualified Health Claims, and Nutrient Content Claims

The rules discussed above with respect to conventional food health, qualified health, and nutrient content claims apply equally to dietary supplements.

18.1.3.2 *Additional Regulatory Considerations*

As with food products, manufacturers and marketers of dietary supplements must ensure their products are safe and not adulterated and adhere to reporting requirements for serious adverse events. Manufacturers must also adhere to GMPs and marketers must ensure their products are properly labeled, including by, among other things, listing the product's statement of identity, *e.g.*, dietary supplement or calcium supplement, and the requisite disclaimer.[74] FDA has provided detailed guidance for GMPs[75] and labeling[76] which, while not binding, companies are encouraged to follow to ensure compliance with applicable laws and regulations.

18.1.4 Drugs

"Drugs" are defined in the Act, in relevant part, as "articles intended for use in the diagnosis, cure, mitigation, treatment, or prevention of disease..." and "articles (other than food) intended to affect the structure or any function of the body of man or other animals."[77] Biological products, including LBPs, which contain viruses, serums, or toxins applicable to the prevention, treatment or cure of disease or a health-related condition[78] are regulated as drugs under the Act.[79]

"New drugs" are defined as those that are not generally recognized as safe and effective (GRASE) by experts qualified by scientific training and experience to evaluate the drugs as safe and effective for use under conditions prescribed, recommended, or suggested on the label.[80] To achieve GRASE status, a drug must satisfy the following three criteria:

1. The particular drug product must have been subjected to adequate and well-controlled clinical investigations that establish it is safe and effective;
2. Those investigations must have been published in scientific literature available to qualified experts; and
3. Experts must generally agree, based on published studies, that the product is safe and effective for its intended uses. At a minimum, the general acceptance of the product as GRASE must be supported by the same quality and quantity of scientific and/or clinical data necessary to support the approval of a new drug application.

All drugs marketed and sold in the U.S. must be pre-approved by FDA.

18.1.4.1   Drug Approval Process

FDA approves drugs through a number of regulatory pathways, the most relevant to probiotics being: (1) Investigational New Drug (IND) applications; (2) New Drug Applications (NDA); and (3) Biologics License Applications (BLA).[81]

18.1.4.1.1   Investigational New Drug Applications

New drugs, including biological products and LBPs, that are neither GRAS nor GRASE, are subject to rigid pre-market clearance requirements, which begin with a sponsor, usually the drug manufacturer or potential marketer, submitting an IND to FDA seeking approval to begin human clinical trials on an experimental drug and allow for shipment of the drug across state lines.[82] The IND must include the following information:

- Animal Pharmacology and Toxicology Studies. This includes pre-clinical data that permits FDA to assess whether the product is reasonably safe for initial testing in humans, and includes information about previous experience with the drugs in humans.
- Manufacturing Information. This information pertains to the composition, stability, and controls used for manufacturing the drug substance and product. FDA assesses the information to ensure the sponsor can adequately produce and supply consistent batches of the drug.
- Clinical Protocols and Investigator Information. Sponsors must submit detailed protocols for the proposed clinical studies to assess whether the initial-phase trials will expose subjects to unnecessary risks. Information submitted should include the qualifications of the clinical investigators overseeing the administration of the drug to allow FDA to assess whether they are qualified to fulfill their clinical trial duties, as well commitments by the sponsor to obtain informed consent from research subjects, review of the study by an institutional review board (IRB), and adherence to investigational new drug regulations.

The IND phase of the drug approval process involves three distinct phases. During Phase I, researchers test the experimental drug or treatment in a small group of people (30-80) for the first time to evaluate the treatment's safety, determine a safe dosage range, and identify side effects. Phase II involves giving the experimental drug to a larger group of people (a few dozen to about 300) to further evaluate its safety and see if it is effective. During Phase III, the drug is given to large groups of people (between several hundred to 3,000) to confirm its effectiveness, monitor side effects, compare it to commonly used treatments, and collect information that will ensure the experimental drug is used safely.[83]

After submitting an IND to FDA, sponsors must wait 30 calendar days before initiating any clinical trials in order to allow for FDA review. FDA has issued numerous guidance documents to help industry determine whether human research studies can be conducted on new drugs without an IND and to assist companies in preparing and submitting an INDs.[84]

18.1.4.1.2   New Drug Applications

Once a sponsor believes it possesses sufficient evidence of a new drug's safety and effectiveness sufficient to meet FDA's requirements during Phase I, the sponsor can submit an NDA to FDA. The purpose of the NDA is to provide enough information to permit FDA to reach the following key decisions:

- Whether the drug is safe and effective for its proposed use(s), and whether the benefits of the drug outweigh the risks;
- Whether the drug's proposed labeling (including package insert) is appropriate, and what it should contain; and
- Whether the methods used in manufacturing the drug and the controls used to maintain the drug's quality are adequate to preserve its identity, strength, quality, and purity

NDA is the vehicle by which a sponsor tells FDA a comprehensive story about its new drug, including:

- Results of clinical tests
- Drug ingredients
- Animal studies' results
- Documentation of drug behavior in the human body
- Drug manufacturing, processing, labeling, and packaging information.

After FDA receives an NDA, the Agency has 60 days to decide whether to file the NDA so it can be reviewed. If accepted for filing, an FDA review team is assigned to evaluate the sponsor's research on the drug's safety and effectiveness. FDA also reviews all the information that goes on the drug's professional labeling, e.g., the carton and container labeling, prescribing information, medication guides, and instructions for use. The Agency also inspects the facilities where the drug will be manufactured. Upon completion of its review, FDA will either approve the NDA or issue a complete response letter advising the sponsor of the basis for its decision not to approve the new drug.[85]

18.1.4.1.3   Biologics License Applications

Biological products are a subset of drugs regulated under the Act and are licensed under the PHS Act. Section 351 of the PHS Act defines biological products as a virus, therapeutic serum, toxin, antitoxin, vaccine, blood, blood component or derivative, allergenic product, or analogous product applicable to the prevention, treatment or cure of a disease or condition of human beings.[86] In contrast to chemically synthesized small molecular weight drugs, which have well-defined structures and can be thoroughly characterized, biological products are generally derived from living material (human, animal, or microorganism), are complex in structure, and not usually fully characterized. FDA regulations and policies have established that biological products include, among other things, products containing microorganisms.

Biological products that meet the definition of new drugs are subject to licensure requirements of the PHS Act.[87] To obtain a BLA, sponsors must first obtain approval of an IND[88] and then demonstrate the product is "safe, pure, and potent" and that the facility in which the biological product is manufactured, processed, packaged, and held meets standards designed to ensure the product continues to be safe, pure, and potent. A finished biological product is "pure" if it is free from extraneous matter, including residual moisture and other volatile and pyrogenic substances, and "potent" if it has the ability or capacity to yield a given result when used as indicated.

FDA approves BLAs by issuing a biological license as part of an approval letter, which includes a biologics license number. The biologics license number must be clearly marked on each package, along with the proper name of the biological product, the name and address of the product's manufacturer, and the product's manufacture date.[89]

18.1.4.2 Additional Regulatory Considerations

The Act imposes certain requirements relating to drug registration and product listing, labeling, post-market reporting, and good manufacturing practices, among others. FDA's website has a series of industry guidance documents discussing these and other drug and biological product requirements.[90]

18.1.5 Cosmetics

"Cosmetics" are defined in the Act as "(1) articles intended to be rubbed, poured, sprinkled, or sprayed on, introduced into, or otherwise applied to the human body or any part thereof for cleansing, beautifying, promoting attractiveness, or altering the appearance, and (2) articles intended for use as a component of any such articles; except that such term shall not include soap."[91]

To qualify as a cosmetic, and not veer into the realm of drugs, cosmetic products cannot claim to affect the structure or function of the body, or claim, whether express or implied, to cure, treat, or prevent any disease or health-related condition. Here (Table 18.5) are some examples of cosmetic claims and similar claims that render the products drug:

Table 18.5 Cosmetic v. drug claims.

Cosmetic claim	Drug claim
Reduces the appearance of fine lines and wrinkles	Removes fine line and wrinkles
Reduces the appearance of blemishes	Treats or prevents acne
Reduces the appearance of redness	Prevents the outbreak of eczema and rosacea
Helps moisturize the skin	Helps treat irritated skin

The key to formulating cosmetic claims is to focus on how a product makes one feel and look and avoiding reference to disease or health-related conditions.

The Act does not require pre-market approval of cosmetics, but it does prohibit the marketing of adulterated or misbranded cosmetics. A cosmetic is adulterated if it bears or contains any poisonous or deleterious substance that may render it injurious to users under the conditions of use prescribed on the label.[92] A cosmetic is generally considered adulterated if the product label or labeling is false or misleading in any way and if the label fails to comply with appropriate labeling regulations.[93]

There are scores of topical cosmetic probiotic skin care products marketed and sold in the U.S., and the number continues to grow. While there is no restriction on including probiotics in cosmetic products, and FDA pre-market approval is not required, companies must still ensure their products are safe before they are marketed to consumers. In addition to testing for safety, products that include live microorganisms should be tested to ensure stability for the anticipated life of the product under normal use indications. FDA continues to evaluate scientific data on the safety of probiotics, but, as of the date of publication, has not issued any guidance documents addressing the use of such ingredients in cosmetics.

As with any other cosmetic product, companies that market topical probiotic skin care products are proscribed from claiming the product affects the structure or function of the body; such claims effectively convert a product from a legally marketed cosmetic into an unapproved drug. For example, claims that a probiotic skin care product can reverse the signs of aging, stimulate the growth of collagen and elastin, or treat acne are structure/function claims that cannot be used to legally market cosmetics in the U.S. While a number of companies market probiotic cosmetic products making such claims, they do so at their peril and run the risk FDA will categorize the products as unapproved adulterated drugs that cannot lawfully be marketed in the U.S. without pre-market approval. To avoid regulatory challenges and possible product recall, companies marketing probiotic skin care products should ensure all product claims are truthful and not misleading and refrain from making structure/function or disease claims on the product label or labeling accompanying the product, as well as on company web sites and social media accounts.

18.2   Summary of Product Categorization and Regulatory Requirements

The chart below summarizes the parameters that govern the categorization of products, requisite regulatory requirements, Federal agencies with oversight responsibility, and permissible claims (Table 18.6).

Table 18.6 Product and regulatory summary.

Product category	Foods	Dietary supplements	Drugs	Biological products	Cosmetics
Definition	All food and drink products, including chewing gum, and articles used as components in such products.	Products taken by mouth that contain a "dietary ingredient," including vitamins, minerals, amino acids, and herbs or botanicals, as well as other substances used to supplement the diet.	A substance intended to diagnose, cure, mitigate, or treat, or prevent disease; a substance (other than food) intended to affect the structure or function of the body.	Large complex molecules produced through biotechnology in a living system, such as a microorganism.	Products (excluding pure soap) intended to be applied to the human body for cleansing, beautifying, promoting attractiveness, or altering the appearance of the body.
FDA Regulatory Center	Center for Food Safety and Applied Nutrition (CFSAN)	CFSAN	Center for Drug Evaluation and Research (CDER)	Center for Biologics Evaluation and Research (CBER)	CFSAN

(Continued)

Table 18.6 Product and regulatory summary. (*Continued*)

Product category	Foods	Dietary supplements	Drugs	Biological products	Cosmetics
Regulatory requirements	Must meet safety and labeling requirements; no pre-market approval required, except for those foods that contain non-approved food additives.	Must meet safety and labeling requirements, including statement of identity and requisite disclaimer; pre-market approval recommended for products containing live microbial dietary ingredients.	Pre-market approval required; must comply with safety, labeling, and manufacturing standards.	Pre-market approval required; must comply with product and manufacturing facility licensing requirements, product safety standards and testing requirements.	Must meet safety and labeling requirements.

(*Continued*)

Table 18.6 Product and regulatory summary. (*Continued*)

Product category	Foods	Dietary supplements	Drugs	Biological products	Cosmetics
Permissible product claims	Structure/function claims relating to taste, aroma, and nutritive value; Health claims permissible if approved by FDA or other recognized body; Qualified health claims with proper notice to FDA and requisite disclaimer language; Nutrient content claims not permitted without FDA determination of established daily value.	Structure/function, health, qualified health, and nutrient content claims permissible without pre-market approval provided regulatory requirements satisfied.	Claims approved by FDA.	Claims approved by FDA.	Cleansing and appearance claims; structure/function not permitted.

18.3   Resources

- For foods and food additives: Office of Food Additive Safety (HFS-200), Center for Food Safety and Applied Nutrition, Food and Drug Administration, 5100 Paint Branch Parkway, College Park, Maryland 20740-3835; Telephone: (301)-436-1200.
- For dietary supplements: Division of Dietary Supplement Programs (HFS-810), Office of Nutritional Products, Labeling, and Dietary Supplements, Center for Food Safety and Applied Nutrition, Food, and Drug Administration, 5100 Paint Branch Parkway, College Park, Maryland 20740; Telephone: (301)-436-2375.
- For human drugs: Division of Drug Information (HFD-240), Center for Drug Evaluation and Research, Food and Drug Administration, 5600 Fishers Lane, Rockville, Maryland 20857; Telephone: 1-(888)-463-6332 or (301)-827-4570. Electronic mail inquiries can also be sent to druginfo@cder.fda.gov.
- For biological products: Manufacturers Assistance and Technical Training Branch, Office of Communications, Training & Manufacturers Assistance (HFM-40), Center for Biologics Evaluation and Research, Food and Drug Administration, 1401 Rockville Pike, Rockville, Maryland 20852-1448; Telephone: 1-(800)-835-4709 or (301)-827-1800.
- For cosmetics: Office of Cosmetics and Colors, Center for Food Safety and Applied Nutrition, College Park, Maryland 20740; Telephone: (301)-436-1130.

18.4   Endnotes

[1] FDA, an agency within the U.S. Department of Health and Human Services (HHS), is the primary agency charged with oversight of food, dietary supplements, drugs, and cosmetics, among other product categories. The U.S. Federal Trade Commission (FTC) has a role in regulating certain aspects of product advertising and marketing.

[2] *See e.g.*, FDA Draft Guidance for Industry on Complementary and Alternative Medicine Products and Their Regulation by the Food and Drug Administration, available at https://www.fda.gov/media/76323/download. FDA recognizes a definition of "prebiotics" as nondigestible food ingredients that beneficially affect the host by selectively stimulating the growth and/or activity of one or a limited number of bacteria in the colon. *Id.* Other agencies within HHS have defined "probiotics" as supplements or food that contain viable microorganisms that alter the microflora of the host, "prebiotics" as supplements

or foods that contain non-digestible ingredients that selectively stimulates the growth and/or activity of indigenous bacteria, "postbiotics" as non-viable bacterial products or metabolic byproducts from probiotic microorganisms that have biologic activity in the host, and "symbiotic" as a product that contains both probiotics and prebiotics. The term "probiotics" as used in this chapter encompasses all of these organisms.

3   Additional factors that may influence a probiotic's categorization include the product's formulation (*e.g.*, capsules and pills are not conventional foods), route of administration (food and dietary supplements must be administered orally), the manner in which consumers are targeted, and safety.

4   A product is deemed "misbranded" under the Act if its labeling is false or misleading in any particular.

5   An "adulterated" product is one where the methods used in, or the facilities or controls used for, its manufacture, processing, packing, or holding fail to conform with existing good manufacturing practices to assure that the product meets the Act's requirements for product safety or the product identity and strength fail to meet stated quality and purity characteristics.

6   15 U.S.C. §§ 41-58.

7   Dietary Supplements: An Advertising Guide for Industry is available at https://www.ftc.gov/system/files/documents/plain-language/bus09-dietary-supplements-advertising-guide-industry.pdf.

8   15 U.S.C. §§ 1451-1461.

9   Public Law 101-535, 104 Stat 2353.

10   *See* FDA Guidance for Industry: Food Labeling Guide (Food Labeling Guide), available at https://www.fda.gov/ media/81606/download; *see also* 21 CFR §§ 101 *et seq.*

11   FDA regulates tampons as medical devices. Although probiotic tampons are sold outside the U.S., as of the date of publication, such products are not approved for sale in the U.S.

12   U.S. also regulates "medical foods" and "foods for special dietary use." Medical foods are foods that are formulated to be consumed or administered enterally under the supervision of a physician and which are intended for the specific dietary management of a disease or condition for which distinctive nutritional requirements, based on recognized scientific principles, are established by medical evaluation. *See* 21 U.S.C. § 360ee(b)(3). "Foods for special dietary use" is a narrow category of foods defined as "foods that are specially formulated to meet a special dietary need, such as a food allergy or difficulty in swallowing, but that provide nutrients intended to meet ordinary nutritional requirements." *See e.g.*, 21 CFR § 105. As probiotics are currently unlikely to fall within either category, regulatory requirements for these products are not discussed herein.

13   21 U.S.C. § 321(f).

14   21 U.S.C. § 201(s).

15   21 CFR §§ 131, 160, and 131.162.

16   21 CFR § 133.

17   21 CFR § 136.110.

18   21 CFR §§ 131.200, 131.203, and 131.206.

19   21 CFR § 133.

20   21 CFR § 160.145.

21   A list of food additives permitted for direct addition to food for human consumption is available at 21 CFR Part 172, §§ 172.5 *et seq.*

²² For a full list of approved food additives derived from microorganisms *see* 21 CFR §§ 172 and 173.

²³ FDA response letters to GRAS notifications and other information about GRAS notices are available on FDA's website, at https://www.fda.gov/food/generally-recognized-safe-gras/gras-notice-inventory

²⁴ For a full list of approved food additives derived from microorganisms *see* 21 CFR § 184.

²⁵ For a complete list of GRAS approved microorganisms for indirect use in food *see* 21 CFR § 186.

²⁶ For a list of foods for human consumption that contain or are derived from microorganisms *see* 21 CFR §§ 131, 133, 136, and 137.

²⁷ FDA guidance documents do not establish legally enforceable responsibilities, but are instead the Agency's then-current thinking on a topic and should be viewed only as recommendations, unless specific regulatory or statutory requirements are cited.

²⁸ *See* Substantiation of Structure/Function Claims Made in Infant Formula Labels and Labeling: Guidance for Industry Draft Guidance (September 2016), available at file:///C:/users/RS2/Work%20Folders/Downloads/Draft_Guidance_for_Industry_on_Substantiation_for_Structure_Function_Claims_in_Infant_Formula_Labels_and_Labeling.pdf.

²⁹ As used herein, the term "disease" refers to both diseases and health-related conditions, and is defined as damage to an organ, part, structure, or system of the body such that it does not function properly (*e.g.*, cardiovascular disease) or a state of health leading to such dysfunctioning (*e.g.*, hypertension). 21 CFR § 101.14(a)(5).

³⁰ 21 CFR § 101.14(a)(1).

³¹ 21 CFR § 101.14(c).

³² 21 U.S.C. § 343(r)(3)(C).

³³ *See* Guidance for Industry: Notification of a Health Claim or Nutrient Content Claim Based on an Authoritative Statement of a Scientific Body (June 1998), FDA Docket Number FDA-2013-0610, available at https://www.fda.gov/regulatory-information/ search-fda-guidance-documents/guidance-industry-notification-health-claim-or-nutri-ent-content-claim-based-authoritative-statement.

³⁴ *See* Guidance for Industry: Evidence-Based Review System for the Scientific Evaluation of Health Claims (January 2009), Docket Number: FDA-2007-D-0371, available at https://www.fda.gov/regulatory-information/search-fda-guidance-documents/guidance-industry-evidence-based-review-system-scientific-evaluation-health-claims.

³⁵ *See* https://www.fda.gov/food/food-labeling-nutrition/authorized-health-claims-meet-significant-scientific-agreement-ssa-standard.

³⁶ Additional examples of approved health claims are available in the Food Labeling Guide.

³⁷ *See* Guidance for Industry: Interim Procedures for Qualified Health Claims in the Labeling of Conventional Human Food and Human Dietary Supplements (July 2003), FDA Docket Number FDA-2013-0610, available at https://www.fda.gov/regulatory-information/search-fda-guidance-documents/guidance-industry-interim-procedures-qualified-health-claims-labeling-conventional-human-food-and.

³⁸ For a list of Letters of Enforcement Discretion for qualified health claims, *see* https://www.fda.gov/food/food-labeling-nutrition/qualified-health-claims-letters-enforcement-discretion. For additional information about qualified health claims including letters of denial, *see* https://www.fda.gov/food/food-labeling-nutrition/qualified-health-claims.

³⁹ *See* Food Labeling Guide, Appendix D, for additional examples of qualified health claims.

⁴⁰ 21 CFR § 101.13.

⁴¹ 21 CFR § 101.13(h)(1).

[42] *See* 21 CFR § 101.13(q)(3)(ii).

[43] *See* 21 CFR § 101.13; *see also* Food Labeling Guide, Appendix A.

[44] *See* 32 CFR § 110; *see also* Current Good Manufacturing Practices (CGMPs), available at https://www.fda.gov/food/guidance-regulation-food-and-dietary-supplements/current-good-manufacturing-practices-cgmps, and Good Manufacturing Practices for the 21st Century for Food Processing (2004 Study) Section 1: Current Good Manufacturing Practices (August 9, 2004), available at https://www.fda.gov/food/current-good-manufacturing-practices-cgmps/good-manufacturing-practices-21st-century-food-processing-2004-study-section-1-current-food-good.

[45] *See* Current Good Manufacturing Practice and Hazard Analysis and Risk-Based Preventive Controls for Human Food, 78 Fed. Reg. 3646 (proposed Jan. 16, 2013); *see also* https://www.fda.gov/food/guidance-regulation-food-and-dietary-supplements/hazard-analysis-critical-control-point-haccp.

[46] In May 2016, FDA published Food Labeling: Revision of the Nutrition and Supplement Facts Labels, Final Rule amending labeling regulations for foods to provide updated nutrition information. The compliance date for the Final Rule for companies with revenues of $10 million or more in annual food sales (including dietary supplements) was January 1, 2020; for companies with less than $10 million in annual food sales, the compliance date is January 1, 2021. FDA issued Industry Resources on the Changes to the Nutrition Facts Label, available at https://www. fda.gov/food/food-labeling-nutrition/industry-resources-changes-nutrition-facts-label. For labeling requirements unrelated to nutrition facts, *see also* Food Labeling Guide.

[47] A 'vitamin' is an organic substance that is a minor component of foods, essential for normal physiological functions (*e.g.*, maintenance, growth, or development), normally not produced endogenously (within the body) in amounts adequate to meet normal physiologic needs, and causes, by its absence or underutilization, a clinically defined deficiency syndrome.

[48] A "mineral" is a substance of defined chemical composition that provides a form or source of inorganic elements to the diet. An "element" is one of a class of substances that cannot be separated into simpler substances by chemical means. Examples include calcium, iodine, and zinc.

[49] A "dietary substance" is a substance that is commonly used as human food or drink.

[50] A "metabolite" is a product of metabolism. In the dietary supplement context, a metabolite of a dietary ingredient is a molecular intermediate that incorporates structural elements of the ingested dietary ingredient and whose flux or net production in the human body increases upon ingestion of the dietary ingredient. A metabolite can be part (or an intermediate part) of the catabolic or metabolic pathway of a dietary ingredient.

[51] A "constituent" is an article that is a physical part of the whole and can be isolated from the whole.

[52] An "extract" is a product consisting of a solvent (menstruum) combined with a dietary substance or botanical biomass by a process that physically separates constituents from the dietary substance or botanical and dissolves them into the solvent. The extract can be further concentrated through drying to a dry powder or semi-solid form.

[53] The Act expressly excludes from the definition of dietary supplement any article authorized for investigation as a new drug for which substantial clinical investigations have been instituted and for which the existence of such investigations has been made public, unless the article was marketed as a dietary supplement or a conventional food before an investigational new drug (IND) application became effective. 21 U.S.C. § 321(ff)(3)(B)(ii).

[54] 42 U.S.C. § 262.

55 2 U.S.C. §§ 321(ff)(2)(A)(i) and 350(c)(1)(B)(i).

56 21 U.S.C. §§ 321(ff)(2) and 350(c)(1)(B)(ii).

57 *See* Dietary Supplement and Nonprescription Drug Consumer Protection Act of 2006, P.L. 109-462 for serious adverse events reporting requirements.

58 Not all bacterial microorganisms are dietary ingredients, and a microorganism that is not a dietary supplement cannot be an NDI. For example, pathogenic species of bacteria, such as *Salmonella* species or *Escherichia* coli, are not dietary ingredients even though they may have been inadvertently present in food as contaminants. Bacteria that have never been consumed as food are unlikely to be dietary ingredients.

59 21 U.S.C. § 359b(d).

60 *See* U.S.C. § 350b and 21 U.S.C. § 342(f).

61 *See* 21 CFR § 190.6 (the "NDI regulation"); *see also* New Dietary Ingredients in Dietary Supplements – Background for Industry, available at https://www.fda.gov/food/new-dietary-ingredients-ndi-notification-process/new-dietary-ingredients-dietary-supplements-background-industry, New Dietary Ingredients (NDI) Notification Process, available at https://www.fda.gov/food/dietary-supplements/new-dietary-ingredients-ndi-notification-process, and Draft Guidance for Industry: New Dietary Ingredient Notifications and Related Issues (October 2016), available at https://www. fda.gov/regulatory-information/search-fda-guidance-documents/draft-guidance-industry-new-dietary-ingredient-notifications-and-related-issues.

62 "Live microbial dietary ingredient" is defined as a single-celled prokaryotic or eukaryotic microorganism that is intended to be viable at the point of ingestion.

63 *See* Dietary Supplements: New Dietary Ingredient Notifications and Related Issues: Guidance for Industry (August 2016), pp. 65-66, 86-87.

64 Since companies are not required to provide notice to FDA before marketing their products, the Agency does not have a list of dietary supplements marketed in the U.S. FDA's website references the Agency has taken actions against dietary supplements it deems unsafe. *See e.g.*, Dietary Supplement Products & Ingredients, available at https://www.fda. gov/food/dietary-supplements/dietary-supplement-products-ingredients, and Dietary Supplement Ingredient List Advisory List, available at https://www.fda.gov/food/ dietary-supplement-products-ingredients/dietary-supplement-ingredient-advisory-list.

65 21 U.S.C. § 343(r)(6).

66 21 U.S.C. § 343(r)(6)(A); *see also* 21 CFR § 101.93.

67 The notification must include the name and address of the manufacturer, the text of the claim, the name of the ingredient for which the claim is being made, and the name of the dietary supplement. The notification must attest that the manufacturer has substantiation that the claim is truthful and not misleading and be signed by a person who can certify the accuracy and completeness of the information. 21 CFR § 101.93(a)(2).

68 21 CFR § 101.93(c)(1).

69 21 U.S.C § 343(r)(6). A "nutritional deficiency" claim is a statement that claims a benefit related to a classical nutritional deficiency disease and discloses the prevalence of such disease in the U.S.; a "structure/function" claim describes the role of a nutrient or dietary ingredient intended to affect the structure or function in humans and characterizes the documented mechanism by which a nutrient or dietary ingredient acts to maintain such structure or function; and a general well-being claim describes general well-being from consumption of a nutrient or dietary ingredient. 42 U.S.C. § 343(r)(6)(A).

[70] *See* Guidance for Industry: Substantiation for Dietary Supplement Claims Made Under Section 403(r)(6) of the Federal Food, Drug, and Cosmetic Act, January 2009 (403 Guidance), available at https://www.fda.gov/regulatory-information/search-fda-guidance-documents/guidance-industry-substantiation-dietary-supplement-claims-made-under-section-403r-6-federal-food.

[71] FTC has also adopted a standard of "competent and reliable scientific evidence" to substantiate claims about the benefit and safety of dietary supplements. *See, e.g.*, https://www.ftc.gov/tips-advice/business-center/guidance/dietary-supplements-advertising-guide-industry.

[72] *See, e.g. In Re Schering Corp.*, 118 F.T.C. 1030, 1123 (1994); *see also* 403 Guidance.

[73] *See* 403 Guidance.

[74] In September 2018, FDA issued a Draft Guidance Policy Regarding Quantitative Labeling of Dietary Supplements Containing Live Microbials: Guidance of Industry, available at https://www.fda.gov/media/115730/download, expressing the Agency's intention to exercise its enforcement discretion with respect to the declaration of live microbial quantity in colony forming units (CFUs), in addition to the quantitative amount by weight declaration as required by regulation within the Supplement Facts of a dietary supplement label, provided certain conditions are met.

[75] *See* Current Good Manufacturing Practices (CGMPs) for Dietary Supplements, available at https://www.fda.gov/food/current-good-manufacturing-practices-cgmps/current-good-manufacturing-practices-cgmps-dietary-supplements; *see also* Small Entity Compliance Guide: Current Good Manufacturing Practice in Manufacturing, Packaging, Labeling or Holding Operations for Dietary Supplements (Small Entity Compliance Guide), available at https://www.fda.gov/regulatory-information/search-fda-guidance-documents/small-entity-compliance-guide-current-good-manufacturing-practice-manufacturing-packaging-labeling.

[76] The Dietary Supplement Labeling Guide is available at https://www.fda.gov/food/dietary-supplements-guidance-documents-regulatory-information/dietary-supplement-labeling-guide; *see also* Small Entity Compliance Guide. Companies should also comply with FDA Final Rule on Food Labeling: Revision of the Nutrition and Supplement Facts Labels, *see* endnote 46.

[77] 21 USC § 201(g)(1).

[78] 21 U.S.C. § 262.

[79] The U.S. Public Health Service (PHS) Act defines a "biological product" as a "virus, therapeutic serum, toxin, antitoxin, vaccine, blood, blood component or derivative, allergenic product, or analogous product...applicable to the prevention, treatment, or cure of a disease or condition of human beings." 42 U.S.C. § 351(i). The term "virus" includes a broad spectrum of microorganisms that cause an infectious disease and includes bacteria. 21 CFR § 600.3(h)(1). Pursuant to FDA regulations and policies, biological products include, among other things, products containing cells or microorganisms and meet the definition of drugs under the Act.

[80] *See* 21 U.S.C. § 321(p).

[81] Additional regulatory pathways for approval of new drugs include Abbreviated New Drug Applications (ANDA) and Over-the-Counter (OTC) monographs. ANDA is the process for FDA approval of generic drugs. These applications are abbreviated because they generally do not require the submission of pre-clinical (animal) and clinical (human) studies to establish safety and efficacy. Instead, the sponsor is required to establish that the generic is the bioequivalent of the innovator drug. OTC are non-prescription drugs that are marketed consistent with a monograph, or "rule book," covering acceptable ingredients, uses (indications), doses, formulations, labeling, and testing. An OTC drug marketed consistent with the conditions set forth in a final monograph and all other applicable OTC's requirements is generally

considered GRASE and appropriate for marketing in the U.S. As of publication, FDA has not approved any probiotic drugs and there are no monographs governing their manufacturing, marketing, or use.

[82] Additional information about the Phase I clinical research phase is available on FDA's website at https://www.fda.gov/patients/drug-development-process/step-3-clinical-research.

[83] During a fourth and final Phase, post-market studies are conducted after a drug is approved for use by FDA to provide additional information, including relating to the drug's risks, benefits, and best use.

[84] See Guidance for Clinical Investigators, Sponsors, and IRBs Investigational New Drug Applications (INDs) – Determining Whether Human Research Studies Can Be Conducted Without an IND (September 2013) (September 2013 IND Guidance), available at https://www.fda.gov/media/79386/download; see also Investigational New Drug Applications Prepared and Submitted by Sponsor-Investigators Guidance for Industry (May 2015), available at https://www.fda.gov/media/92604/download. See also Guidance for Industry, Investigators, and Reviewers, Exploratory IND Studies, January 2006, available at https://www.fda.gov/media/72325/download; Guidance for Industry Q&A Content and Format of INDs for Phase I Studies of Drugs, Including Well-Characterized, Therapeutic, Biotechnology Derived Products, October 2000, available at https://www. fda.gov/media/72284/download; and Guidance for Industry Content and Format of Investigational New Drug Applications (INDs) for Phase I Studies of Drugs, Including Well-Characterized, Therapeutic, Biotechnology Derived Products, November 1995, available at https://www.fda.gov/media/71203/download.

[85] Additional information about FDA's drug approval process is available at https://www.fda.gov/drugs/drug-information-consumers/fdas-drug-review-process-ensuring-drugs-are-safe-and-effective.

[86] PHS Act § 351.

[87] 42 U.S.C. § 262.

[88] FDA issued a guidance for industry setting forth recommendations regarding IND submissions for early clinical trials with LBPs, including LBPs lawfully marketed as conventional foods and dietary supplements. See Early Clinical Trials with Live Biotherapeutic Products: Chemistry, Manufacturing, and Control Information Guidance for Industry (February 2012, Updated June 2016), available at https://www.fda.gov/media/82945/download. The guidance addresses the chemistry, manufacturing, and control (CMC) information that sponsors should include with an IND for an LBP.

[89] 42 U.S.C. § 262(a)(1).

[90] See CMC and GMP guidance documents, available at https://www.fda.gov/vaccines-blood-biologics/general-biologics-guidances/cmc-and-gmp-guidances.

[91] 21 U.S.C. § 201(i).

[92] 21 U.S.C. § 361.

[93] 21 U.S.C. § 362. For guidance on cosmetic labeling regulations see FDA Cosmetic Labeling Guide, available at https://www.fda.gov/cosmetics/cosmetics-labeling-regulations/cosmetics-labeling-guide.

19

A Future Research Perspective

Is There a Connection Between Sun Exposure, Microbiome and Skin Cancer?

Nava Dayan

Dr. Nava Dayan LLC, New Jersey, USA

Abstract

This chapter is written merely as a theoretical thinking exercise. My path in research of the skin microbiome began more than a decade ago when investigating skin barrier and innate immunity and capturing the skin barrier not merely as a physical barrier but also as a biological entity. This research resulted in a book that I edited in collaboration with Prof. Phil Wertz and was published by Wiley and Sons in 2012. From inception, it was clear to me that our understanding of the microbiome is incomplete and that a meta-analysis approach to connecting elements is essential. Observations in two dimensions connecting the microbiome community and behavior to one module at a time will not assist us in navigating the maze of its complexity since a key aspect of the effect of biota on the human body biology is its function. Most of the current research on the skin microbiome is focused on its mapping and identification while only a fraction is aimed at understanding its means of communication with human cells. Moreover, the acknowledgment that human cell effectors influence the microbiome as well is only beginning to settle in. While working on the innate immunity and microbiome projects, separately, I studied the effect of visible light on skin. This is a part of the sun spectrum that is only partially investigated and to a less extent when compared to our knowledge about UVB and UVA exposure wavelengths. I designed and executed an experiment to explore the impact of this light on various skin biomarkers and cascades and the particular effect of light on chromophores in skin cells [1, 2].

Keywords: Skin microbiome, immunosuppression, impaired barrier, UV exposure, chromophores, mutagenic, carcinogenic

Email: nava.dayan@verizon.net

Nava Dayan (ed.) Skin Microbiome Handbook: From Basic Research to Product Development, (377–388) © 2020 Scrivener Publishing LLC

19.1   Introduction

The skin microbiome includes bacteria, yeast, mites and viruses.

Studying the role of the skin microbiome in health and disease is an area that requires multiple disciplines. Therefore, when working on such projects, it is imperative that teams are built which include, for example, microbiologists, physicians, pharmacists and pharmacologists. This chapter is aimed at sharing a few observations on the imminent effect of sunlight on the skin microbiome and potential relation to skin cancer. When adding the effect of sunlight to skin microbiome, it is highly recommended that physicists are added to the investigative team as well.

Our skin can be perceived as an ecosystem since it hosts various populations of microbial entities. These seem to differ in their type and distribution depending on skin site characteristics and topography [3]. The majority of the microbiome entities are relatively permanent, but some are transient. Factors known to affect the nature and distribution of the microbiome on skin include humidity, temperature, pH, lipid and sebum content as well as antimicrobial lipids and peptides. Among environmental impacts, is sun exposure affecting the skin microbiome?

I would like to share a few interesting aspects that attempt to make a three-dimensional connection between ultraviolet radiation exposure, skin microbiome and skin cancer. The connection between these factors is not clear and key gaps are yet to be explored, but we can begin to make sense of it and to possibly connect the dots in what research reveals thus far.

19.2   Ultraviolet Light (UV) – The Skin Microbiome and Cancer

It is important to explore the interaction of UV with the microbiome and its possible relation to cancer because the direct effects of UV on skin cells only partially explains the initiation, progression, development and prevalence of skin cancer. Attributing it solely to immunosuppression and direct mutagenicity did not yield end-to-end causation; therefore, strategies for prevention and treatment are limited. For example, some skin diseases, such as psoriasis and atopic dermatitis, include immunosuppression elements, but the prevalence of skin cancer in patient populations and how it differs among different communities is not clear [4]. While some information reveals the effect of sunlight on the conditions of these diseases, the connection to its biota dysbiosis is not fully understood. One key question related to the initiation of carcinogenesis is the threshold of its triggering, meaning, at which point and under which conditions radiation that is "educating" the immune system changes its cause and becomes mutagenic. I am therefore suggesting that we try to expand our thinking by adding another dimension, an innate part of our body, by studying the role of the microbiome in this context.

It is well established that UV radiation imparts immunosuppression to skin. Some of the mechanisms involved include oxidative stress and inflammation, direct effects on the DNA and cell cycle, which lead to carcinogenesis [5, 6]. It is also known that these interactions are mediated by specific molecules in the skin that are spread within its layers in various cells (such as melanin in melanocytes) and systems (such as hemoglobin in the vascularized dermis), as well as other molecules that interact with radiation at the molecular and/or quantum level. These molecules are named chromophores.

Interestingly, chromophores are also present in some bacteria that reside on our skin, and there are structural similarities between those that are produced by our cells to those that are produced by biota. For example, *Cutibacterium acnes* produces porphyrins that are similar in structure to hemoglobin [7], and *Malassezia furfur* (MF) produces pityriacitrin with a structure that exhibits some similarity to melanin [8]. Who taught who in the evolutionary process? Did we learn from the microbiome to protect our cells or vice versa? Or perhaps both protection strategies were developed in parallel. Do chromophores protect us and the bacteria or do they harm us? The same as with human cells where chromophores can be occasionally protecting and sometimes mediators for destruction, various microbiome populations can either benefit or be destroyed by the chromophores of their own production. I will share some evidence on these processes later in this chapter.

Our cells contain the genome that we inherited from our parents. The biota community that we acquire in early life is a result of the environment we are exposed to, including our parents or caregivers that come in physical contact with us during the first two weeks after birth.

While the skin microbiome is relatively stable, persistent change in the environment can alter it. Just as bacteria can alter immunological and physiological functions, the human body can alter the microbiome community. Factors such as nutrients, pH, barrier strength, hygiene, exposure to chemicals and radiation, overall health condition and stress levels can allow certain microbial species to supersede others if the environment supports their survival or vice versa. UV exposure can be considered among the environmental factors.

Prof. Peter Elias and colleagues who have studied atopic dermatitis and skin barrier for many years, suggested the hypothesis that a contributing factor to the rise in the prevalence of the disease is due to the dramatically reduced exposure to UV in urban higher-class society. They argue, for example, that the higher population of *Staphylococcus aureus* in these patients may be controlled, at least in part, by attenuated exposure to sunlight, thereby not only reducing the levels of the bacteria but as a result, reducing its secretion of toxins, supporting antimicrobial elements and innate immunity of skin. This can be critical in early life because of the imbalance existing on the newborn skin, mostly the relatively basic pH being a dominant factor [9].

The connection between impaired immunity and overpopulation of pathogens on skin is further expressed in patients who underwent organ transplantation and took immunosuppressing drugs on a chronic basis. It was shown that in such cases, not only do excess pathogens live on the skin, but they are more invasive, taking advantage of the impaired barrier by developing means to penetrate the tissue by secreting catabolic enzymes [10].

To further elaborate on the conditions that will alter skin health associated with dysbiosis, it can be explained that both resident and transient biota exist on our skin regularly. There are two key controlling factors of the skin microbiome: our immunity and the composition of the biota community. It will be challenging for resident biota to protect an immunocompromised skin and transient opportunistic bacteria will most likely not induce disease when the barrier is healthy and intact. This understanding dampens our human classification of microbiome being "good" or "bad" because the agenda for biota communities is distinct: survival and proliferation. It is the condition of our health that dictates its behavior towards us. Presence of transient bacteria is not necessarily associated with clinical manifestation of disease and resident species can become pathogenic. Resident bacteria become pathogenic due to trauma, injury and when the host becomes immunocompromised. Skin biota, skin integrity and the immune system work coherently to control cutaneous function and prevent disease.

So, what creates the shift from health to disease?

Time and exposure patterns are most likely key factors. Chronic dysbiosis allows crossing the line between health and disease. Persistent communication of biota secreted elements to human cells establishes an epigenetic change in our own cellular behavior that is difficult to reverse, such as chronic disease or cancer. Tissue injury and chronic inflammation increase the risk of developing cancer. For example, 2% of burn scars undergo malignant transformation, and squamous cell carcinoma (SCC) is the most common form of cancer that develops from such lesions. Specific bacteria that have been demonstrated to be present in excess in cancer lesions are: *S. aureus* in cutaneous T-cell lymphoma, *Chlamydophila pneumoniae* in cutaneous T-cell lymphoma and *Borrelia burgdorferi* in cutaneous T-cell lymphoma. It is thought that transient extreme episodes of exposure to sun which provoke sunburn and inflammation, if occurring in relapse throughout our life span, cause skin inflammation and elevate the odds of developing skin cancer [11]. Is this exposure changing the skin, attenuating its immune strength, hence allowing opportunistic transient biota to thrive; or perhaps sun exposure changes the biota, directly transforming it into becoming mutagenic for human cells.

Is cancer association with biota direct or indirect? Science demonstrates that it can be direct. In 2008, Harald zur Hausen, a German virologist, received the Nobel Prize for his discovery that human papilloma viruses cause cervical cancer [12]. While it can be argued that technically, viruses do not meet the definition of "living" they are perceived as part of the microbiome community since they interact and alter living bacteria and human cells behavior. Moreover, they have the ability to relatively quickly adapt to new challenging conditions that will enhance their survival chances.

The award was given to him because he went against the existing dogma and postulated that oncogenic human papilloma virus (HPV) caused cervical cancer, the second most common cancer among women. He realized that HPV-DNA could exist in a non-productive state in the tumors, and should be detectable by specific searches for viral DNA. He found HPV to be a heterogeneous family of viruses. Only some HPV types cause cancer. His discovery has led to characterization of the natural history of HPV infection, an understanding of mechanisms of HPV-induced carcinogenesis and the development of prophylactic vaccines against HPV acquisition.

This discovery further supported epigenetics in microbiome-human cells relationships, anchoring the idea that environment dictates behavior.

A few important conclusions are drawn from this exploration:

- Biota can directly interact with human DNA.
- Strains may differ in their activity.
- Metabolic state of the biota is important—it's not sufficient to identify the strain. We need to know if it's is alive, dead or dormant.
- An understanding of the circumstances at which the specific strain is activated and how is key.
- Normally, the virus is retained in the cytoplasm and only under certain conditions does it penetrate the cell nucleolus.

How does HPV, a virus triggering cervical cancer, relate to skin cancer? Unraveling the viral mode of action that was mutagenic in cervical cells, pointed to a global mechanism that may be utilized by viruses in other organs, including the skin. In skin microbiome research, similar to other research areas, the availability of tools and methods dictates the selection of studies to be conducted. Since viruses cannot be cultivated and do not portray consensus sequences to be detected by molecular methods, most microbiome investigations are bacteria and not virus related. When observing the various lesions, the clinical manifestation of viral infection on skin often appears as a tumor with an excess of tissue extending from the organ.

In 2015, a team of U.S. scientists together with a biochemist from the FDA published a hypothesis linking HPV to malignant melanoma. The basis for their hypothesis was evidence found by clinicians to the significant presence of HPV strains in skin melanoma lesions [6].

The following HPV strains were found in more than 50% of patients with the following skin cancers: HPV-38 and 16/18 in melanomas, HPV-77 in non-melanoma skin cancers. They also eluded to the potential mode of action of HPV as a carcinogen unraveling specific HPV secreted proteins that inactivate the cancer protective gene p53. P53 is a fidelity gene that protects cells from cancerous mutations. Upon activation it may trigger three potential paths: apoptosis, cellular senescence or cell replication arrest combined with the activation of DNA repair enzymes. As such, when inactivated, its protection from cancer is halted. Another interesting finding was that a population-based case control study suggested that the association of HPV with SCC was greater in those using glucocorticoids (i.e., immunosuppressed individuals).

An additional example is provided for Merkel cell carcinoma (MCC), which is a rare, highly aggressive primary neuroendocrine carcinoma of the skin that usually affects elderly Caucasians on sun-exposed regions of the face, neck and head. Merkel cell polyomavirus was found to contribute to the development of the majority of MCCs. In fact, about 80% of MCCs have this virus clonally integrated into the cancerous cells. This virus is considered a persistent resident of skin microbiome, but immunosuppressed patients are more prone to develop MCC [13].

Healthy skin harbors resident and short-lived viruses. Papillomaviruses (α-HPV, β-HPV, γ-HPV) are present on and within the upper layers of human skin. UV-R is known to be a stimulus for the skin resident herpes simplex virus (HSV), activating the viral promotor and transcription factors.

Does this mean that viruses are the "skin carcinogens" among the microbiome? Viruses may act as contributing factors but not all strains are mutagenic and the condition of the skin plays a pivotal role in their ability to harm. Human HPVs, especially the epidermodysplasia verruciformis (EV) types, are known to be widespread on human skin and have been linked to skin carcinogenesis in the genetic disease of EV. Interestingly, EV HPV strains are found in hair follicles of psoriasis patients, in particular of those treated with PUVA (a combination of psoralen application and ultraviolet A therapy) whereas its expression was not observed in patients who had received no treatment. This observation requires further investigation into exploring the interconnection between PUVA treatment and the dysbiosis of EV HPV in psoriatic skin [14].

The knowledge that viruses have the ability to penetrate a cell and alter its DNA gave rise to a new class of drugs in the biologic's classification. In 2015, the FDA approved the first oncolytic virus as a drug to treat melanoma [15]. This drug developed by Amgen Pharmaceuticals is a genetically engineered virus that replicates in cancer cells, causing them to burst. It is indicated for local treatment of unresectable cutaneous, subcutaneous, and nodal lesions in patients with melanoma recurrent after initial surgery. With this drug, Amgen used the virulence of herpes virus as a vector to target melanoma lesions and genetically engineered it. The genes that were deleted from the virus were those that shut down cellular defenses and those that assist the virus to escape the immune system. In such a way, cells infected by the virus were eradicated by the patient's own immune system. The added gene was granulocyte-macrophage colony-stimulating factor (GM-CSF), a gene that promotes the proliferation and differentiation of hematopoietic progenitor cells and the generation of neutrophils, eosinophils, and macrophages. The naive herpes virus therefore expresses two sets of functional genes: one that allows it to penetrate the human cell and proliferate there and the second that is deceiving our immune system, thereby preventing it from acting against the virus. The oncolytic drug sustained the first type of genes while manipulating the second type of genes. The result changes the power relationship between the virus and our immune system, creating an advantage for our own immunity, and making it effective at identifying the virus as hostile and triggering cell lysis of cancer infected cells.

What may be the additional factors that affect the skin biota population and what can we learn from chronic skin disease that exhibits genetic predisposition but is also impacted by environmental factors?

In psoriasis, the direct link between biota dysbiosis and the pathogenesis of the disease is under exploration. Apart from improving the course of psoriasis, selective modulation of the microbiota may increase the efficacy of medical treatments as well as attenuate a drug's side effects. When PUVA was suggested as a treatment for severe psoriasis its mode of action was not fully understood, and it was believed to induce cell death and attenuate cell proliferation [16]. With our expanded knowledge on the involvement of the microbiome in chronic inflammatory disorders, it will not be surprising to find that irradiation with light activates antimicrobial agents. Psoralen, the drug applied to skin before irradiation in PUVA therapy is present in parsley. Parsley contains photoactive compounds called furocoumarins. Interestingly, it was demonstrated that parsley leaves inhibited a DNA repair-deficient *Escherichia coli* in a photobiological assay; therefore, it is possible that the combination used in PUVA is, essentially, antimicrobial. Additional studies should be conducted to understand the effect of the PUVA on the skin microbiome [17].

While affecting the microbiome, PUVA may also be boosting the skin's immunity by accelerating the production of vitamin D in skin. Synthetic vitamin D3 derivative ointments have been commercialized for topical dermatological use. Does vitamin D affect the microbiome population?

Vitamin D production in the skin is induced by both sunlight as well as pathogens [18]. Lipopolysaccharides are glycolipids found in the outer membrane of some types of Gram-negative bacteria, such as *Escherichia* and *Pseudomonas* strains. These trigger the production of Toll-like receptors (TLR) and inflammatory cytokines that, in turn, induce the production of vitamin D. Additional cascades that are initiated when the skin is exposed to light or infected with pathogenic bacteria relate to the production of antimicrobial lipids and peptides that induce cellular autophagy, all aimed at restoration of biota homeostasis.

The intensity of exposure to sun is most likely similar for commensal bacteria as well as skin keratinocytes in the epidermis. In a study conducted in 2013 at the University of California, San Diego, the effect of UVB exposure on *C. acnes* has been investigated. This study revealed a dose-dependent decrease in the bacterial porphyrins, suggesting the responsiveness of facial bacteria to UV radiation. As such, *C. acnes* may respond to UVB before significant skin damage is detected. Researchers concluded that the concept of detecting the changes in the porphyrin profile of *C. acnes* as a reflection of human responses to environments can be applied to the development of various disease monitors [19].

Both UV and a pathogenic microbiome population have key roles in educating our skin's immunity, so it is trained to draw its weapon upon a threat. Figure 19.1 is a simplified illustration of some mechanisms involved in this education pattern. Both UV and bacterial infection induce vitamin D production as well as inflammation. When the secretion of TLRs is under control, the immune system is activated as part of its training and various

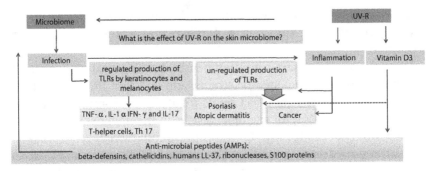

Figure 19.1 Both microbiome and UV-R educate the skin's immune system.

cytokines allow recruitment of specific T cells. But when the secretion of TLRs is out of control due to persistent exposure to threat, inflammation becomes persistent too, with no resolution and healing, and therefore may trigger mutagenicity, chronic or autoimmune disease. Antimicrobial peptides such as β-defensins, cathelicidins, human's LL-37, ribonucleases, and S100 proteins where shown to be responsible for the balance of this system. Keratinocytes and melanocytes, the main cell types involved in melanoma and nonmelanoma skin cancers, express TLRs that induce inflammatory responses against invading pathogens. Nevertheless, uncontrolled activation of TLRs leads to chronic inflammation that may give rise to skin cancer.

Remarkably, melanoma and basal cell carcinoma have been found to be successfully treated by TLR agonists targeting TLR7, TLR8 and TLR9. Unregulated inflammation in addition to microbiome dysbiosis may increase the risk for carcinogenesis.

The direct effect of UV on the skin microbiome can be either beneficial or detrimental to the biota community. In the case of MF, for example, a resident fungus that is thought to be associated with dandruff and seborrheic dermatitis, the initial exposure of MF to UV halts its growth. However, after adaptation it produces a UV filter, pityriacitrin. This UV filter protects the fungus and sustains its population in exposure to UV. But MF may not be protecting only itself. It may be protecting our skin as well since it produces another protective agent malassezin, that was shown to induce apoptosis in skin melanocytes, thereby preventing the accumulation and survival of defective cells [20]. Is this the nature of the symbiotic relationship between our skin cells and MF? Is it "paying" us back for our hospitality by eliminating mutagenic cells and preventing cancer?

A damaging effect of UV to bacteria is demonstrated with C. acnes. As previously explained, porphyrins are UV filters that are produced by these bacteria [21, 22]. However, here, unlike in the case of MF, exposure to UV is associated with both reduction in porphyrins as well as in the *C. acnes* population.

When we try and arrange skin commensals by their location in the skin and prospective effect on specific strains, and add to it the ability of the strain to mitigate the light effect by its innate UV absorbing agents, we find no correlation. MF, for example, resides in the upper skin layers and its count does not change with UV exposure. Similarly, *Staphylococcus epidermidis* resides deeper in the skin. Counts for both *S. aureus* and *C. acnes* decline after exposure to UV, although *C. acnes* contains UV-absorbing agents and *S. aureus* does not.

19.3 Conclusion

In summary, while the connection between sun exposure and skin immunosuppression is known, in recent years, scientists have developed an understanding that such a connection is complicated and may depend on patterns of exposure as well as on other factors. Here I suggest that the skin microbiome may be a contributing factor to skin health and disease directly and indirectly in connection with exposure to sunlight. These relationships are complicated. In recent years there has been increasing evidence indicating a key role of the involvement of biota in carcinogenesis. In addition, there is accumulating evidence for the direct and indirect effects of sun exposure on the skin microbiome.

Many questions are open for discussion and exploration. An interesting question relates to those with chronic inflammatory skin disorders who are more susceptible to cancer. Such questions will be hard to study because many of these patients are treated with drugs, therefore control groups of untreated patients are limited.

Nevertheless, the information shared here will hopefully provoke thoughts about the potential connected contributions of skin microbiome and UV to carcinogenesis.

Acknowledgment

The author would like to acknowledge Phil Wertz PhD, Professor Emeritus, The University of Iowa, for his kind contribution to the review and advice on the manuscript.

References

1. Dayan, N., Ballantyne, T., Ngo, T., Peterson, A., Larsen, K., Knaggs, J., Gallas, J.A., Melanin Derivative to Shield the Skin from High Energy Visible Light. *C&T Mag.*, 126, 3, 2011, 186–193. 2013. https://www.cosmeticsand toiletries.com/formulating/function/uvfilter/premium-a-melanin-derivative-to-shield-the-skin-from-high-energy-visible-light-211002591.html.

2. Patent: Compound, composition, and method for protecting skin from high energy visible light. https:patents.google.com/patent/WO2011112414A3/en.

3. Grice, E.A., Kong, H.H., Conlan, S., Deming, C.B., Davis, J., Young, A.C., Bouffard, G.G., Blackesley, R.W., Murray, P.R., Green, E.D., Turner, M.L., Segre, J.A., Topographical and temporal diversity of the human skin microbiome. *Science*, 324, 1190–1192, 2009.

4. Sherwani, M.A., Tufail, S., Muzaffar, A.F., Yusuf, N., The skin microbiome and immune system: Potential target for chemopreventiom? *Photodermatol. Photoimmunol. Photomed.*, 34, 1, 25–34, 2018.

5. Hart, P.H. and Norval, M., Ultraviolet radiation-induced immunosuppression and its relevance for skin carcinogenesis. *Photochem. Photobiol.*, 17, 1872, 2018.

6. Merrill, S.J., Ashrafi, S., Subramanian, M., Godar, D.E., Exponentially increasing incidences of cutaneous malignant melanoma in Europe correlates with low personal annual UV doses and suggests 2 major risk factors. *Dermatoendocrinol.*, 27, 7, 1, e1004018, 2015.

7. Patwardhan, S.V., Richter, C., Vogt, A., Blume-Peytavi, U., Canfield, D., Kottner, J., Measuring acne using Coproporphyrin III, Protoporphyrin IX, and lesion-specific inflammation: An exploratory study. *Arch. Dermatol. Res.*, 309, 159–167, 2017.

8. Machowinski, A., Kramer, H.W., Hort, W., Mayser, P., Pityriacitrin – a potent UV filter produced by Malassezia furfur and its effect on human skin microflora. *Mycoses*, 49, 388–392, 2006.

9. Thyssen, J.P., Zirwas, M.J., Elias, P.M., Potential role of reducing environmental UV exposure as a driver of the current epidemic of atopic dermatitis. *J. Allergy Clin. Immunol.*, 136, 1163–1169, 2015.

10. Fishman, J.A., Opportunistic infections – coming to the limits of immunosuppression? Cold Spring Harb. *Perspect. Med.*, 1, 3, 10, a015669, 2013.

11. Gul, U. and Klc, A., Squamous cell carcinoma developing on burn scar. *Annals Plast. Surg.*, 56, 406–408, 2006.

12. Nour, N.M., Cervical cancer: A preventable death. *Rev. Obstet. Gynecol.*, 2, 240–244, 2009.

13. Becker, C.J., Stang, A., DeCaprio, J.A., Cerroni, L., Lebbe, C., Veness, M., Nghiem, P., Merkel cell carcinoma. *Nat. Rev. Dis. Primers*, 3, 17077, 2107.

14. Benhadou, F., Mintoff, D., Schnebert, B., Thio, H.B., Psoriasis and microbiota: 14A systematic review. *Diseases*, 2, 6, 2, pii: E47, 2018.

15. https://www.amgen.com/media/news-releases/2015/10/fda-approves-imlygic-talimogene-laher-parepvec-as-first-oncolytic-viral-therapy-in-the-us/.

16. Chuang, T.-Y., Heinrich, L.A., Schultz, M.D., Reizner, G.T., Kumm, R.C., Cripps, D.J., PUVA and skin cancer. *J. Amer. Acad. Dermatol.*, 26, 173–177, 1992.

17. Manderfeld, M.M., Schafer, H.W., Davidson, P.M., Zottola, E.A., Isolation and identification of antimicrobial furocoumarins from parsley. *J. Food Prot.*, 60, 72–77, 1996.

18. Lagishetti, V., Liu, N.Q., Hewison, M., Vitamin D metabolism and innate immunity. *Mol. Cell. Endocrinol.*, 347, 97–105, 2011.

19. Shu, M., Kuo, S., Wang, Y., Jiang, Y., Liu, Y.T., Garrl, R.L., Huang, C.M., Porphyrin metabolisms in human skin commensal Propionibacterium acnes bacteria: Potential application to monitor human radiation risk. *Curr. Med. Chem.*, 20, 562–568, 2013.

20. Gaitanis, G., Magiatis, P., Hantschke, M., Bassukas, I.D., Velegraki, A., The Malassezia genus in skin and systemic diseases. *Clin. Microbiol. Rev.*, 1, 106–41, 2012.

21. Ashkenazi, H., Malik, Z., Harth, Y., Nitzan, Y., Eradication of Propionibacterium acnes by its endogenic porphyrins after illumination with high intensity blue light. *FEMS Immunol. Med. Microbiol.*, 35, 17–24, 2003.

22. Wang, Y., Zhu, W., Shu, M., Jiang, Y., Gallo, R.L., Liu, Y.T., Huang, C.M., The response of human skin commensal bacteria as a reflection of UV radiation: UV-B decreases porphyrin production. *PLoS One*, 7, 10, e47798, 2012.

Glossary

A

Nα-Acylglutamine aminoacylase: Bacterial enzyme responsible for mediating the release of malodorous medium-chain VFAs, including 3H3MH and 3M2H, from their non-odorous precursors. (James G.).

Acne: (1). Acne is a disease of the pilosebaceous unit (sebaceous follicle) producing clinical manifestations of non-inflammatory (comedones) and inflammatory skin lesions (papules, pustules and cystic nodules) that can result in scarring of the face and upper trunk. Acne onset and persistence range for pre-teen years to young adulthood. (Lessin S.R. and Leyden J.J.). (2). Acne is a skin condition that occurs when hair follicles become plugged with oil and dead skin cells. (Farahmand S.).

Antibiotic: An antibiotic is a drug used to treat bacterial infections that inhibits the growth of or destroys the microorganisms. (Lessin S.R. and Leyden J.J.).

Antibody drug complex: Molecular complex composed of an antibody linked to a biologically active and potent drug directed to a specific site, particularly specific types of cancer cells. (Strobel S.L.).

Antigen presenting cells: Cells that ingest microbes, process their components and present them to the acquired immunity system. (Blumenberg M.).

Antimicrobial: An antimicrobial is an agent that disrupt and prevent the growth of microorganisms. (Lessin S.R. and Leyden J.J.).

Antimicrobial lipid: Endogenously produced sebaceous and stratum corneum derived lipids which display antimicrobial activity against non-commensal bacteria and fungi. (Samaras S. and Hoptroff M.).

Antimicrobial peptide: Skin or microbiome derived peptides which form part of the innate immune system and which are selectively antimicrobial against non-commensal bacteria, fungi and viruses. (Samaras S. and Hoptroff M.).

Antimicrobial proteins: Polypeptides that discourage microbial growth, often by act largely by disrupting the structure or function of microbial cell membranes. (Blumenberg M.).

Atopic dermatitis: (1). A chronic inflammatory skin condition character-ized by relapsing inflamed and pruritic skin lesions. (Cheng J. and Hata T.). (2). Atopic dermatitis is a common skin pathology with pruritus and eczematous lesions that affects mainly children and it is characterized by three different host and environmental factors that are linked together, establishing a vicious cycle, leading to the allergic disease: dysregu-lated immune response, barrier dysfunction, and *S. aureus* infection. (Meloni M. and Balzaretti S.). (3). Atopic dermatitis is a chronic pruritic inflammatory skin disease of unknown origin that usually starts in early infancy, but also affects a substantial number of adults. (Farahmand S.). (4). Atopic dermatitis (AD, or eczema), is a chronic, pruritic, inflamma-tory skin disease common in children and is characterized by dry, scaly, itchy skin. (Whitfill T. and Dube G.R and Oh J.).

B

Bacterial communication: Signaling molecules secreted by one microbe that influence growth and gene expression of another microbe. (Buerger S. and Huber M.).

Bacteriome: Bacteria members of the microbiome. (Buerger S. and Huber M.).

Biologics: Biologics, also known as biological products, are products that replicate natural substances such as enzymes, antibodies, or hormones in the human body. Biologics can be composed of sugars, proteins, or nucleic acids, or a combination of these substances. They may also be living entities, such as cells and tissues. (Schmelz R. M.).

C

Carbon-sulphur β-lyase: Abbreviated as C-S β-lyase, a bacterial enzyme responsible for mediating the release of thioalcohols including 3M3SH from their non-odorous precursors. (James G.).

Center for Biologics Evaluation and Research (CBER): The Center within the FDA that regulates biological products for human use. (Schmelz R. M.).

Center for Drug Evaluation and Research (CDER): The Center within the FDA that regulates over-the-counter and prescription drugs, includ-ing biological therapeutics and generic drugs. (Schmelz R. M.).

Center for Food Safety and Applied Nutrition (CFSAN): A branch of the FDA that regulates foods, dietary supplements, and cosmetics. (Schmelz R. M.).

Ceramide: A lipid consisting of a fatty acid amide-linked to a long-chain base. (Fischer C.L. and Wertz P.W.).

[22] For a full list of approved food additives derived from microorganisms *see* 21 CFR §§ 172 and 173.

[23] FDA response letters to GRAS notifications and other information about GRAS notices are available on FDA's website, at https://www.fda.gov/food/generally-recognized-safe-gras/gras-notice-inventory

[24] For a full list of approved food additives derived from microorganisms *see* 21 CFR § 184.

[25] For a complete list of GRAS approved microorganisms for indirect use in food *see* 21 CFR § 186.

[26] For a list of foods for human consumption that contain or are derived from microorganisms *see* 21 CFR §§ 131, 133, 136, and 137.

[27] FDA guidance documents do not establish legally enforceable responsibilities, but are instead the Agency's then-current thinking on a topic and should be viewed only as recommendations, unless specific regulatory or statutory requirements are cited.

[28] *See* Substantiation of Structure/Function Claims Made in Infant Formula Labels and Labeling: Guidance for Industry Draft Guidance (September 2016), available at file:///C:/users/RS2/Work%20Folders/Downloads/Draft_Guidance_for_Industry_on_Substantiation_for_Structure_Function_Claims_in_Infant_Formula_Labels_and_Labeling.pdf.

[29] As used herein, the term "disease" refers to both diseases and health-related conditions, and is defined as damage to an organ, part, structure, or system of the body such that it does not function properly (*e.g.*, cardiovascular disease) or a state of health leading to such dysfunctioning (*e.g.*, hypertension). 21 CFR § 101.14(a)(5).

[30] 21 CFR § 101.14(a)(1).

[31] 21 CFR § 101.14(c).

[32] 21 U.S.C. § 343(r)(3)(C).

[33] *See* Guidance for Industry: Notification of a Health Claim or Nutrient Content Claim Based on an Authoritative Statement of a Scientific Body (June 1998), FDA Docket Number FDA-2013-0610, available at https://www.fda.gov/regulatory-information/ search-fda-guidance-documents/guidance-industry-notification-health-claim-or-nutri-ent-content-claim-based-authoritative-statement.

[34] *See* Guidance for Industry: Evidence-Based Review System for the Scientific Evaluation of Health Claims (January 2009), Docket Number: FDA-2007-D-0371, available at https://www.fda.gov/regulatory-information/search-fda-guidance-documents/guidance-industry-evidence-based-review-system-scientific-evaluation-health-claims.

[35] *See* https://www.fda.gov/food/food-labeling-nutrition/authorized-health-claims-meet-significant-scientific-agreement-ssa-standard.

[36] Additional examples of approved health claims are available in the Food Labeling Guide.

[37] *See* Guidance for Industry: Interim Procedures for Qualified Health Claims in the Labeling of Conventional Human Food and Human Dietary Supplements (July 2003), FDA Docket Number FDA-2013-0610, available at https://www.fda.gov/regulatory-information/search-fda-guidance-documents/guidance-industry-interim-procedures-qualified-health-claims-labeling-conventional-human-food-and.

[38] For a list of Letters of Enforcement Discretion for qualified health claims, *see* https://www.fda.gov/food/food-labeling-nutrition/qualified-health-claims-letters-enforcement-discretion. For additional information about qualified health claims including letters of denial, *see* https://www.fda.gov/food/food-labeling-nutrition/qualified-health-claims.

[39] *See* Food Labeling Guide, Appendix D, for additional examples of qualified health claims.

[40] 21 CFR § 101.13.

[41] 21 CFR § 101.13(h)(1).

...lels: *In Vitro* Reconstructed ... representative of the skin ...clinical testing and research

...host without causing disease ... and Hata T.).

...mmunity of skin-associated ...tionship with skin. (Samaras

...species in which one obtains ...or benefiting it to be distin-...: (Blumenberg M.).

...associated with changes in ...:ratum corneum proteins and ...idermal water loss (TEWL), ...ased hydration and abnormal ...ed by exogenous factors such ...ses such as atopic dermatitis.

...authorship fixed in a tangible

...rial genera colonising axillary ...the generation of underarm ...that are aerobic gram-positive ...ormal skin microbiota (Chung

...d in the FDCA as "(1) articles ..., or sprayed on, introduced into, ...or any part thereof for cleansing, ...or altering the appearance, and ...nent of such articles; except that ...:.C. § 321(i). (Schmelz R. M.).

...found on human skin. It is a ...ated with hair follicles. (Fischer ...*opionibacterium acnes (P. acnes)* ...ic dipheroid that is a part of the ...d in the pathogenesis of inflam-...:.J.).

...nformation between cells, often ...cellular protective mechanisms.

D

Dandruff: Dandruff is a skin condition that mainly affects the scalp leading to flaking and sometimes mild itchiness. (Farahmand S.).

Demodex: A microscopic, obligate cutaneous ectoparasite ubiquitous in mammals. Two species exist in humans, D. folliculorum and D. Brevis. (Strobel S.L.).

Diaper dermatitis: Diaper dermatitis is inflammation of the skin under a diaper as a result of irritation from urine and feces. (Farahmand S.).

Dietary Supplement Health and Education Act (DSHEA): The Dietary Supplement Health and Education Act of 1994 (DSHEA) is a U.S. law that amends the FDCA by, among other things, affirms the status of dietary supplements as a category of food and creates a specific definition of dietary supplements, and requires companies to comply with good manufacturing practices for dietary supplements. (Schmelz R. M.).

Dietary supplements: A dietary supplement is a product taken by mouth that contain a "dietary ingredient." Dietary ingredients include vitamins, minerals, amino acids, and herbs or botanicals, as well as other substances that can be used to supplement the diet. (Schmelz R. M.).

Directive: EU Directives require EU countries to achieve a certain result, but leave them free to choose how to do so. (von Wright A.).

Diversity (microbial): The diversification among microorganisms on the basis of their structure and/or function; quantitatively microbial diversity can be estimated with the Shannon or the Simpson indices. Diversity takes into account both the microbial richness and the evenness of the relative abundances. (Stamatas G.N.).

Drug: A drug is defined in the FDCA as "(A) articles recognized in the official United States Pharmacopoeia, official Homeopathic Pharmacopeia of the United States, or official National Formulary, or any supplement to any of them; and (B) articles intended for use in the diagnosis, cure, mitigation, treatment, or prevention of disease in man or other animals; (C) articles (other than food) intended to affect the structure or any function of the body of man or other animals; and (D) articles intended for use as a component of any article specified in (A), (B), or (C). 21 U.S.C. § 321(g). (Schmelz R. M.).

Dysbiosis: (1). An imbalance between the types of organisms present in a person's normal microbial. community, often associated with disease (Cheng J. and Hata T.). (2). Dysbiosis is a term for a microbial imbalance or maladaptation on or inside the body, such as an impaired microbiota. (Farahmand S.). (3). As an alteration of the microbiome away from steady-state conditions and is generally associated with disease states and shifts in microbial communities. (Whitfill T. and Dube G.R.

e, Appendix A.
cturing Practices (CGMPs), available at
od-and-dietary-supplements/current-
Manufacturing Practices for the 21st
: Current Good Manufacturing Practices
a.gov/food/current-good-manufacturing-
st-century-food-processing-2004-study-

nd Hazard Analysis and Risk-Based
g. 3646 (proposed Jan. 16, 2013); *see also*
food-and-dietary-supplements/hazard-

vision of the Nutrition and Supplement
tions for foods to provide updated nutri-
nal Rule for companies with revenues of
ling dietary supplements) was January 1,
n annual food sales, the compliance date
es on the Changes to the Nutrition Facts
od-labeling-nutrition/industry-resources-
irements unrelated to nutrition facts, *see*

r component of foods, essential for normal
1, or development), normally not produced
uate to meet normal physiologic needs, and
ally defined deficiency syndrome.
mposition that provides a form or source of
e of a class of substances that cannot be sepa-
Examples include calcium, iodine, and zinc.
only used as human food or drink.
e dietary supplement context, a metabolite of
that incorporates structural elements of the
et production in the human body increases
olite can be part (or an intermediate part) of
ngredient.
f the whole and can be isolated from the whole.
ent (menstruum) combined with a dietary
at physically separates constituents from the
m into the solvent. The extract can be further
r semi-solid form.
of dietary supplement any article authorized
tantial clinical investigations have been insti-
estigations has been made public, unless the
a conventional food before an investigational
21 U.S.C. § 321(ff)(3)(B)(ii).

and Oh J.) (4). an imbalance in the composition and subsequent metabolic activity of a community of microorganisms, leading to systemic diseases. (Drake D.).

E

Ectoparasites: Parasitic organisms that exist on or in the skin. (Strobel S.L.)

European Food Safety Authority (EFSA): is one of the agencies of the EU with a special task to perform independent risk assessment and advice in aspects related to the food chain. (von Wright A.).

European Union (EU): The European Union is a political and economic union of 28 European member states that act as a one economic unit in the world economy. (von Wright A.).

Exposome: The exposome is the measure of all the exposures of an individual in a lifetime and how those exposures relate to health. (Farahmand S.).

F

Federal Food, Drug and Cosmetic Act (FDCA): The United States (U.S.) Federal Food, Drug, and Cosmetic Act (FDCA) is a set of laws initially passed by the U.S. Congress in 1938 giving authority to the U.S. Food and Drug Administration (FDA) to oversee the safety of food, drugs, medical devices, and cosmetics. The FDCA prohibits the movement of adulterated or misbranded food, drugs, devices, and cosmetics in interstate commerce and for other purposes. Among other things, the FDCA requires premarket approval by FDA for new drugs, authorizes regulation of foods, prohibits false therapeutic claims, authorizes factory inspections. The FDCA has been amended many times, including in 1994 with the Dietary Supplement Health and Education Act (DSHEA). (Schmelz R. M.).

Federal Trade Commission (FTC): The FTC is an independent federal agency of the U.S. government whose mission is to protect U.S. consumers and competition by preventing anticompetitive, deceptive, and unfair business practices through law enforcement, advocacy, and education without unduly burdening legitimate business activity. (Schmelz R. M.).

Food: The term "food" is defined in the FDCA as "(1) articles used for food or drink for man or other animals, (2) chewing gum, and (3) articles used for components of any such article." 21 U.S.C. § 321(f). (Schmelz R. M.).

Food additives: A food additive is any substance the intended use of which results or may reasonably be expected to result – directly or indirectly – in its becoming a component or otherwise affecting the characteristics of any food. Food additives include any substance used in the production, processing, treatment, packaging, transportation, or storage of food. The definition of food additives excludes ingredients whose use is generally recognized as safe, those ingredients approved for use by FDA or the U.S. Department of Agriculture prior to the food additive provisions of U.S. law, and color additives or pesticides where other legal pre-market approval requirements apply. (Schmelz R. M.).

Food and Drug Administration (FDA): The FDA is the federal agency within the U.S. Department of Health and Human Services responsible for protecting the public health by ensuring the safety, efficacy, and security of human and veterinary drugs, biological products, dietary supplements, and medical devices, and the safety of the U.S. food supply, cosmetics, and products that emit radiation. FDA is responsible for enforcing and carrying out the purpose of the FDCA. (Schmelz R. M.).

G

Gram-positive anaerobic cocci: Abbreviated as GPAC, a heterogeneous group of bacteria latterly shown to be significant colonisers of axillary skin. The main genera present are *Anaerococcus* and *Peptoniphilus* (James G.).

Gut microbiome: the community of microorganisms and their combined genetic material inhabiting the intestinal tract. (Drake D.).

H

Hand dermatitis: Hand dermatitis is a common condition caused by genetics, contact allergens and/or irritating substances. The symptoms include redness, itching, blisters, dryness, cracks, flaking and pain. (Farahmand S.).

I

Infant skin maturation: The dynamic changes that take place in infant skin and relate to its structure, function and composition. (Stamatas G.N.).

Intellectual property: Laws and regulations linked to creations of the mind. (Mills J.K.).

Intertriginous: two skin areas that may touch or rub together (Chung J., Strober B.E., Weinstock G.M.).

Irritant contact dermatitis: Irritant contact dermatitis is a form of contact dermatitis, in which the skin is injured by friction, environmental factors such as cold, over-exposure to water, or chemicals such as acids, alkalis, detergents and solvents. (Farahmand S.).

L

Lauric acid: A twelve carbon, straight-chained fatty acid. (Fischer C.L. and Wertz P.W.).

Long-chain base: An aliphatic lipid containing an amino group on the second carbon and hydroxyl groups on the first and third carbons. If there are no other functional groups it is a dihydrosphingosine. If an additional hydroxyl group is added to carbon 4 it is a phytosphingosine. If a *trans* double bond is introduced between carbons 4 and 5 it is a sphingosine. If there is a double bond between carbons 4 and 5 and a hydroxyl group is introduced on carbon 6 it is a 6-hydroxysphingosine. (Fischer C.L. and Wertz P.W.).

M

Marassezia spp: Related species of yeast found on human skin, especially on the scalp. (Fischer C.L. and Wertz P.W.).

Medical device: Any instrument, apparatus, implement, machine, appliance, implant, reagent for *in vitro* use, software, material or other similar or related article used to treat, alleviate or diagnose a disease or injury, and not acting by pharmacological, immunological or metabolic means, in or on the human body. (von Wright A.).

Metagenomics: application of genomics techniques to analyze mix microbial samples collected from the environment or patients. While genomics refers to the study of the genome from one species, metagenomic samples contain the genomes from more than one species. (O'Hara N.B.).

Microbiome: (1). The microorganisms in a particular environment (including the body or part of the body) (Cheng J. and Hata T.). (2). Combined genetic material of the microorganisms in a particular environment, here the human skin. (Blumenberg M.). (3). The microbial community associated a particular environmental niche (including the body or a part of the body). (Samaras S. and Hoptroff M.) *Microbiome:* the community of microorganisms and their combined genetic material in a particular environment (Drake D.).

MRSA: methicillin-resistant *Staphylococcus aureus.* (O'Hara N.B.).

Mycobiome: Fungal members of the microbiome. (Buerger S. and Huber M.).

N

NGS: Next generation sequencing is a high-throughput sequencing technology that allows for the generation of millions or billions of DNA strands data through sequencing in parallel. (O'Hara N.B.).

Novel foods: In the EU "Novel Foods" are defined as foods that have not been consumed to a significant degree by humans in the EU before 15 May 1997, when the first Regulation on novel food came into force. (von Wright A.).

O

Oral microbiome: (1). Microbial community in the oral cavity. (Buerger S. and Huber M.) (2) The community of microorganisms and their combined genetic material inhabiting the oral cavity. (Drake D.).

P

Patent: a contract with the United States government that allows the holder to exclude someone from making, using, selling, or offering to sell, what is claimed in the document. (Mills J.K.).

Pathogen: A disease-causing bacterium, virus, or other microorganism. (Samaras S. and Hoptroff M.).

Pharmaceuticals: Pharmaceuticals (medicines, drugs) are substances used to treat or alleviate an illness, and typically acting on the metabolic, physiological, immunological or molecular functions of the body, or a pathogenic target organism. (von Wright A.).

Pilosebaceous unit: The complex within the skin composed of the hair shaft, hair follicle, arrector pili muscles and sebaceous gland. (Strobel S.L.).

Psoriasis: (1). Psoriasis is a chronic skin condition that speeds up the life cycle of skin cells. It causes cells to build up rapidly on the surface of the skin. The extra skin cells form scales and red patches that are itchy and sometimes painful. (Farahmand S.); (2). Common chronic inflammatory skin disease that causes red patches on the skin (Chung J., Strober B.E., Weinstock G.M.).

Q

Qualified Presumption of Safety (QPS): A generic safety evaluation concept for microorganisms in the EU. If an assessment of a group of microorganisms concludes that they do not raise safety concerns, the group is granted "QPS status". (von Wright A.).

Quorum sensing: Bacterial communication reliant on cell density. (Buerger S. and Huber M.).

R

Regulation: EU Regulations are legal acts that apply automatically and uniformly to all EU countries as soon as they enter into force, without needing to be transposed into national law. (von Wright A.).

Regulatory T cells: a subpopulation of T lymphocytes that modulate the immune system. Formerly known as suppressor T cells. (Drake D.).

Richness (microbial): The number of distinct groups at a given phylogenetic level in a microbiological community; typical estimators of microbial richness are the ACE and Chao1 indices. (Stamatas G.N.).

S

Sapienic acid: A sixteen carbon fatty acid with a *cis* double bond between carbons 6 and 7. (Fischer C.L. and Wertz P.W.).

Seborrheic dermatitis: Seborrheic dermatitis is a common skin condition that affects scalp or oily areas of body and causes scaly patches, red skin and dandruff. (Farahmand S.).

Sebum: A mixture of oily lipids produced in sebaceous glands and secreted onto the skin surface. (Fischer C.L. and Wertz P.W.).

Skin infections: Condition usually caused by bacterial infection and characterized by inflammation, pain, and swelling. (Whitfill T. and Dube G.R and Oh J.).

Skin microbiome: Microbial community on the skin. (Buerger S. and Huber M.).

Skin microbiota: the ensemble of microorganisms which reside on the skin and its annexes, composed of about 1,000 species from nineteen phyla. (Meloni M. and Balzaretti S.).

*Staphylococcus***:** The other main bacterial genera colonizing axillary skin, the most abundant species being *Staphylococcus epidermidis*. (James G.).

*Staphylococcus aureus***:** (1). A Gram-positive bacterium commonly found on the skin of patients with atopic dermatitis (Cheng J. and Hata T.). (2). A Gram-positive, round-shaped bacterium that is often associated with a number of skin diseases. (Whitfill T. and Dube G.R. and Oh J.) (3). A spherical Gram-positive bacterium that causes a variety of skin infections. (Fischer C.L. and Wertz P.W.) (4). It is a pathogen bacterium frequently isolated from skin lesions, expressing several molecules that contribute to the intensity of symptoms, including α-toxin and protein A which damages keratinocytes and trigger inflammatory responses. Moreover, its secreted proteases contribute to disruption of the epidermal barrier. (Meloni M. and Balzaretti S.).

*Staphylococcus epidermidis***:** it is a coagulase-negative staphylococcal species, which is predominant on normal human skin. It can produce proteins that work together with endogenous host antimicrobial peptides (AMPs) to provide direct protection against infectious pathogens. (Meloni M. and Balzaretti S.).

Staphylococcus hominis: The second most abundant *Staphylococcus* species colonising axillary skin. Recently heavily implicated in the generation of thioalcohol-based malodour. (James G.).

Staphylococcal diseases: Diseases driven by infection by *Staphylococcus* spp., particularly *S. aureus*. (Whitfill T. and Dube G.R and Oh J.).

T

Taxonomy: Classification of living things. (Buerger S. and Huber M.).

Thioalcohol: The other primary class of compounds responsible for axillary malodour, the most important example being 3-methyl-3-sulfanyl-hexan-1-ol (3M3SH) (James G.).

Trade secret: confidential information, not known the public, from which a company derives and economic or business advantage. (Mills J.K.).

Trademark: Any word, name, symbol, device, or combination, used to identify and distinguish the goods or services of one seller or provider from those of another. (Mills J.K.).

Triglyceride: A lipid consisting of three fatty acids ester-linked to glycerol. (Fischer C.L. and Wertz P.W.)

V

Virome: Viral members of the microbiome. (Buerger S. and Huber M.).

Volatile fatty acid: Abbreviated as VFA, one of the primary classes of compounds responsible for axillary malodour. The most important examples are the medium-chain VFAs 3-hydroxy-3-methylhexanoic acid (3H3MH) and 3-methyl-2-hexenoic acid (3M2H) (James G.).

VRSA: vancomycin-resistant *Staphylococcus aureus* (O'Hara N.B.).

Index

Also by Nava Dayan

Handbook of Formulating Dermal Applications

A Definitive Practical Guide

2018, 698 pages ISBN: 9781119363620

The conceptualization and formulation of skin care products intended for topical use is a multifaceted and evolving area of science. Formulators must account for myriad skin types, emerging opportunities for product development as well as a very temperamental retail market.

Originally published as "Apply Topically" in 2013 (now out of print), this reissued detailed and comprehensive handbook offers a practical approach to the formulation chemist's day-to-day endeavors by:

- Addressing the innumerable challenges facing the chemist both in design and at the bench, such as formulating with/for specific properties; formulation, processing and production techniques; sensory and elegancy; stability and preservation; color cosmetics; sunscreens
- Offering valuable guidance to troubleshooting issues regarding ingredient selection and interaction, regulatory concerns that must be addressed early in development, and the extrapolation of preservative systems, fragrances, stability and texture aids
- Exploring the advantages and limitations of raw materials
- Addressing scale-up and pilot production process and concerns
- Testing and measurements methods.

The 22 chapters written by industry experts such as Roger L. McMullen, Paul Thau, Hemi Nae, Ada Polla, Howard Epstein, Joseph Albanese, Mark Chandler, Steve Herman, Gary Kelm, Patricia Aikens, and Sam Shefer, along with many others, give the reader and user the ultimate handbook on topical product development.

www.scrivenerpublishing.com